CLEAN SIMPLE EATS

A MACRO-BASED COOKBOOK

The ideas, concepts and opinions expressed in all Clean Simple Eats meal plans, books and other media are intended to be used for educational purposes only. The books and meal plans are sold with the understanding that authors and publisher are not rendering medical advice of any kind, nor are the books or meal plans intended to replace medical advice, nor to diagnose, prescribe or treat any disease, condition, illness or injury. By my use of any of the products and/or programs of Clean Simple Eats, I am agreeing to assume all of the risks associated with such use. I further agree to waive, release, and discharge Clean Simple Eats from any and all liability arising from its negligence or fault.

It is imperative that before beginning any diet or exercise program, including any aspect of the Clean Simple Eats program, you receive full medical clearance from a licensed physician.

Authors and publisher claim no responsibility to any person or entity for any liability, loss or damage caused or alleged to be caused directly or indirectly as a result of the use, application or interpretation of the material in the books or meal plan.

The Food and Drug Administration has not evaluated the statements contained in any Clean Simple Eats books, meal plans, or other media.

This book, and any other Clean Simple Eats seasonal meal plan or book, is protected under copyright laws and may not be duplicated, shared, copied or plagiarized, under any circumstance, in digital or bound form.

Author: Erika Peterson
Food Photography: Erika Peterson
Lifestyle Photography: Jessica Janae

©2022 CLEAN SIMPLE EATS, INC
ITEM NOT FOR RESALE OR DISTRIBUTION

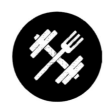

Dedicated to our family,
friends and CSE Squad!

Thank you for always believing
in and supporting us.

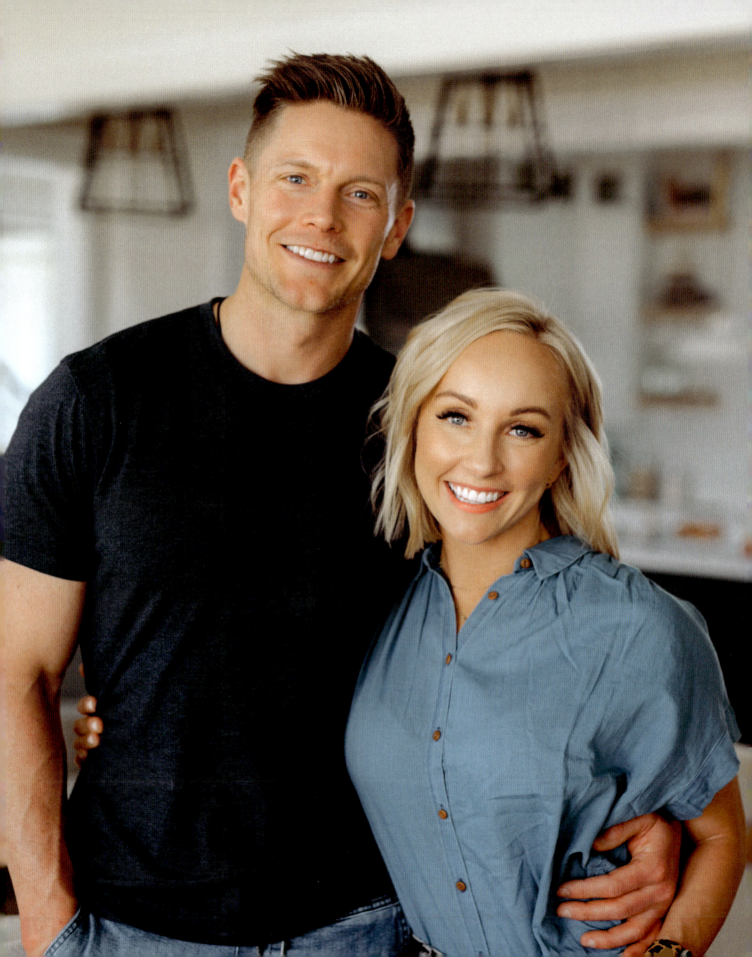

WELCOME TO CLEAN SIMPLE EATS

Hi! We're JJ and Erika, the husband and wife team behind Clean Simple Eats! We are passionate about helping others elevate their lives through food and fitness, and we are here to prove that clean eating can be simple, fun and satisfying. That's why we've put a healthy, macro-balanced spin on delicious comfort food recipes that we all know and love.

Frustrated by bland and boring diet food, we started experimenting in our own kitchen, subbing in simple, healthier ingredients and before we knew it, Clean Simple Eats was born! Our recipes have proven to please even the pickiest of eaters (aka our four kiddos), so we had to share these recipe creations with the world, and we guarantee that you will love them too.

Aside from our recipes, we've also created our own line of clean and delicious protein powders, supplements, and gourmet nut butters. Our goal was to create the best-tasting, highest quality products on the market, and we honestly believe we've done just that!

This CSE Best of Book is a compilation of our very favorite recipes, carefully handpicked from our library of thousands of macro-balanced meals! An amazing feature of this book is that whether you're enjoying pizza, waffles or salad, the macros will stay the same. It's like magic! Each breakfast, snack and entree has the perfect balance of protein, fat and carbs to keep your body fueled and satisfied.

We dedicate this book to our amazing community, the CSE Squad. They are everything to us! There is something powerful about belonging to a community that supports you; there are tens of thousands of amazing people throughout the world who have shaped Clean Simple Eats into what it is today, and we are excited you are here and can't wait to be a part of your health and fitness journey! It's been a great adventure, but the very best part is watching others take control of their narrative, reach their goals, find inner confidence and transform their lives. This is why we do what we do!

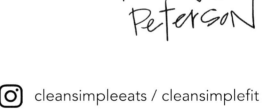

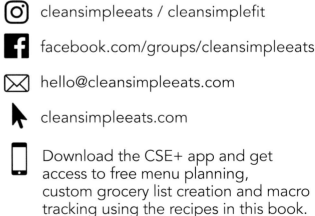

cleansimpleeats / cleansimplefit

facebook.com/groups/cleansimpleeats

hello@cleansimpleeats.com

cleansimpleeats.com

Download the CSE+ app and get access to free menu planning, custom grocery list creation and macro tracking using the recipes in this book.

RECIPE INDEX

BREAKFASTS

Shakes & Smoothies — 11
Almond Joy Protein Shake — 13
Butterfinger Shake — 15
Chocolate Lover's Açaí Bowl — 17
Chocolate Peanut Butter Cup Shake — 19
Chocolate Speckled Frosty — 21
CSE Hot Cocoa — 23
Hulk Power Shake — 25
Mint Cookies & Cream Shake — 27
Orange Julius (Post-Workout) — 29
PB&J Breakfast Shake — 31
Peanut Butter Caramel Milkshake — 33
Peanut Butter Cookie Breakfast Shake — 35
Snickers Shake — 37
Strawberry Colada — 39
Sweet Cherry Almond Freeze — 41

Oatmeals — 43
Almond Joy Oatmeal — 45
Banana Bread Oatmeal — 47
Cinna-Berry Breakfast Squares — 49
Cinnamon Bun in a Bowl — 51
Cookie Crumb Granola — 53
Hot Apple Pie Oats — 55
Ooey-Gooey Breakfast Brownies — 57
Peach Cobbler Overnight Oats — 59
Peanut Butter Overnight Oats — 61
Raspberry Almond Oats — 63
Superfoods Breakfast Bowl — 65

Pancakes & Waffles — 67
Banana Macadamia Nut Pancakes — 69
German Pancakes — 71
Hot Cocoa Pancakes — 73
Lemon Chia Pancakes — 75
Blueberry PB Power Waffles — 77
Caramel Apple Pie Waffles — 79
Chocolate Waffles — 81
Pumpkin Protein Waffles — 83
Baked Cinnamon Roll French Toast — 85
Strawberry Cream French Toast — 87
Chocolate Banana Crepes — 89
Lemon Raspberry Flourless Crepes — 91

Savory — 93
BLTA Waffle Sandwich — 95
Breakfast Burritos — 97
Breakfast Taquitos — 99
Brekkie Bruschetta — 101
Cheesy Sausage Egg Bake — 103
Country Breakfast Skillet — 105
Egg White, Pepper Jack & Avocado Sandwich — 107
Loaded Breakfast Burrito Bowl — 109
Savory Stuffed Waffles — 111

SNACKS

Crunchy & Savory — 115
Caprese Crunch Snack — 117
Chips & Cheesy Chile Dip — 119
Kickin' Avo Toast — 121
Open-Faced Turkey & Veggie Sandwich — 123
Pretzel Snap Dip — 125

Parfaits & Fruit Dips — 127
Banana Cream Pie Parfait — 129
Birchgrove Muesli — 131
Caramel Apple Dip — 133
Chocolate Fondue Power Dip — 135
Chunky Monkey Bowl — 137
Creamy Cinnamon Sugar Apple Bowl — 139
Dark Chocolate Mousse — 141
Strawberry Cheesecake Bowl — 143

Muffins — 145
Apple Crumb Muffins — 147
Banana Chocolate Chip Muffins — 149
Blueberry Muffin & Eggs — 151
Chocolate PB Swirl Muffins — 153
Mini Pumpkin Chocolate Chip Muffins — 155

Power Bites — 157
Almond Joy Cookie Dough Bites — 159
Crispy Chocolate PB Bites — 161
Dark Chocolate Peanut Butter Bites — 163
Lemon Coconut Bliss Bites — 165
Salted Caramel Bites — 167
Snickers Power Bites — 169
Thin Mint Cookie Bites — 171

Recipe Key

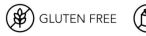 GLUTEN FREE   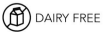 DAIRY FREE

RECIPE INDEX

ENTREES

Soups, Salads & Sandwiches — 175
Best Ever Chili — 177
Creamy Chicken Corn Chowder — 179
Creamy Chicken Noodle Soup — 181
Pasta e Fagioli — 183
Taco Soup — 185
Thai Chicken Soup — 187
BBQ Chicken Chopped Salad — 189
Green Goddess Salad — 191
Harvest Cobb Salad — 193
Thai Crunch Salad — 195
Turkey Sub Salad — 197
Hot Turkey & Swiss — 199
Homemade Honey-Wheat Bread — 201
Meatball Subs — 203
Mediterranean Meatball Gyro — 205
Pesto Chicken Panini — 207

Tex-Mex — 209
Black Bean Tostadas — 211
Buffalo Chicken Tostadas — 213
Cashew Sour Cream — 215
Chicken & Rice Enchiladas — 217
Chicken Burrito Bowl — 219
Grilled Lime Salmon Tacos — 221
Honey Garlic Chicken Tacos — 223
Honey-Lime Chicken Enchiladas — 225
Loaded Chicken Quesadillas — 227
Marinated Steak Tacos — 229
Mexican Tortilla Pizza — 231
Queenstown Nachos — 233
Taco Fries — 235

Pizza & Pasta — 237
BBQ Chicken Pizza — 239
Buffalo Chicken Pizza — 241
Garden Veggie Pizza — 243
Grilled Bruschetta Pizza — 245
Pepperoni Pizza Pinwheels — 247
Stacked Supreme Pizza Bites — 249
Caprese Pasta Bowl — 251
Chicken Fettuccine Alfredo — 253
Chicken Pad Thai — 255
One Pan Cheddar Beef Rotini — 257
Turkey Sausage Lasagna — 259

Comfort Food — 261
Aloha Chicken Kabobs — 263
Apple Chicken Hash — 265
BBQ Ranch Grilled Bounty Bowl — 267
Boss Baked Mac & Cheese — 269
Buffalo Chicken Waffle Fries — 271
Cajun Chicken Sausage Jambalaya — 273
Cashew Kung Pao Chicken — 275
Cheddar Ranch Chicken & Potatoes — 277
Chili-Lime Junkyard Fries — 279
Crispy Chicken Nuggets — 281
Grilled Coconut-Lime Curry Chicken — 283
Guacamole Turkey Burger — 285
Lemon Butter Chicken — 287
Meatballs & Mashed Potatoes — 289
Mustard-Fried Bacon Burger — 291
Parmesan Chicken — 293
Sesame Chicken Bowl — 295
Turkey Pot Pies — 297

DESSERTS

Breads & Rolls — 301
Chocolate Chip Banana Bread Squares — 303
Double Chocolate Banana Bread — 305
Sweet Honey Cinnamon Rolls — 307
Zesty Orange Sweet Rolls — 309

Brownies & Bars — 311
Banana Cheesecake Cups — 313
Blueberry Crumble Bars — 315
Chovocado Brownies — 317
Crispy Caramel Butterscotch Bars — 319
Scotcharoo Bars — 321

Cakes & Crumbles — 323
Berry Cobbler Crumble — 325
Caramel Apple Cake — 327
Chocolate Zucchini Cake — 329
Double Chocolate Cake Donuts — 331
Lemon Pound Cake — 333
Peach Crisp — 335

Cookies — 337
Gingerbread Chocolate Chip Cookies — 339
Ice Cream Cookie Sandwiches — 341
Lemon Drop Cookies — 343
Mint Chocolate Cookies — 345
Oatmeal PB Chocolate Chip Cookies — 347
Pumpkin Chocolate Chip Cookies — 349

Party Treats — 351
Brownie Batter Buddies — 353
Raspberry Oreo Ice Cream — 355
White Chocolate Cinnamon Puppy Chow — 357
Zebra Caramel Corn — 359

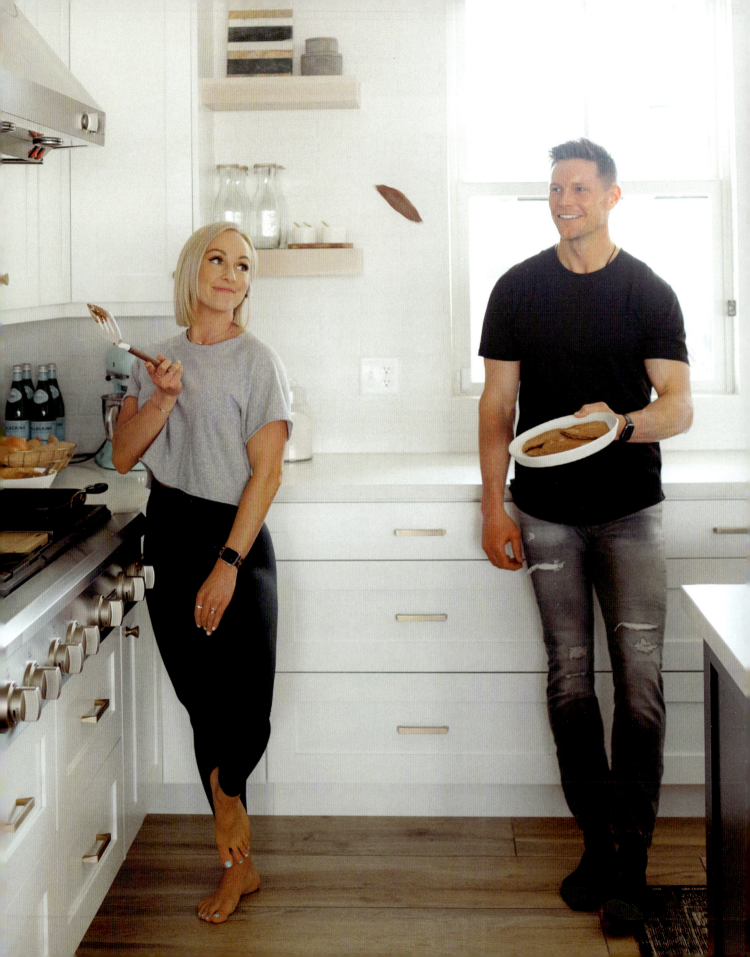

BREAKFAST

Brekkie just got an upgrade because we are covering ALL the bases! Shake up your breakfast (literally) with one of our delicious **Shakes or Smoothies** and take it on-the-go! Not in a hurry? Take your morning slow and sit down with a fresh stack of protein-packed **Pancakes & Waffles**. Maybe you're into that **Savory** vibe… grab a Breakfast Burrito or cook up the Country Skillet! And then there's our personal weekday staple, **Oatmeal**! Hot or cold, we've got you! We truly put the GOOD in 'good morning'!

SHAKES & SMOOTHIES

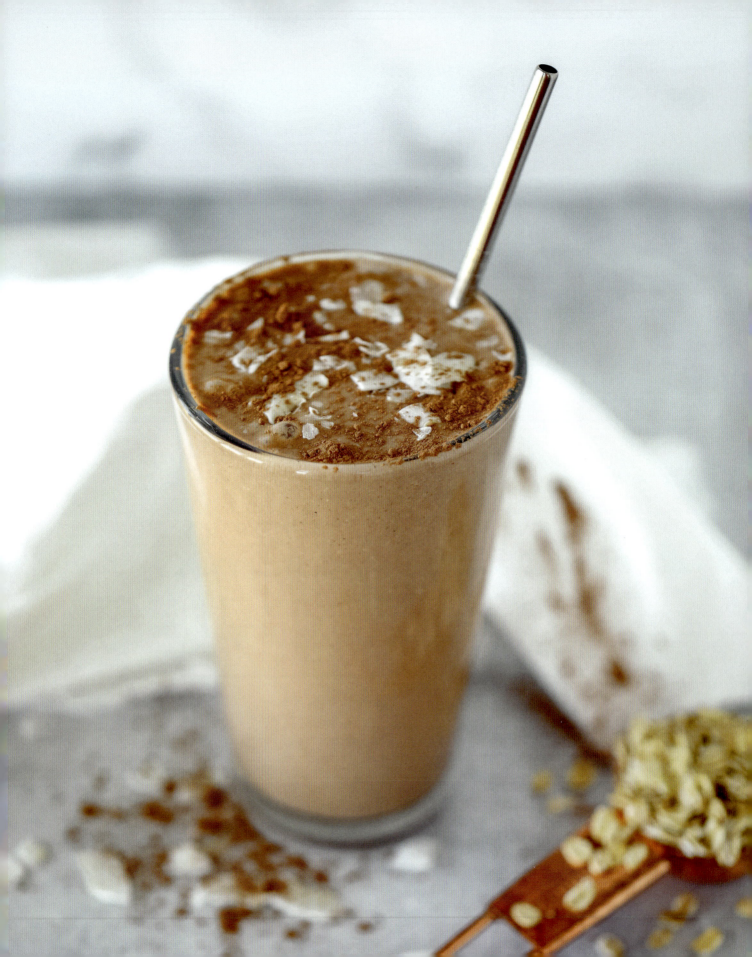

ALMOND JOY PROTEIN SHAKE
Makes 1 serving
345 calories / 11.5F / 34.5C / 25.5P

___

Prep: 5 min

1 cup unsweetened almond milk
1 serving CSE Chocolate Brownie Batter Protein Powder
2 Tbs. old-fashioned rolled oats
60g frozen banana slices
1 Tbs. cocoa powder
1 Tbs. unsweetened shredded coconut
½ Tbs. CSE Midnight Almond Coconut Butter
    or natural almond butter
½ tsp. vanilla extract
½ tsp. coconut extract
6-8 (120g) ice cubes

1. Add all of the ingredients to a high-powered blender. Blend until smooth. Enjoy!

___

PRO TIPS: Try it with half CSE Chocolate Brownie Batter Protein Powder and half CSE Coconut Cream Protein Powder for an extra boost of coconut!

Prep a bunch of these ahead of time for a quick breakfast or snack option. Measure all of the ingredients out into individual zip top bags or containers, excluding the almond milk, and store in the freezer. When ready to use, dump the contents of the bags into the blender with the almond milk. Blend until smooth.

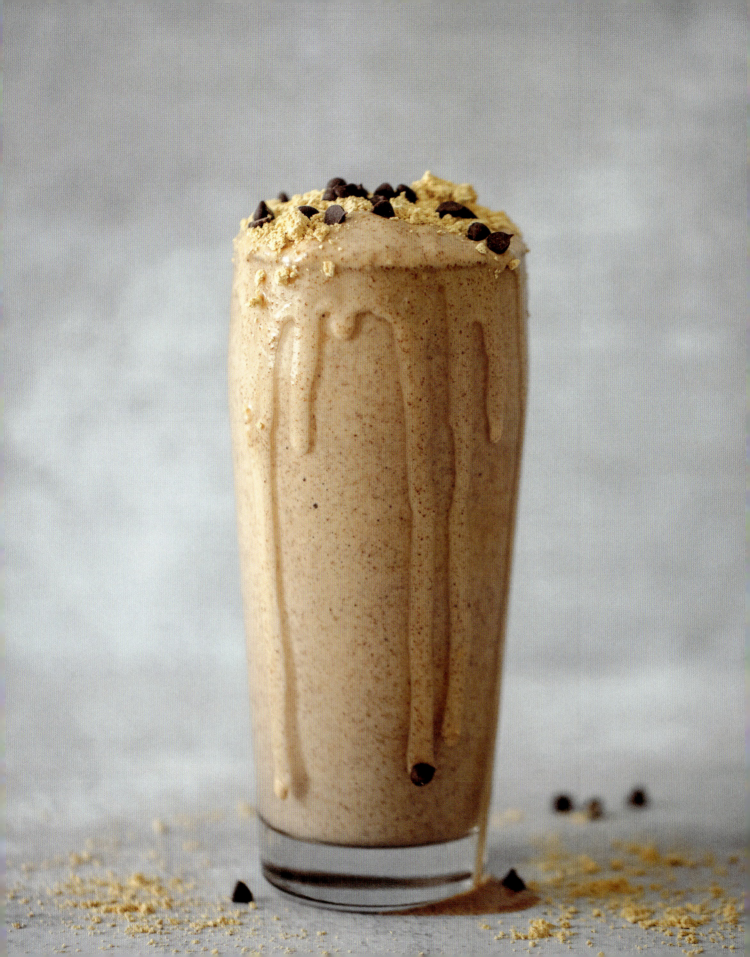

BUTTERFINGER SHAKE
Makes 1 serving
350 calories / 11.5F / 36C / 27P

Prep: 5 min

1 cup unsweetened almond milk
¾ serving CSE Simply Vanilla Protein Powder
30g frozen banana slices
10g CSE Chocolate Peanut Butter Cup, Sweet Classic Peanut Butter
    or natural peanut butter
10g butterscotch pudding mix
10g semi-sweet chocolate chips
120g ice cubes
Topping:
2 Tbs. (16g) CSE Powdered Peanut Butter

1. Add all of the ingredients to a high-powered blender and blend until smooth.

2. Pour into a cup. Top with powdered peanut butter and stir into the shake. Enjoy!

PRO TIP: Prep a bunch of these ahead of time for a quick breakfast or snack option. Measure all of the ingredients out into individual zip top bags or containers, excluding the almond milk and topping, and store in the freezer. When ready to use, dump the contents of the bag into the blender with the almond milk. Blend until smooth.

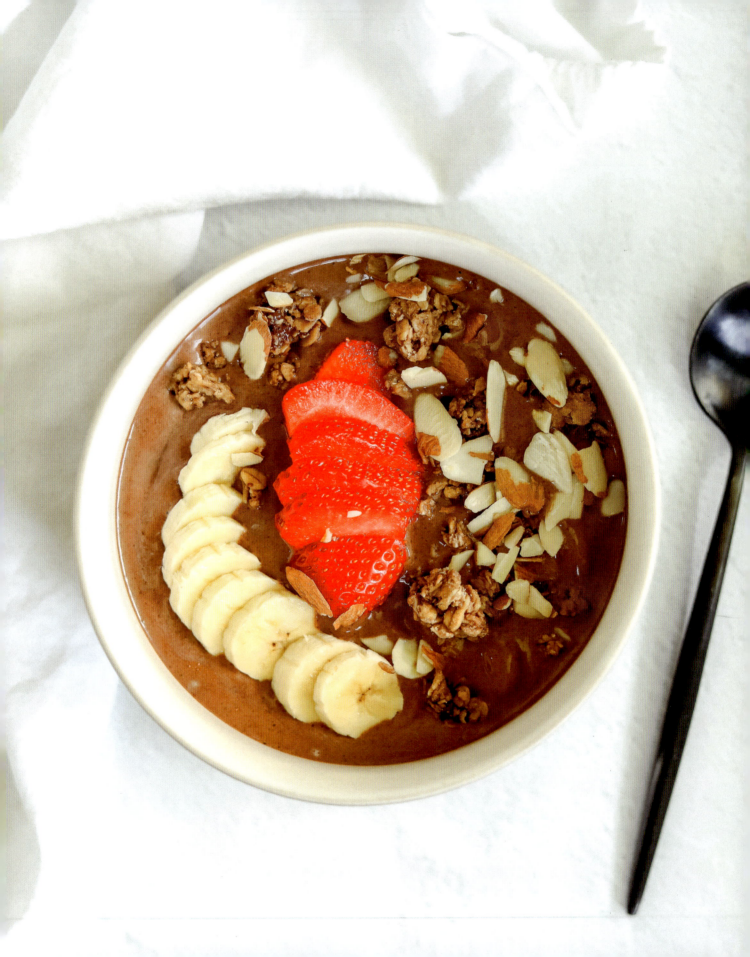

CHOCOLATE LOVER'S AÇAÍ BOWL
Makes 1 serving
355 calories / 12F / 37C / 25P

Prep: 10 min

1 frozen unsweetened Sambazon Açaí pack
¼ cup unsweetened almond coconut milk
40g frozen banana slices
1 serving CSE Chocolate Brownie Batter Protein Powder
1 Tbs. special dark cocoa powder
4-6 (80g) ice cubes
Toppings:
20g banana slices
20g strawberry slices
1 Tbs. sliced almonds
1 Tbs. Dark Chocolate & Red Berries Love Crunch Granola

1. Place frozen açaí in a blender and pulse until broken up. Scrape down the sides of the blender and add the almond coconut milk, frozen bananas, protein powder, cocoa powder and ice. Blend until smooth and thick.

2. Pour into a bowl and top with bananas, strawberries, almonds and granola.

PRO TIP: Make endless varieties by swapping in different protein powder flavors and toppings!

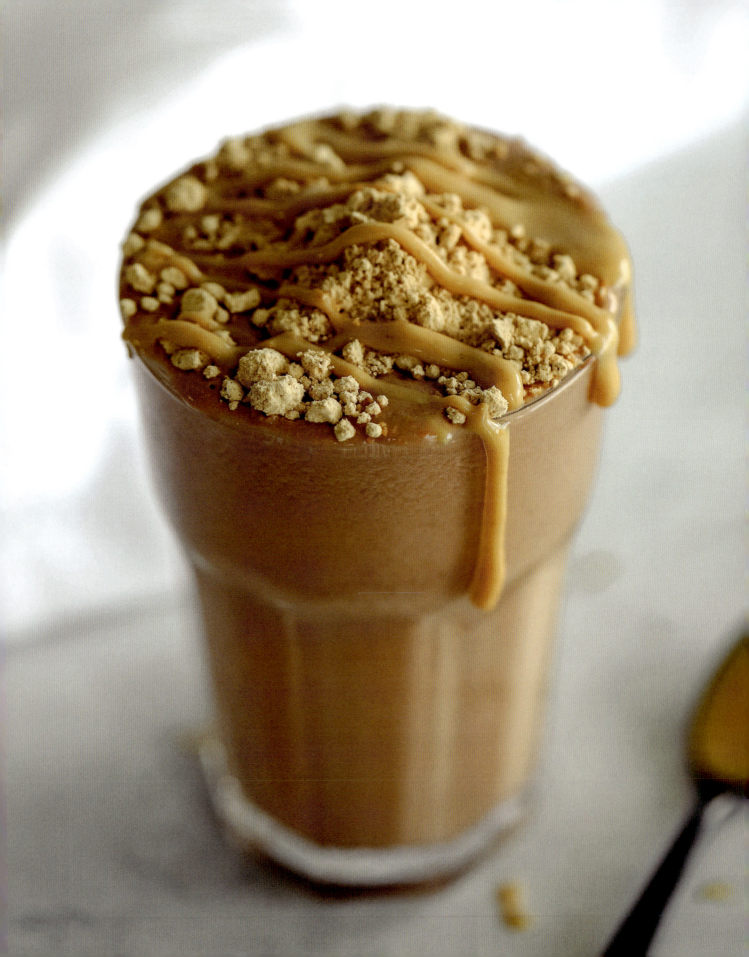

CHOCOLATE PEANUT BUTTER CUP SHAKE
Makes 1 serving
345 calories / 11F / 32C / 29.5P

Prep: 5 min

1 cup unsweetened vanilla almond milk
1 serving CSE Chocolate Peanut Butter Protein Powder
1 Tbs. cocoa powder
14g CSE Sweet Classic Peanut Butter
   or natural peanut butter
60g frozen banana slices
120g ice cubes
Topping:
1 Tbs. CSE Powdered Peanut Butter

1. Add all of the shake ingredients to a high-powered blender. Blend until smooth.

2. Pour into a cup. Top with powdered peanut butter and lightly fold into the shake. Enjoy!

PRO TIP: Make ahead and store in an insulated bottle in the fridge or in a cooler with ice. It will stay fresh, thick and cold for up to 24 hours. Add toppings fresh.

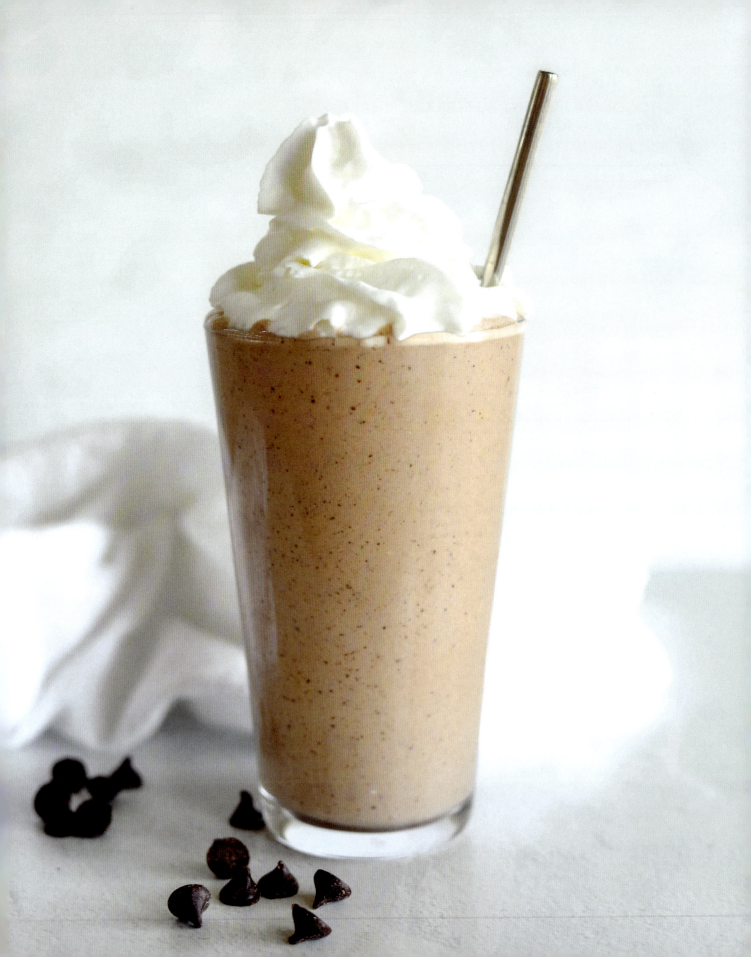

CHOCOLATE SPECKLED FROSTY

Makes 1 serving
240 calories / 7F / 25C / 18.5P

Prep: 5 min

⅔ cup unsweetened almond milk
½ serving (16g) CSE Chocolate Brownie Batter Protein Powder
50g frozen banana slices
¼ cup low-fat cottage cheese
10g dark chocolate chips
1 tsp. cocoa powder
½ tsp. vanilla extract
10-12 (150g) ice cubes
Topping:
2 Tbs. spray whipped cream

1. Add all of the ingredients to a high-powered blender. Blend on high until smooth.

2. Pour into a cup, top with whipped cream and enjoy!

PRO TIP: Serve up in place of dessert!

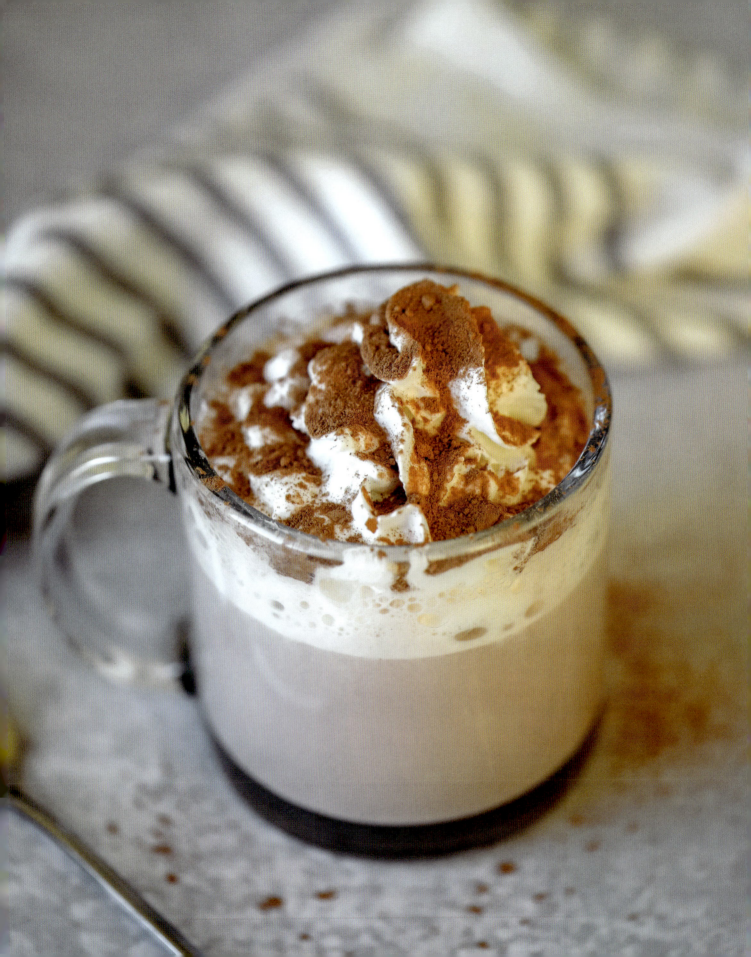

CSE HOT COCOA
Makes 1 serving
245 calories / 2F / 25.5C / 30.5P

Prep: 5 min

1 cup water
1 ½ servings CSE Chocolate Brownie Batter Protein Powder
Topping:
¼ cup spray whipped cream
Side:
50g banana

1. Add water to a mug and microwave for 1-2 minutes or until hot. Let cool for a couple minutes.

2. Add the protein powder and whisk until smooth.

3. Top with whipped cream and enjoy the banana on the side.

PRO TIP: Try swapping in other protein flavors or mix a combination of flavors. Our favorites are Mint Chocolate Cookie mixed with Chocolate Brownie Batter or Coconut Cream mixed with Chocolate Brownie Batter.

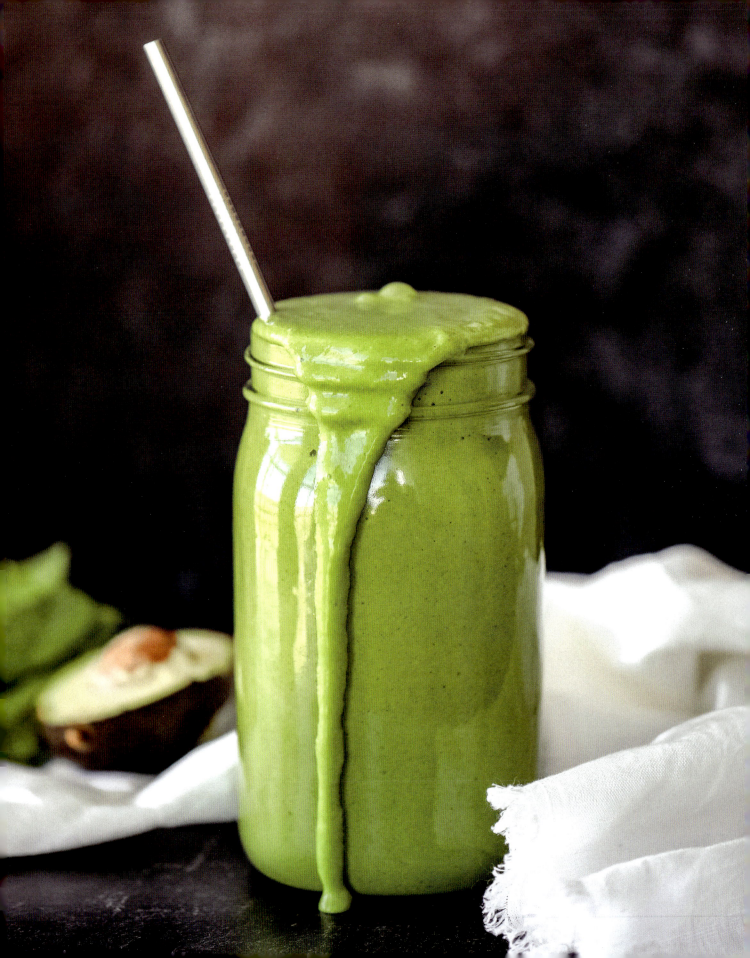

HULK POWER SHAKE

Makes 1 serving
350 calories / 13F / 34C / 25P

Prep: 5 min

1 cup unsweetened almond milk
1 serving CSE Simply Vanilla Protein Powder
80g frozen banana slices
15g avocado
1 Tbs. CSE Butter of choice
  or natural almond butter
1 cup spinach
1 tsp. cinnamon
10 (130g) ice cubes

1. Add all of the ingredients to a high-powered blender. Blend on high until smooth.

2. Pour into a cup and enjoy!

PRO TIP: Add one serving of CSE Super Greens or Peachy Greens Mix for an easy way to increase your daily veggie intake and boost your immunity!

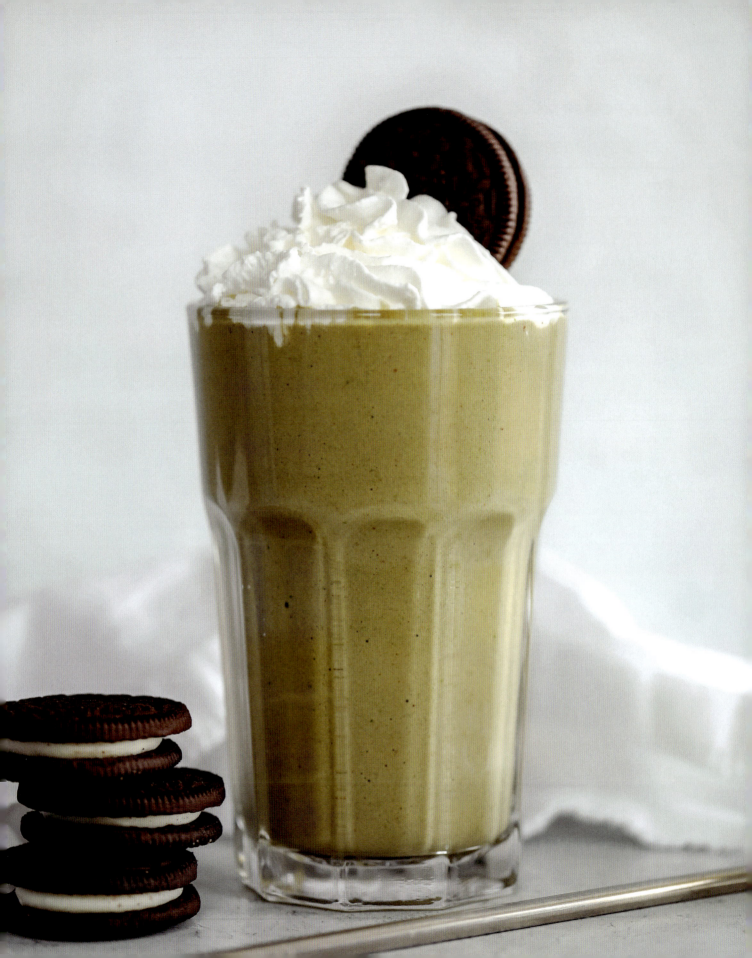

MINT COOKIES & CREAM SHAKE
Makes 1 serving
360 calories / 13.5F / 29C / 27P

Prep: 5 min

   1 cup unsweetened almond milk
   ¾ serving CSE Mint Chocolate Cookie Protein Powder
   ½ Tbs. CSE Mint Chocolate Chip Cookie Butter
      or natural almond butter
   ¼ cup low-fat cottage cheese
   1 cream filled chocolate cookie
   1 cup spinach
   ¼ tsp. xanthan gum
   8-10 (150g) ice cubes

Toppings:
2 Tbs. spray whipped cream
1 cream filled chocolate cookie

1. Add all of the ingredients to a high-powered blender. Blend until smooth and thick.

2. Pour into a cup and top with whipped cream and a crumbled cookie.

PRO TIP: Serve up in place of dessert!

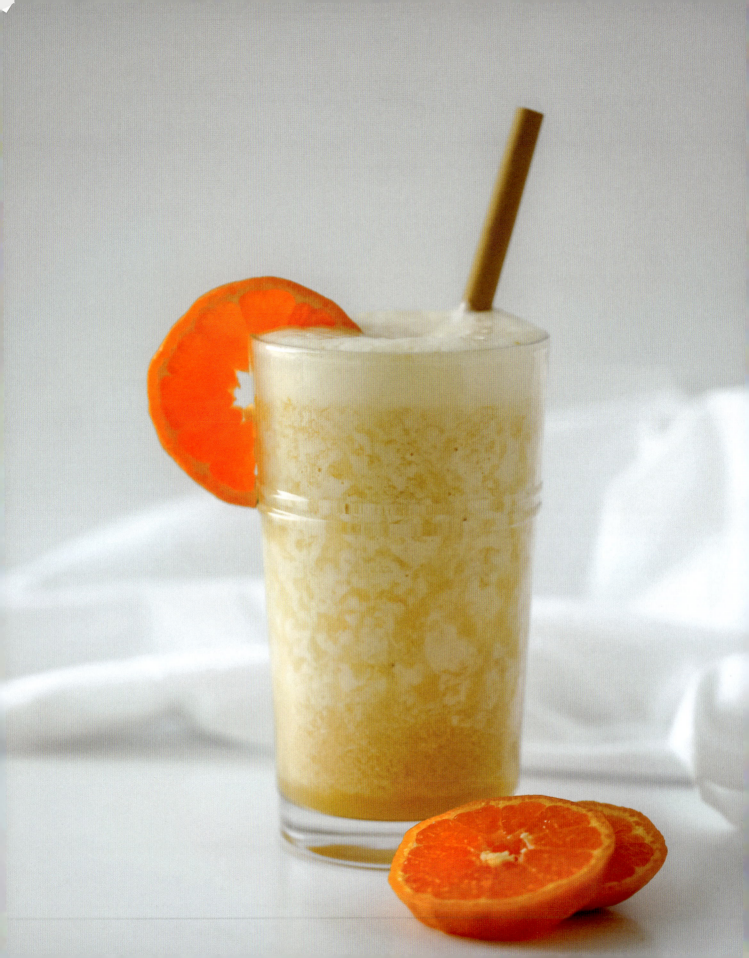

ORANGE JULIUS

Makes 1 serving
250 calories / 1F / 33.5C / 26.5P

Prep: 5 min

½ cup unsweetened cashew milk
½ cup fresh orange juice
1 serving CSE Simply Vanilla Protein Powder
1 serving CSE Peach Mango Super Collagen Mix
30g frozen bananas
6-8 (120g) ice cubes

1. Add all of the ingredients to a high-powered blender. Blend on high until smooth. Pour into a cup and enjoy!

PRO TIP: Enjoy after a workout! The ratio of higher protein and carbs paired with lower fats will help the nutrients act fast in fueling and repairing your muscle.

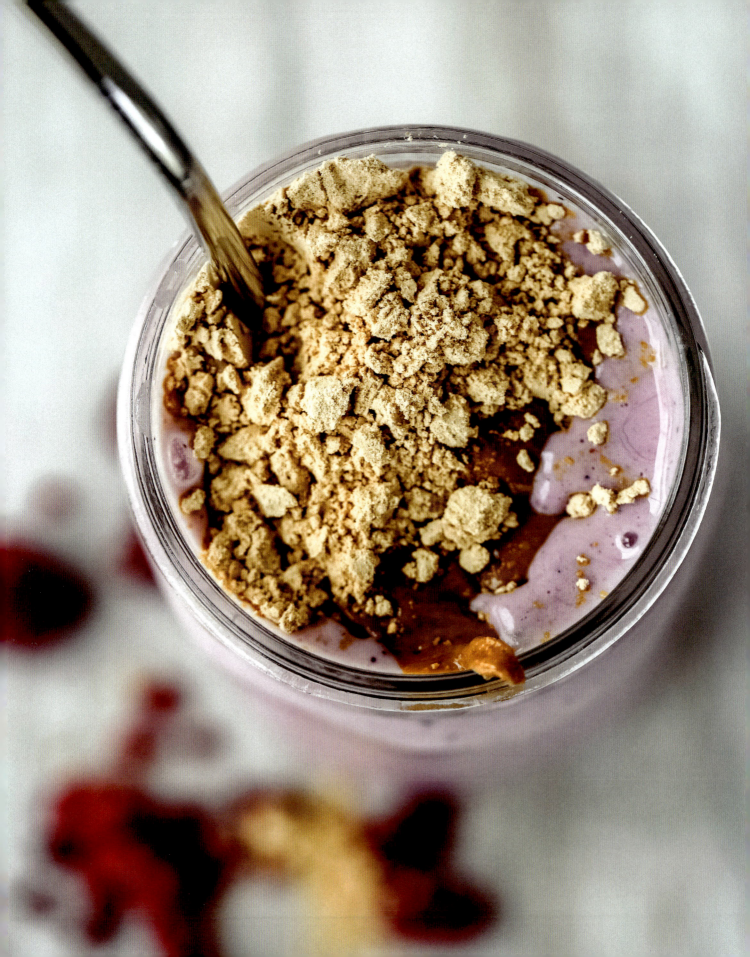

PB&J BREAKFAST SHAKE
Makes 1 serving
316 cal / 9.5F / 30C / 27.5P

___

Prep: 5 min

1 cup unsweetened almond milk
1 serving CSE Simply Vanilla or Strawberry Cheesecake Protein Powder
60g frozen berries
50g frozen banana slices
¼ tsp. xanthan gum, optional for thickness
8-10 (120g) ice cubes
Topping:
1 Tbs. CSE Powdered Peanut Butter

1. Add all of the ingredients to a high-powered blender. Blend until smooth.

2. Pour into a cup. Top with powdered peanut butter and fold into the shake. Enjoy with a spoon or a thick straw.

___

PRO TIP: Add our Super Berry Antioxidant Mix to rev up the flavor and boost your immunity.

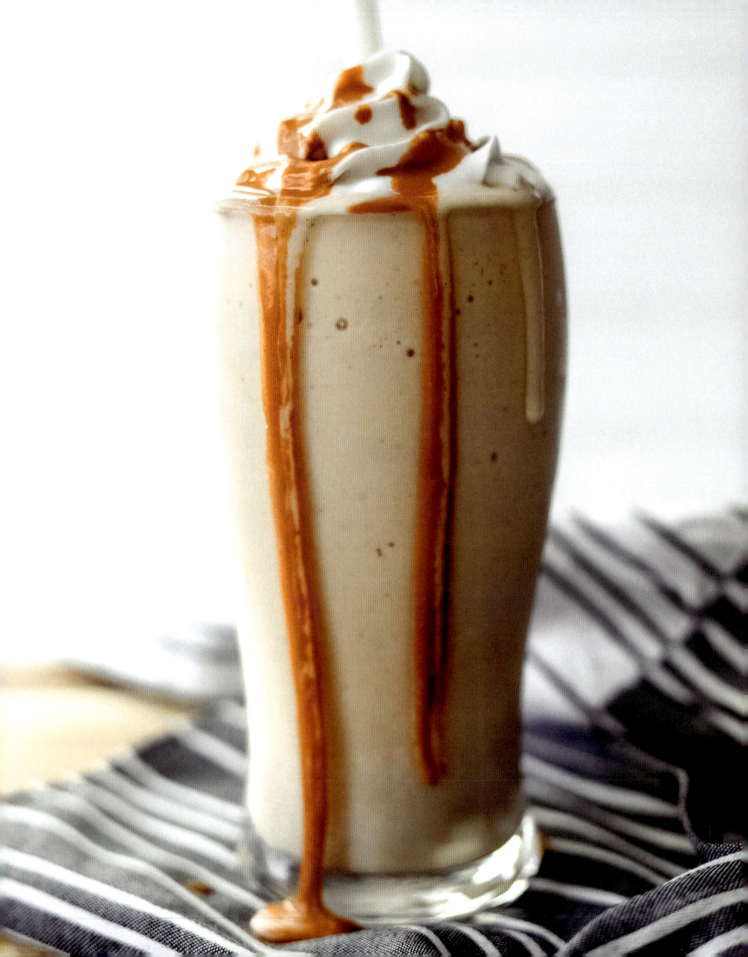

PEANUT BUTTER CARAMEL MILKSHAKE
Makes 1 serving
240 calories / 6.5F / 24C / 20.5P

Prep: 5 min

½ cup fat-free milk
½ cup Sea Salt Caramel or Vanilla Bean Protein Ice Cream
30g frozen banana slices
2 Tbs. CSE Simply Vanilla or Caramel Toffee Protein Powder
½ Tbs. CSE Sweet Classic Peanut Butter
   or natural peanut butter
6-8 (120g) ice cubes
Toppings:
2 Tbs. spray whipped cream
1 tsp. Walden Farms Caramel Syrup

1. Add all of the ingredients to a high-powered blender. Blend on high until smooth.

2. Top with whipped cream and enjoy!

PRO TIP: Serve up in place of dessert!

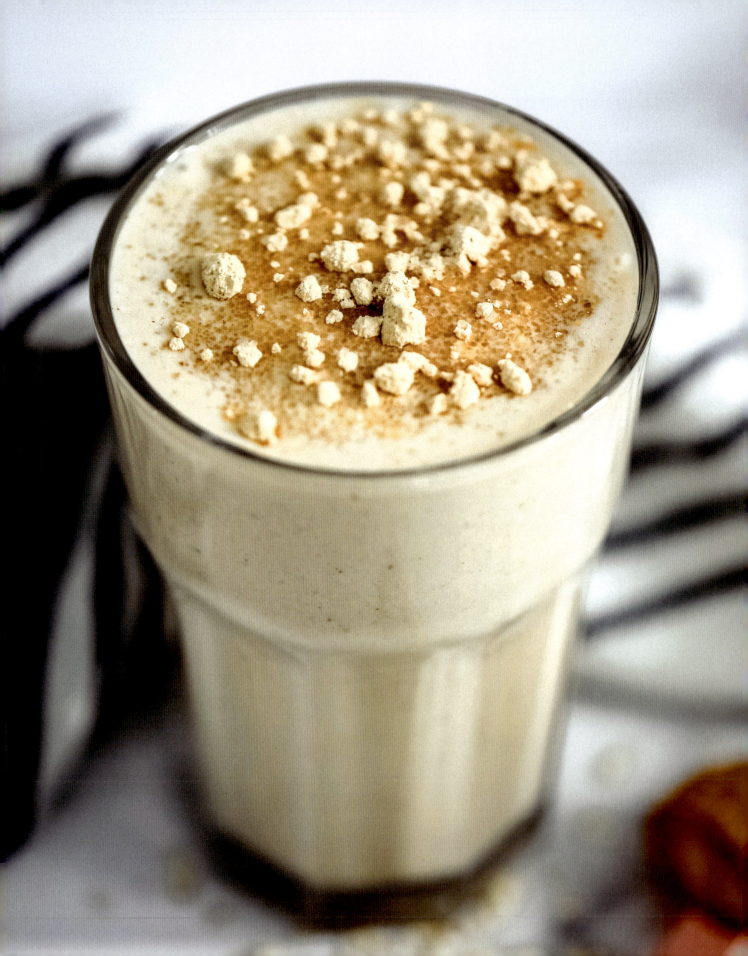

PEANUT BUTTER COOKIE BREAKFAST SHAKE

Makes 1 serving
335 calories / 9F / 33.5C / 30P

Prep: 5 min

1 cup unsweetened almond milk
1 serving CSE Simply Vanilla Protein Powder
2 Tbs. old-fashioned rolled oats
40g frozen banana slices
2 Tbs. CSE Powdered Peanut Butter
1 Tbs. CSE Sweet Classic Peanut Butter
   or natural peanut butter
Dash sea salt
6-8 (120g) ice cubes

Topping:
1 tsp. sugar in the raw

1. Add all of the ingredients to a high-powered blender. Blend on high until smooth.

2. Sprinkle sugar in the raw on top. Enjoy!

PRO TIP: Make ahead and store in an insulated bottle in the fridge or in a cooler with ice. It will stay fresh, thick and cold for up to 24 hours. Add toppings fresh.

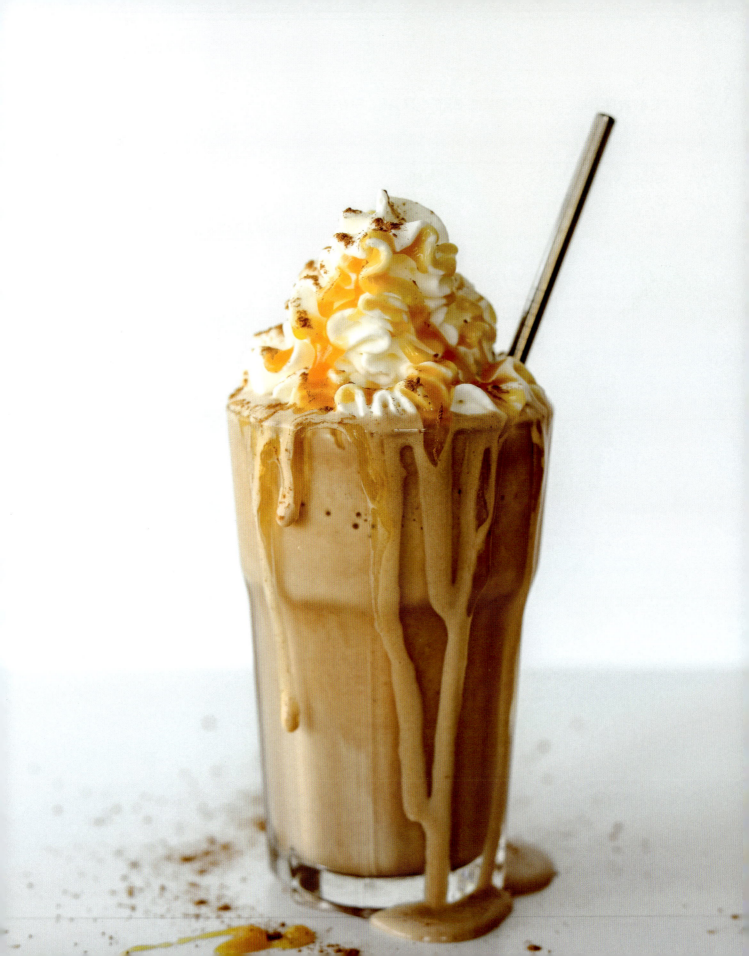

SNICKERS SHAKE
Makes 1 serving
240 calories / 7.5F / 26.5C / 19.5P

Prep: 5 min

¾ cup fat-free milk
½ serving (17g) CSE Chocolate Brownie Batter
   or Caramel Toffee Protein Powder
30g frozen banana slices
1 Tbs. old-fashioned rolled oats
2 tsp. CSE Sweet Classic Peanut Butter, Salted Caramel Butter,
   or natural peanut butter
1 tsp. cocoa powder
6-8 (120g) ice cubes
Toppings:
2 Tbs. spray whipped cream
Walden Farms Caramel Syrup

1. Add all of the ingredients to a high-powered blender. Blend on high until smooth.

2. Pour into a cup. Top with whipped cream and caramel syrup. Enjoy!

PRO TIP: Prep a bunch of these ahead of time for a quick breakfast or snack option. Measure all of the ingredients out into individual zip top bags or containers, excluding the milk and toppings, and store in the freezer. When ready to use, dump the contents of the bag into the blender with the milk. Blend until smooth. Add toppings fresh.

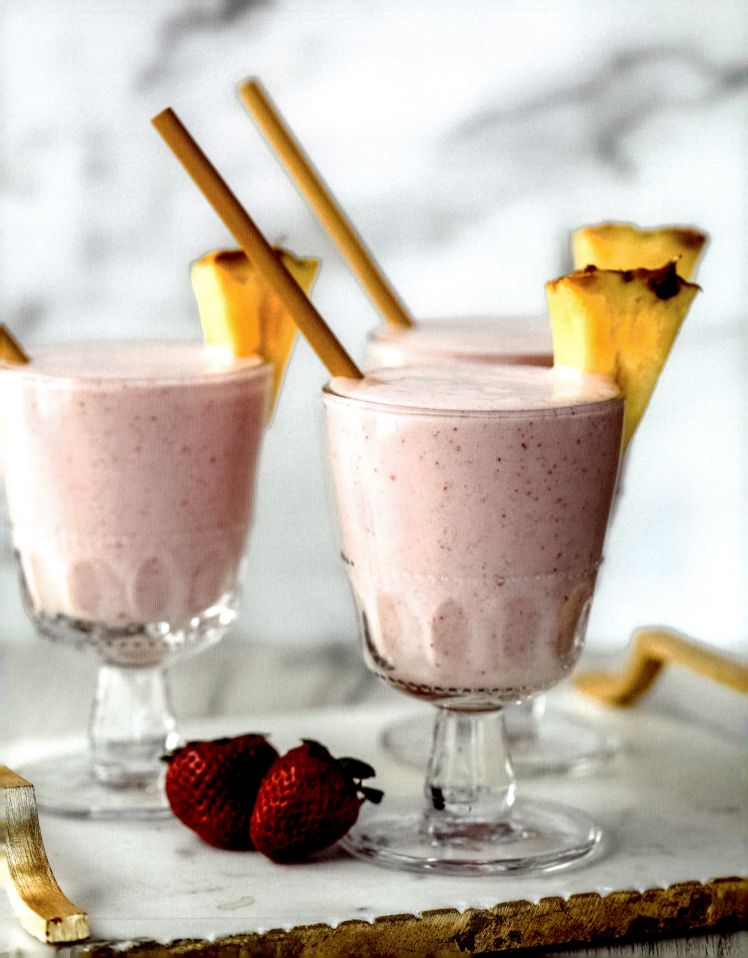

STRAWBERRY COLADA

Makes 1 serving
235 calories / 6F / 28C / 17P

Prep: 5 min

½ cup lite canned coconut milk
½ serving (16g) CSE Simply Vanilla, Strawberry Cheesecake,
   or Coconut Cream Protein Powder
¼ cup nonfat, plain Greek yogurt
½ tsp. coconut extract
75g fresh strawberries
75g frozen pineapple
6-8 (120g) ice cubes

1. Add all of the ingredients to a high-powered blender. Blend on high until smooth.

2. Pour into a cup and enjoy!

PRO TIP: Prep a bunch of these ahead of time for a quick breakfast or snack option. Measure all of the ingredients out into individual zip top bags or containers, excluding the coconut milk, and store in the freezer. When ready to use, dump the contents of the bag into the blender with the coconut milk. Blend until smooth.

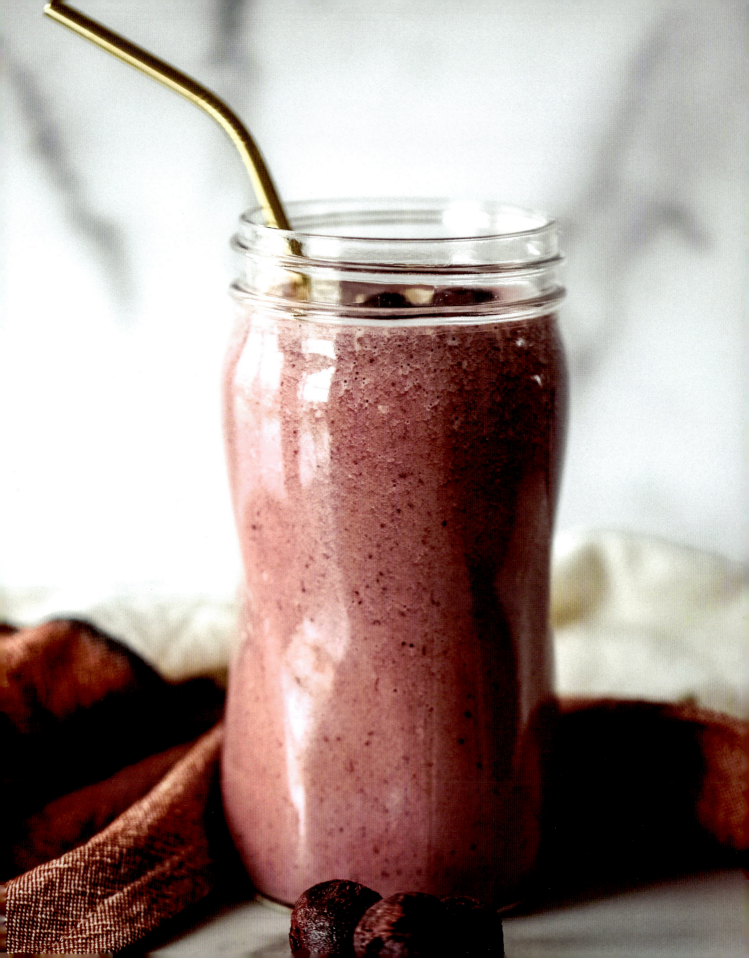

SWEET CHERRY ALMOND FREEZE

Makes 1 serving
350 calories / 13F / 32C / 26P

Prep: 5 min

1 cup unsweetened almond milk
¼ cup nonfat, plain Greek yogurt
130g frozen, pitted dark sweet cherries
¾ serving (24g) CSE Simply Vanilla
   or Chocolate Brownie Batter Protein Powder
1 Tbs. CSE Almond Mocha, Midnight Almond Coconut Butter
   or natural almond butter
½ tsp. almond extract
6-8 (120g) ice cubes

1. Add all of the ingredients to a high-powered blender. Blend on high until smooth.

2. Pour into a cup and enjoy!

PRO TIP: Prep a bunch of these ahead of time for a quick breakfast or snack option. Measure all of the ingredients out into individual zip top bags or containers, excluding the almond milk, and store in the freezer. When ready to use, dump the contents of the bag into the blender with the almond milk. Blend until smooth.

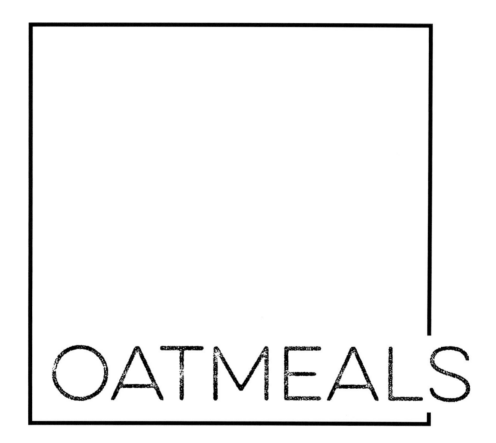

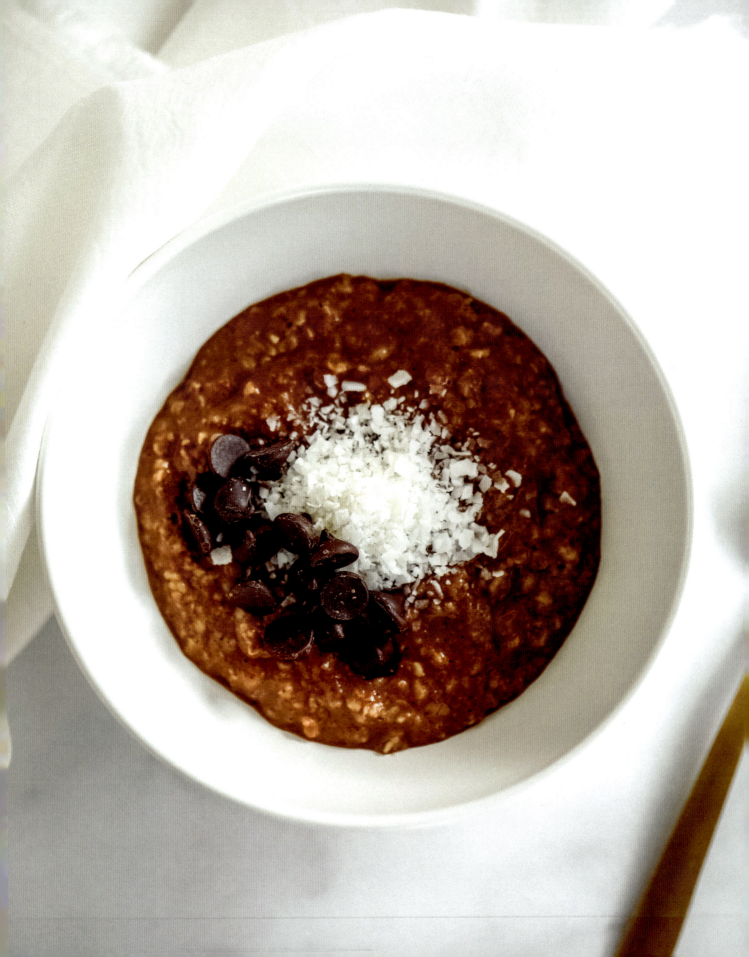

ALMOND JOY OATMEAL

Makes 1 serving
350 calories / 13F / 32C / 26P

Prep: 5 min | **Cook:** 2 min

⅓ cup old-fashioned rolled oats
½ cup water
3 Tbs. liquid egg whites
½ Tbs. CSE Midnight Almond Coconut Butter
 or natural almond butter
¾ serving (25g) CSE Chocolate Brownie Batter Protein Powder
5g unsweetened coconut flakes
10g dark chocolate chips

1. Place the oats, water and egg whites in a microwave-safe bowl. Whisk until the egg whites are well combined.

2. Microwave for 1-2 minutes.

3. Stir in the nut butter and then let cool slightly. Stir in the protein powder and top with the coconut flakes and chocolate chips.

PRO TIPS: To turn this into overnight oats, use almond milk instead of water, remove the egg whites, and add an extra ¼ serving of protein powder. Mix all the ingredients together and store in the fridge overnight. No cooking needed. Stores well in the fridge for up to four days.

How to prepare an easy breakfast in advance for travel: add all the dry ingredients to a zip top bag (omit the egg whites and add an extra ¼ serving of protein powder). When ready to eat, add ½ cup almond milk and nut butter. Stir together and enjoy it cold with a spoon.

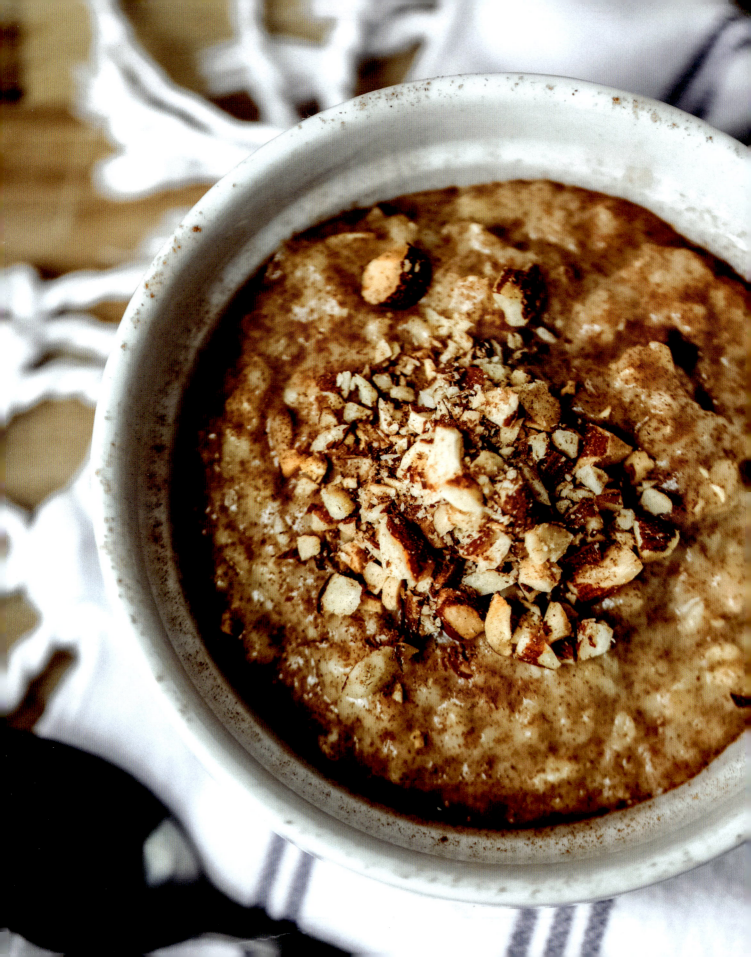

BANANA BREAD OATMEAL
Makes 1 serving
350 calories / 10.5F / 37C / 27P

Prep: 5 min | **Cook:** 2 min

⅓ cup old-fashioned rolled oats
½ cup water
3 Tbs. liquid egg whites
40g mashed banana
Dash sea salt
1 tsp. vanilla extract
2 tsp. CSE Cinnamon Bun, Monkey Business Butter,
 or natural almond butter
¾ serving (25g) CSE Simply Vanilla
 or Bananas Foster Protein Powder

Toppings:
1 Tbs. chopped almonds
Dash cinnamon

1. Combine the rolled oats, water, egg whites, mashed banana, salt and vanilla together in a microwave-safe bowl. Microwave for 1-2 minutes or until oatmeal begins to rise to the top of the bowl.

2. Stir in the nut butter. Let cool for a couple minutes, then stir in the protein powder.

3. Top with chopped almonds and a sprinkle of cinnamon.

PRO TIP: To turn this into overnight oats, use almond milk instead of water, remove the egg whites, and add an extra ¼ scoop of protein powder. Mix all the ingredients together and store in the fridge overnight. No cooking needed. Stores well in the fridge for up to four days.

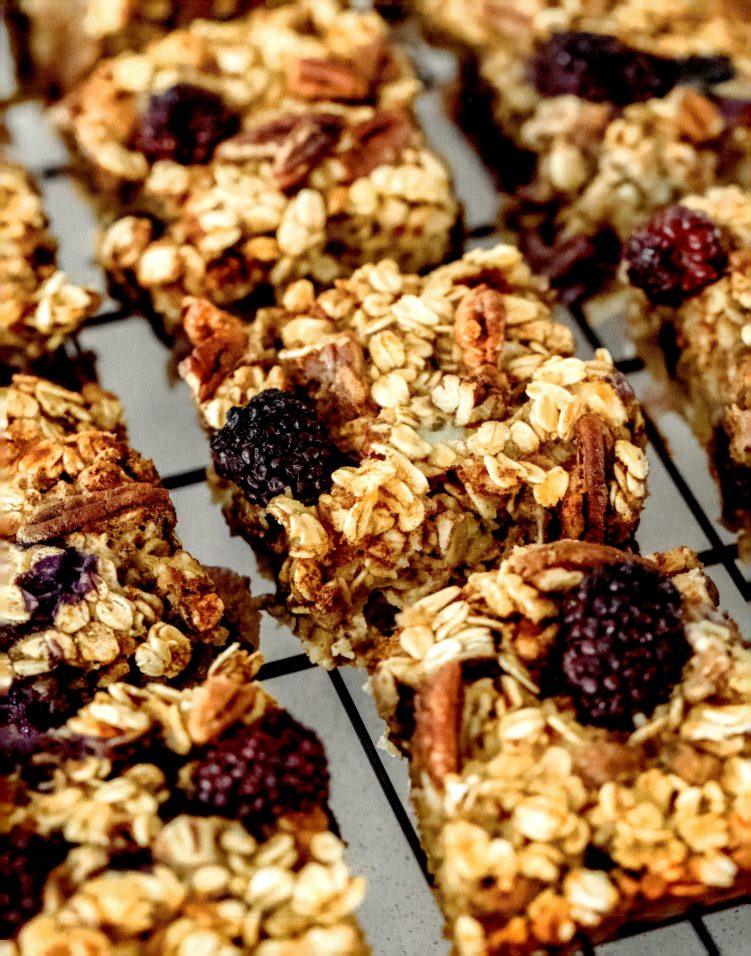

CINNA-BERRY BREAKFAST SQUARES

Makes 12 servings
345 calories / 12F / 34.5C / 24.5P / per serving

Prep: 20 min | **Cook:** 40 min

2 ½ cups old-fashioned rolled oats
½ cup chopped pecans
1 Tbs. cinnamon
1 tsp. baking powder
½ tsp. sea salt
2 cups unsweetened almond milk
2 servings CSE Simply Vanilla
   or Cinnamon Roll Protein Powder
2 large eggs
½ cup raw honey
2 Tbs. unsweetened applesauce

2 tsp. vanilla extract
2 (240g) bananas
1 cup blueberries
½ cup blackberries

Topping per serving:
2 Tbs. spray whipped cream

Side per serving:
1 large egg
3 egg whites (6 Tbs. liquid egg whites)

1. Preheat the oven to 375 degrees.

2. In a large bowl, stir the oats, pecans, cinnamon, baking powder and salt together. Set aside.

3. In a separate bowl, beat the almond milk, protein powder, two eggs, honey, applesauce and vanilla together. Set aside.

4. Grease a 9x13 baking dish. Slice the bananas and place them in a single layer on the bottom of the pan. Layer the blueberries, the dry oat mixture, the wet mixture over the dry and then top with the blackberries. Bake for 40 minutes.

5. Enjoy warm topped with whipped cream.

6. Cook the eggs to your liking and enjoy on the side.

PRO TIP: Make and freeze into individual servings. Thaw in the fridge and microwave or reheat in the oven. Prepare toppings and sides fresh.

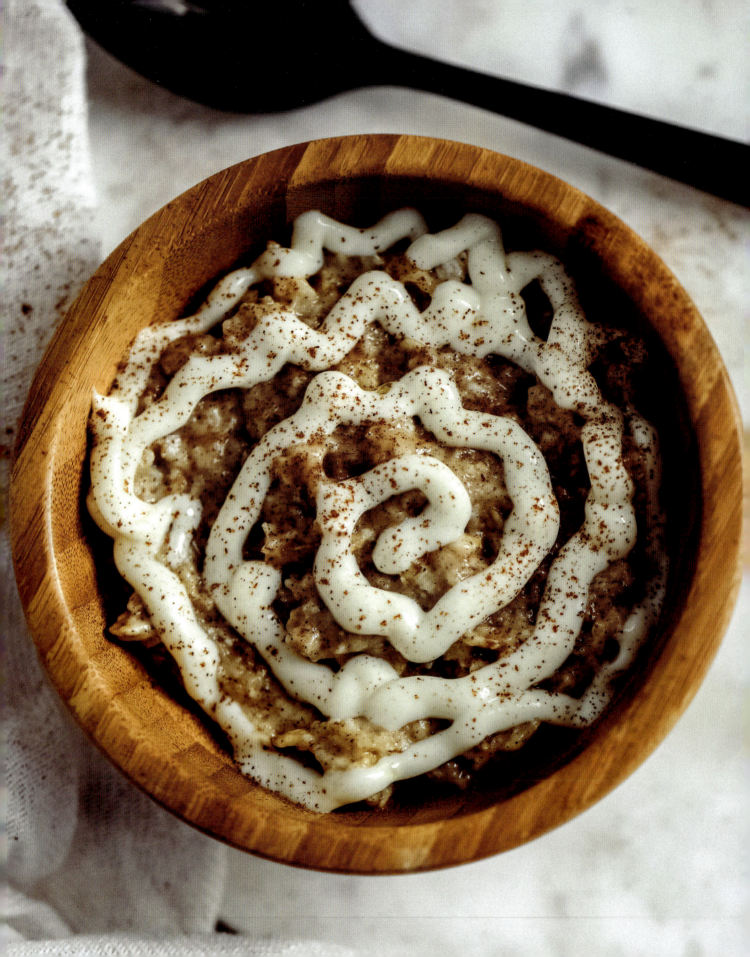

CINNAMON BUN IN A BOWL

Makes 1 serving
350 calories / 13F / 31.5C / 27P

Prep: 10 min | **Cook:** 3 min

⅓ cup old-fashioned rolled oats
½ cup water
2 Tbs. liquid egg whites
1 Tbs. CSE Cinnamon Bun Butter or natural almond butter
½ serving CSE Simply Vanilla
   or Cinnamon Roll Protein Powder
½ tsp. cinnamon
¼ tsp. butter extract
Dash sea salt
Frosting:
1 tsp. melted butter
2 Tbs. nonfat, plain Greek yogurt
¼ tsp. vanilla extract
8g CSE Simply Vanilla or Cinnamon Roll Protein Powder

1. Add the rolled oats, water and egg whites to a bowl. Microwave for 1-2 minutes.

2. Stir in the nut butter. Add ½ serving protein powder, cinnamon, butter extract and sea salt. Stir until well combined.

3. In a separate bowl, add the butter. Microwave for 10-20 seconds or until melted. Stir in the Greek yogurt and vanilla. Add 8g protein powder last and stir until well combined.

4. Drizzle the frosting over the top of the oatmeal and enjoy warm!

PRO TIP: To turn this into overnight oats, use almond milk instead of water, remove the egg whites, and add an extra ¼ scoop of protein powder. Mix all the ingredients together, drizzle the frosting over the top and store in the fridge overnight. No cooking needed. Stores well in the fridge for up to four days.

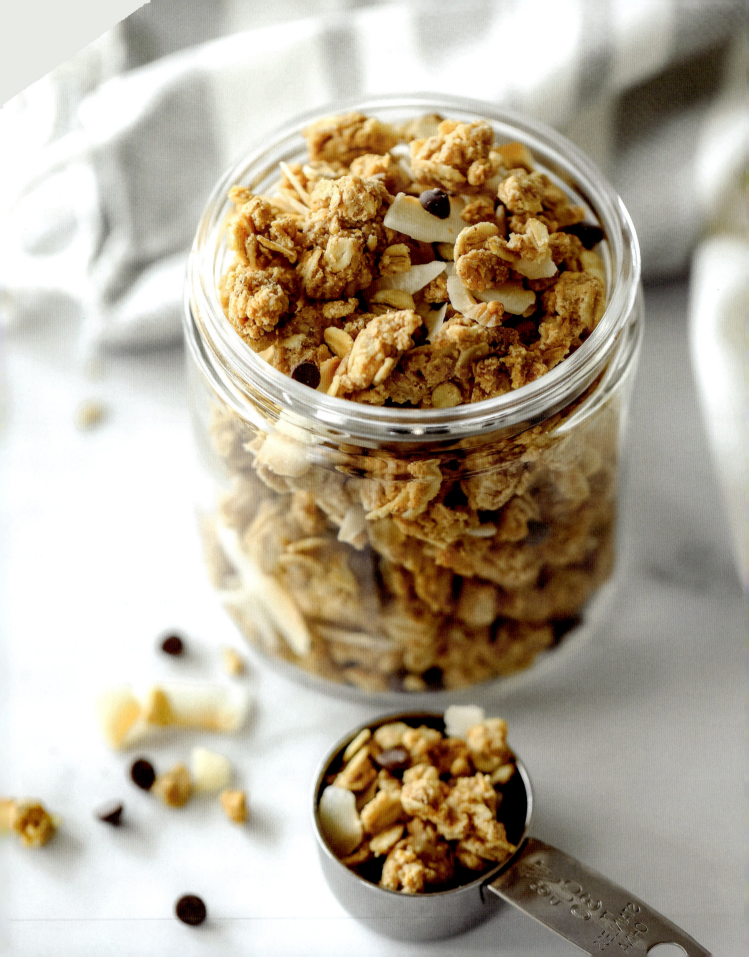

COOKIE CRUMB GRANOLA

Makes 24 servings / about 32g per serving
150 calories / 7.5F / 15C / 5P / per serving

Prep: 15 min | **Cook:** 14 min

- ½ cup CSE Sweet Classic Peanut Butter or natural peanut butter
- ½ cup CSE Butter Salted Caramel Butter or natural almond butter
- ½ cup raw honey
- ½ cup unsweetened flaked coconut
- ¼ cup flaxseed meal
- 2 servings CSE Simply Vanilla Protein Powder
- 2 cups old-fashioned rolled oats
- ½ tsp. sea salt
- ½ tsp. vanilla or almond extract

Topping:
- ¼ cup mini chocolate chips

1. Preheat the oven to 350 degrees.

2. Place all the ingredients into a bowl and mix until combined and crumbly.

3. Spread out onto a baking sheet lined with parchment paper. Bake for 5-7 minutes, then flip and bake for another 5-7 minutes.

4. Let cool on the cookie sheet for 30 minutes before adding the chocolate chips. Sprinkle the chocolate chips on top (they should melt a little) and pour into an airtight container; store in the fridge.

PRO TIP: Make endless varieties by swapping in different protein powder flavors, nut butters and add-ins!

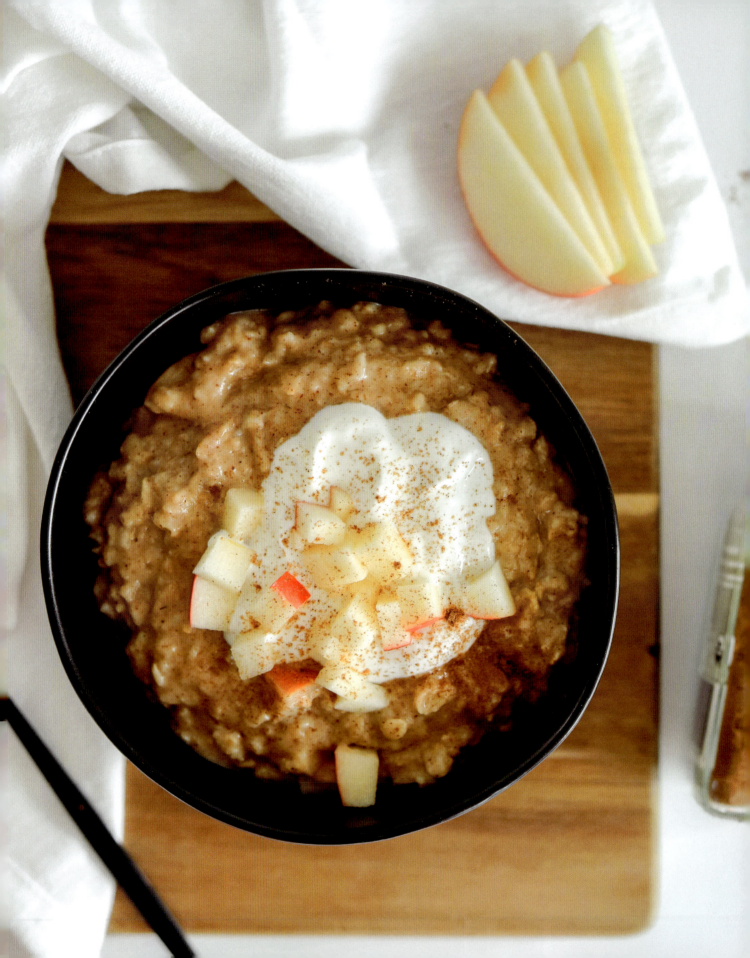

HOT APPLE PIE OATS

Makes 1 serving
330 calories / 11F / 34C / 26P

Prep: 10 min | **Cook:** 2 min

⅓ cup old-fashioned rolled oats
½ cup water
¼ cup liquid egg whites
60g fresh, chopped apples
2 tsp. CSE Cinnamon Bun Butter
   or natural almond butter
1 tsp. grass-fed butter
Dash cinnamon
Dash nutmeg
½ serving (16g) CSE Simply Vanilla or Cinnamon Roll Protein Powder
Toppings:
2 Tbs. nonfat, plain Greek yogurt
Vanilla stevia drops

1. Stir raw oats, water, egg whites and apples together in a bowl. Mix well and microwave for 1-2 minutes. Stir in nut butter, butter, cinnamon and nutmeg. Stir in protein powder last.

2. Stir Greek yogurt and stevia together in a bowl. Top oatmeal with yogurt and enjoy warm.

PRO TIP: To turn this into overnight oats, use almond milk instead of water, remove the egg whites, and add an extra ¼ scoop of protein powder. Mix all the ingredients together, add toppings and store in the fridge overnight. No cooking needed. Stores well in the fridge for up to four days.

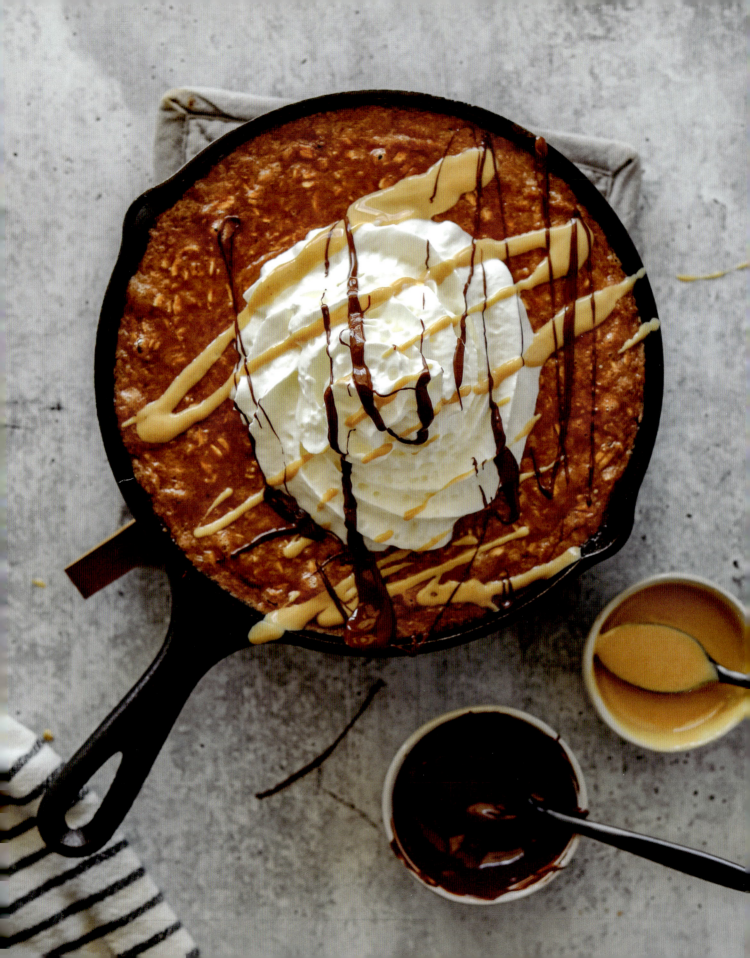

OOEY-GOOEY BREAKFAST BROWNIES

Makes 4 servings
350 calories / 13F / 37C / 25P / per serving

Prep: 15 min | **Cook:** 12 min

1 ½ cups old-fashioned rolled oats
3 servings CSE Chocolate Brownie Batter
   or Chocolate Peanut Butter Protein Powder
1 Tbs. cocoa powder
Dash sea salt
½ tsp. baking powder
¾ cup unsweetened almond milk
½ cup unsweetened applesauce
100g liquid egg whites
50g CSE Sweet Classic Peanut Butter
   or natural peanut butter
½ tsp. vanilla extract

Toppings:
8 Tbs. spray whipped cream
32g dark chocolate chips

1. Preheat the oven to 350 degrees.

2. Add the oats, protein powder, cocoa powder, sea salt and baking powder to a bowl. Stir together.

3. In a separate bowl, add the almond milk, applesauce, egg whites, peanut butter and vanilla. Whisk together until well combined.

4. Add the wet ingredients to the dry ingredients and stir until well coated.

5. Pour into a greased 8x8 baking dish or cast iron skillet of similar size. Bake for 10-12 minutes or to your desired doneness. Divide into four equal servings. Top each serving with two tablespoons of spray whipped cream and 8g chocolate chips.

PRO TIP: Make endless varieties by swapping in different protein powder flavors and nut butters! Serve up as dessert!

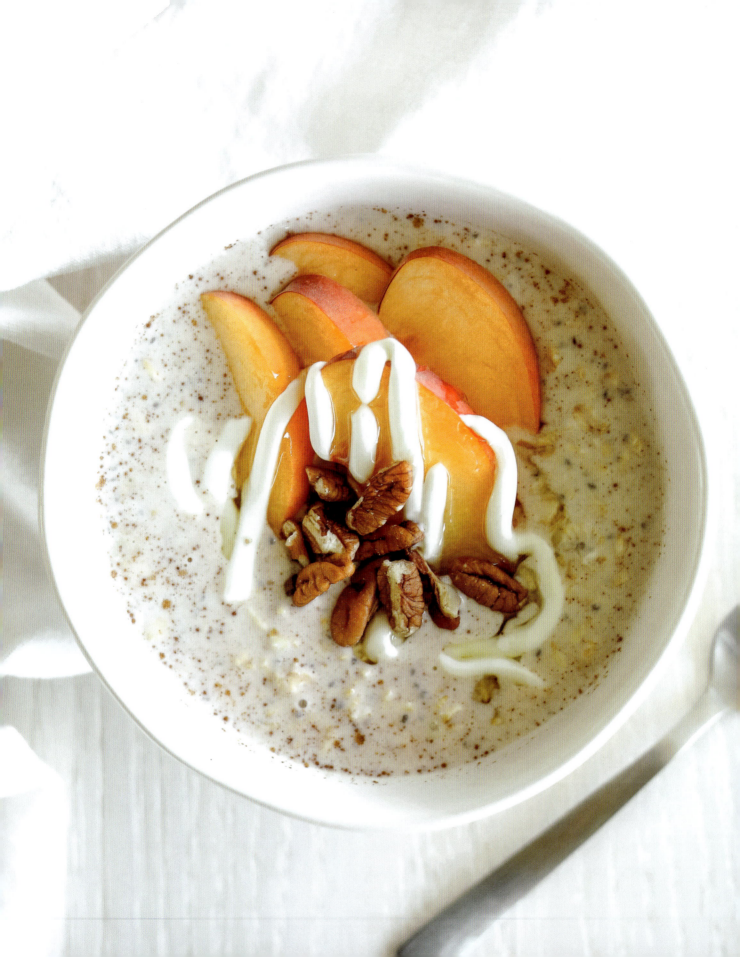

PEACH COBBLER OVERNIGHT OATS
Makes 1 serving
345 calories / 12F / 39C / 22P

Prep: 10 min + refrigeration

⅓ cup old-fashioned rolled oats
⅔ cup unsweetened almond milk
4 Tbs. nonfat, plain Greek yogurt
½ serving CSE Simply Vanilla
   or Peaches & Cream Protein Powder
1 tsp. chia seeds
¼ tsp. ground cinnamon
Dash ground nutmeg
Toppings:
75g fresh, ripe peaches
1 serving vanilla stevia drops
10g chopped pecans
1 tsp. raw honey

1. Stir oats, milk, two tablespoons of yogurt, protein powder, chia seeds, cinnamon and nutmeg together in a jar or container. Store in the fridge overnight.

2. In the morning, sweeten two tablespoons of yogurt with stevia. Top overnight oats with peaches, sweetened yogurt, chopped pecans and a drizzle of honey. Enjoy cold; no cooking necessary. Store in the fridge for up to four days.

PRO TIP: To turn this into a hot peach cobbler, use ½ cup water instead of milk. Add the oats and the water to a bowl. Mix well and microwave for 1-2 minutes. Stir in the yogurt, protein powder, chia seeds, spices and stevia. Top with peaches, pecans and honey.

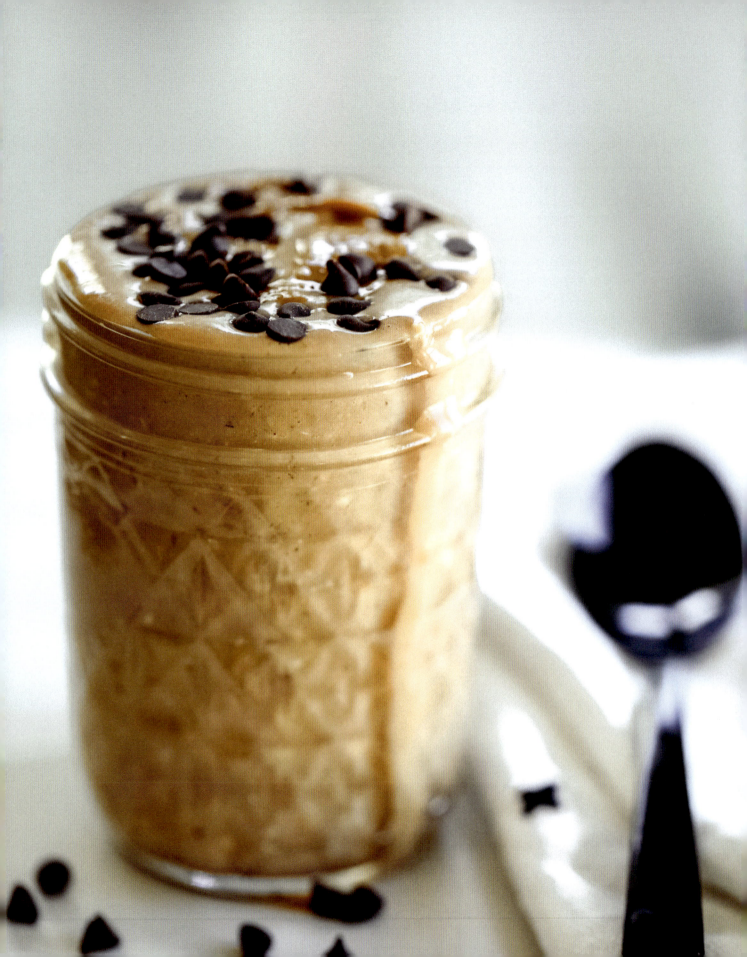

PEANUT BUTTER OVERNIGHT OATS
Makes 1 serving
350 calories / 10.5F / 39C / 25P

Prep: 10 min + refrigeration

⅓ cup old-fashioned rolled oats
½ serving (16g) CSE Chocolate Brownie Batter
  or Chocolate Peanut Butter Protein Powder
⅔ cup unsweetened almond milk
3 Tbs. CSE Powdered Peanut Butter
1 tsp. golden flaxseed meal
25g sliced or mashed banana (or add as a topping)
Toppings:
1 tsp. mini chocolate chips
1 tsp. CSE Sweet Classic Peanut Butter, Candy Bar,
  Buckeye Brownie Peanut Butter or natural peanut butter

1. Add all of the ingredients (except for the toppings) to a jar or container and stir until well combined. Cover and store in the fridge overnight.

2. In the morning, add the chocolate chips and peanut butter. Enjoy cold. No cooking necessary. Store in the fridge for up to four days.

PRO TIPS: To turn this into a hot oatmeal, use ⅔ cup water instead of milk. Add the oats, water and mashed banana to a bowl. Mix well and microwave for 1-2 minutes. Stir in the powdered peanut butter, flaxseed meal, and protein powder. Top with mini chocolate chips and peanut butter.

How to prepare an easy breakfast in advance for travel: add all the dry ingredients to a zip top bag. When ready to eat, add ½ cup almond milk, nut butter and banana. Stir together and enjoy it cold with a spoon.

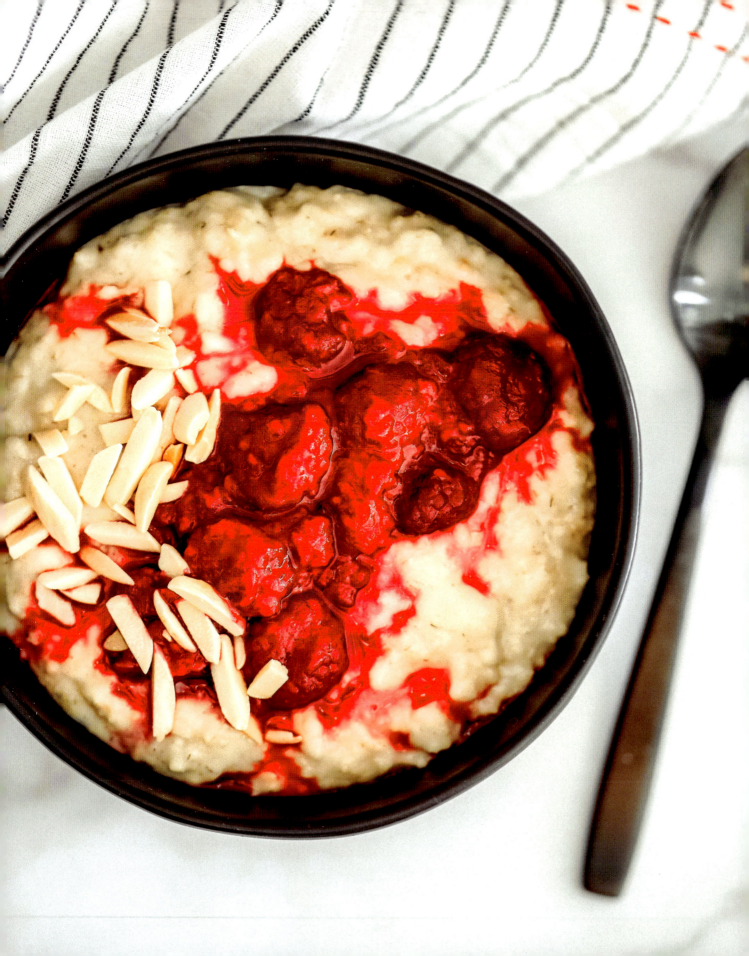

RASPBERRY ALMOND OATS

Makes 1 serving
340 calories / 10.5F / 35C / 26.5P

Prep: 10 min | **Cook:** 3 min

⅓ cup old-fashioned rolled oats
½ cup water
2 Tbs. liquid egg whites
½ Tbs. CSE Salted Caramel Butter
  or natural almond butter
⅛ tsp. almond extract
Vanilla stevia drops, optional
¼ cup nonfat, plain Greek yogurt
½ serving CSE Simply Vanilla Protein Powder
⅓ cup fresh or frozen raspberries
1 Tbs. sliced almonds

1. Mix oats, egg whites and water together in a bowl.

2. Microwave for 1-2 minutes.

3. Stir in the nut butter, almond extract, stevia and Greek yogurt. Add in the protein powder last and mix until well combined.

4. Heat the raspberries in the microwave for 30-60 seconds or in a small saucepan on the stovetop. Cook until melted down and warm. Add to the oatmeal and top with sliced almonds.

PRO TIP: To turn this into overnight oats, use almond milk instead of water, remove the egg whites, and add an extra ¼ scoop of protein powder. Mix all the ingredients together, except for the raspberries and almonds, and store in the fridge overnight. No cooking needed. Add the raspberries and almonds fresh before eating. Stores well in the fridge for up to four days.

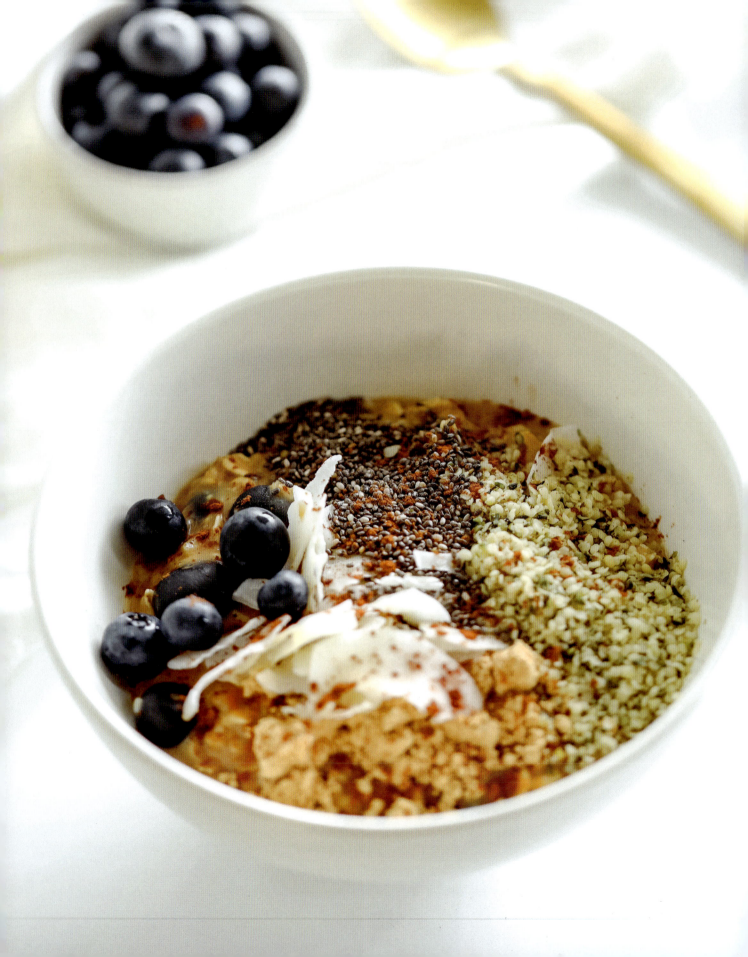

SUPERFOODS BREAKFAST BOWL
Makes 1 serving
350 calories / 13F / 35C / 24P

Prep: 10 min | **Cook:** 2 min

⅓ cup old-fashioned rolled oats
½ cup water
2 Tbs. CSE Powdered Peanut Butter
½ serving (16g) CSE Chocolate Brownie Batter
    or Simply Vanilla Protein Powder
Toppings:
¼ cup fresh blueberries
1 Tbs. unsweetened shredded coconut
1 Tbs. hemp seeds
1 tsp. chia seeds
Dash cinnamon
Splash of unsweetened almond milk, if needed

1. Mix the rolled oats, water and powdered peanut butter together in a bowl. Microwave on high for 1-2 minutes. Let cool for 2 minutes then stir in the protein powder.

2. Top with blueberries, coconut, hemp seeds, chia seeds and cinnamon. If the oatmeal is too thick, add a splash of unsweetened almond milk and stir together.

PRO TIPS: To turn this into overnight oats, use ⅔ cup almond milk instead of water. Mix all the ingredients together, except for the blueberries and store in the fridge overnight. No cooking needed. Add the blueberries fresh before eating. Stores well in the fridge for up to four days.

How to prepare an easy breakfast in advance for travel: add all the dry ingredients to a zip top bag. When ready to eat, add ½ cup almond milk and blueberries. Stir together and enjoy it cold with a spoon.

PANCAKES & WAFFLES

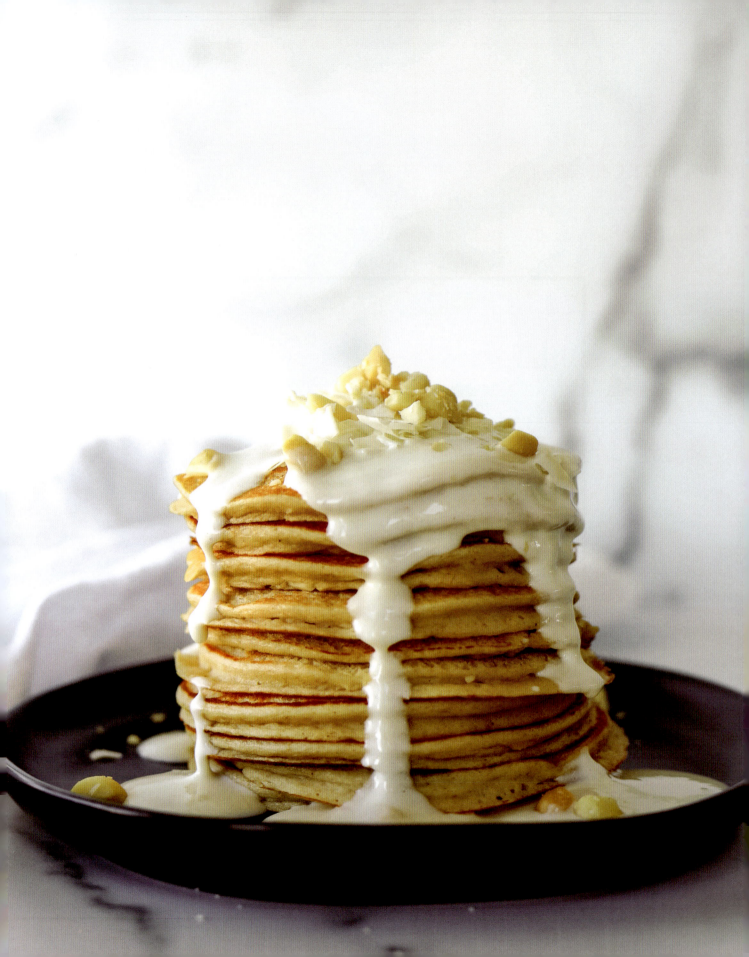

BANANA MACADAMIA NUT PANCAKES

Makes 4 servings
355 calories / 11.5F / 37.5C / 26P / per serving

Prep: 15 min | **Cook:** 15 min

¾ cup water
2 egg whites (¼ cup liquid egg whites)
½ cup low-fat cottage cheese
75g banana
1 ½ cups CSE Buttermilk, Gluten-Free Buttermilk,
  or Vanilla Pancake & Waffle Mix
40g finely chopped macadamia nuts

Coconut Cream Syrup:
½ cup nonfat, plain Greek yogurt
¼ cup unsweetened almond milk
1 Tbs. raw honey
1 serving CSE Simply Vanilla
  or Coconut Cream Protein Powder
2 Tbs. unsweetened shredded coconut
1 tsp. coconut extract, optional

1. Heat griddle to medium heat.

2. Place water, egg whites, cottage cheese, banana and CSE Pancake & Waffle Mix in a blender. Blend on high until smooth. Stir in macadamia nuts.

3. Spray griddle with cooking spray. Using a ¼ measuring cup, pour batter slowly onto the griddle. Once small bubbles form on top of the pancakes, flip and cook on the other side. Weigh the pancakes, and divide the amount by four to get the amount needed to fill one serving.

4. Add all of the Coconut Cream Syrup ingredients to a blender and blend until smooth. Weigh the syrup and divide the weight by four to get the amount needed to fill one serving.

5. Top the warm pancakes with the Coconut Cream Syrup and enjoy!

PRO TIP: Make a double or triple batch, then freeze the pancakes into individual servings. Reheat in the toaster when ready to serve. Make the Coconut Cream Syrup fresh.

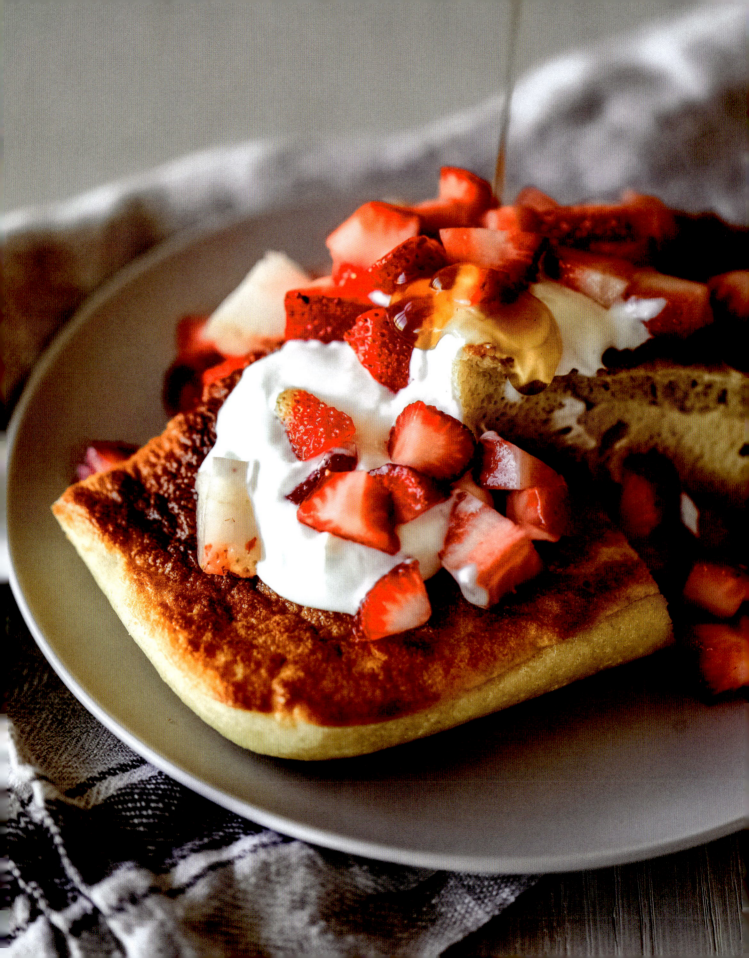

GERMAN PANCAKES

Makes 4 servings
340 calories / 11F / 34C / 27P / per serving

Prep: 15 min | **Cook:** 20 min

2 Tbs. coconut oil
2 large eggs
8 egg whites (1 cup liquid egg whites)
1 ½ cups fat-free milk
1 ½ cups CSE Buttermilk, Gluten-Free Buttermilk,
 or Vanilla Pancake & Waffle Mix
½ tsp. sea salt
½ tsp. vanilla extract

Toppings:
¼ cup nonfat, plain Greek yogurt
Vanilla stevia drops
2 cups chopped strawberries
CSE Maple Syrup or other syrup of choice (not included in macros)

1. Preheat the oven to 425 degrees. Add coconut oil to a 9x13 glass baking dish. Place in the oven until melted, about 5 minutes. Remove from the oven and set aside.

2. Place eggs, egg whites, milk, CSE Pancake & Waffle Mix, salt and vanilla in a blender and blend on medium speed for 5 minutes, no less.

3. Spray the sides of the baking dish with cooking spray and pour mixture into the hot coconut oil. Bake for 20 minutes.

4. Cut the pancake into four equal portions. Sweeten the yogurt with stevia and spoon one tablespoon onto each portion along with a ¼ cup of fresh strawberries and syrup to taste.

PRO TIP: Try swapping in different varieties of fruit for a topping. Our favorites are peaches, blueberries or bananas.

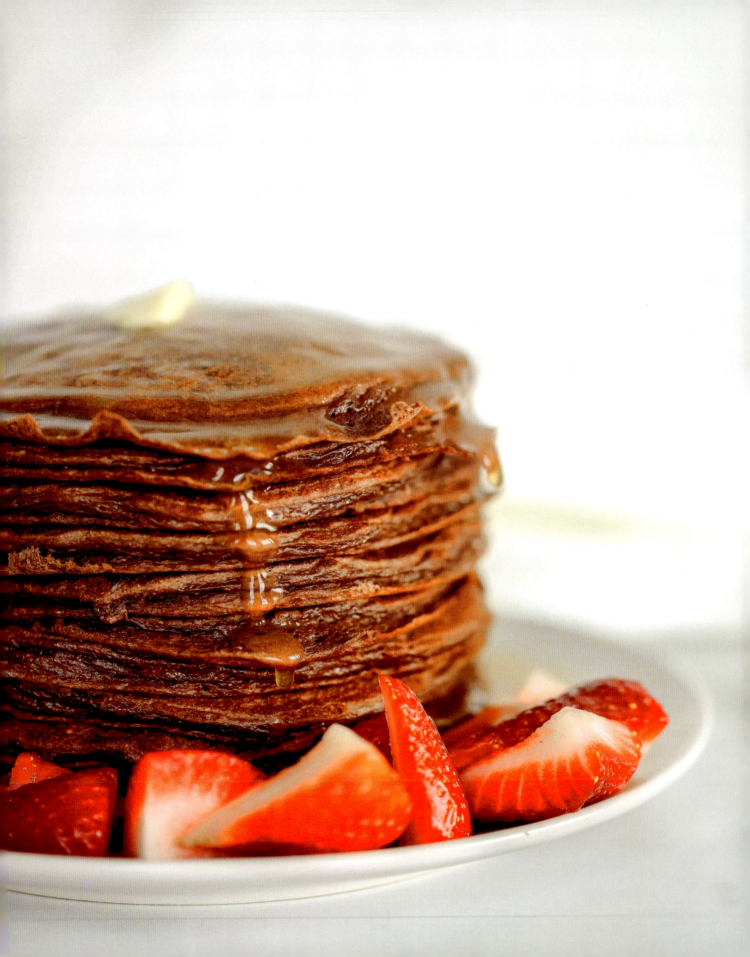

HOT COCOA PANCAKES

Makes 4 servings
350 calories / 11.5F / 36.5C / 26P / per serving

Prep: 15 min | **Cook:** 15 min

½ cup nonfat, plain Greek yogurt
1 cup unsweetened almond milk
3 large eggs
2 tsp. vanilla extract
Vanilla stevia drops, to taste
1 ½ cups CSE Chocolate Chocolate or Gluten-Free Chocolate Chocolate Pancake & Waffle Mix
2 Tbs. cocoa powder
1 serving CSE Chocolate Brownie Batter Protein Powder
Dash sea salt

Toppings per serving:
½ Tbs. grass-fed butter
1 serving CSE Maple Syrup or other syrup of choice
2 Tbs. strawberries

1. Heat griddle to medium heat.

2. Whisk the Greek yogurt, almond milk, eggs, vanilla and stevia together in a bowl; set aside.

3. In a separate bowl, combine the CSE Pancake & Waffle Mix, cocoa powder, protein powder and sea salt together. Add the wet ingredients to the dry ingredients and stir until just combined.

4. Using a ¼ measuring cup, pour the batter onto the greased griddle. Once small bubbles begin to form around the edges, flip and cook on the other side until golden brown. Should make about 16 pancakes; four per serving.

5. Make the CSE Maple Syrup Mix by mixing with water and top each serving of pancakes with ½ tablespoon butter, two tablespoons of prepared syrup and two tablespoons of fresh cut strawberries. Enjoy!

PRO TIP: Make a double or triple batch, then freeze the pancakes into individual servings. Reheat in the toaster when ready to serve. Add the toppings fresh.

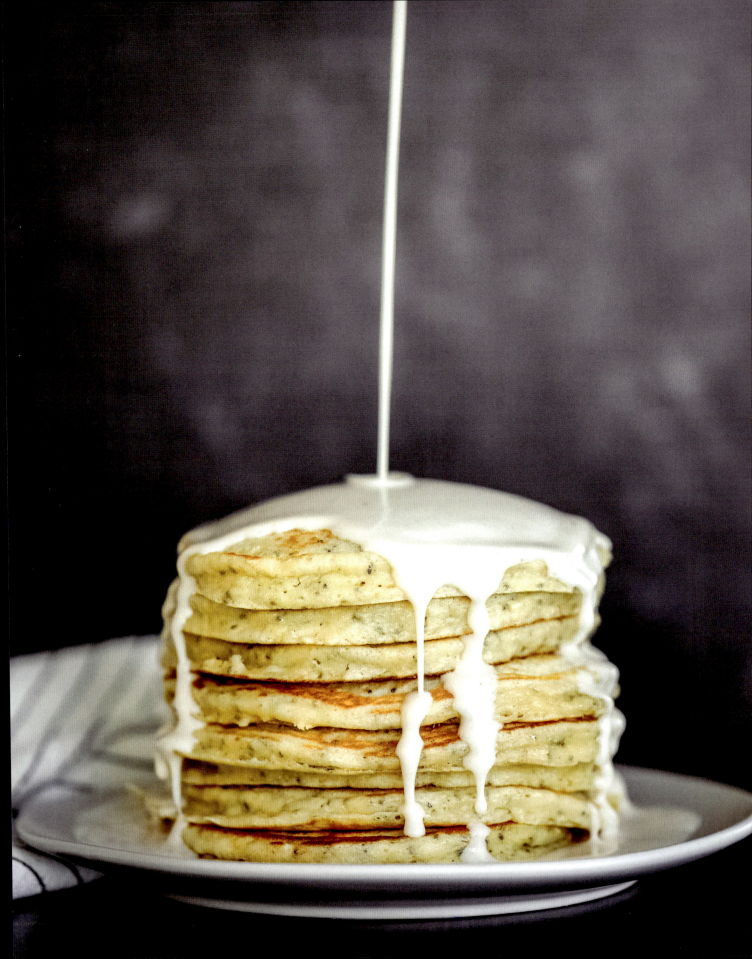

LEMON CHIA PANCAKES

Makes 4 servings
350 calories / 12F / 34.5C / 28.5P / per serving

Prep: 15 min | **Cook:** 15 min

1 ¾ cups CSE Buttermilk, Gluten-Free Buttermilk,
  or Vanilla Pancake & Waffle Mix
⅓ cup water
1 cup nonfat, plain Greek yogurt
4 large eggs
Vanilla stevia drops, optional
1 ½ Tbs. chia seeds
1 lemon, zest of

Toppings per serving:
1 Tbs. nonfat, plain Greek yogurt
½ serving CSE Maple Syrup or other syrup of choice
1 tsp. coconut oil or grass-fed butter

1. Heat a skillet to medium heat.

2. In a large bowl, whisk the CSE Pancake & Waffle Mix, water, yogurt, eggs and stevia together. Once combined, stir in the chia seeds and lemon zest.

3. Pour ¼ cup of the mixture onto the griddle. When small bubbles begin to form on the top, flip the pancakes over. Repeat for the remaining batter. Weigh the pancakes, and divide the amount by four to get the amount needed to fill one serving.

4. Make the CSE Maple Syrup Mix by mixing with water. Stir the Greek yogurt and syrup together in a small bowl. Top each serving with one teaspoon of coconut oil or butter, then drizzle the yogurt/syrup mixture over the top.

PRO TIP: Make a double or triple batch, then freeze the pancakes into individual servings. Reheat in the toaster when ready to serve. Add the toppings fresh.

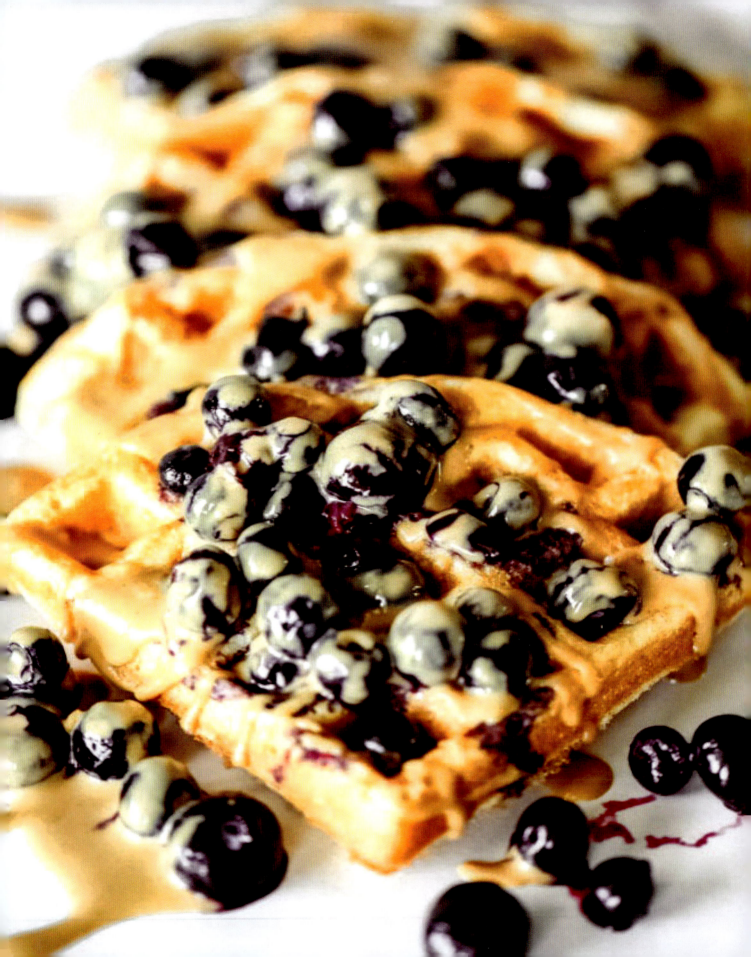

BLUEBERRY PB POWER WAFFLES
Makes 4 servings
350 calories / 11.5F / 34C / 27.5P / per serving

Prep: 15 min | **Cook:** 15 min

1 cup CSE Buttermilk, Gluten-Free Buttermilk, or Vanilla Pancake & Waffle Mix
½ cup water
4 large eggs
½ cup low-fat cottage cheese
Vanilla stevia drops, optional

Peanut Butter Sauce:
½ cup CSE Powdered Peanut Butter
7 Tbs. water
2 Tbs. CSE Sweet Classic Peanut Butter or natural peanut butter
4 tsp. raw honey

Toppings:
1 cup frozen blueberries
Vanilla stevia drops, optional

1. Heat waffle iron to medium heat.

2. Place the CSE Pancake & Waffle Mix, water, eggs, cottage cheese and stevia in a blender; blend until smooth. Once the waffle iron is hot, spray with cooking spray and pour batter inside. Weigh all the waffles and divide the weight by four to get the amount needed to fill one serving.

3. Whisk all the ingredients for the Peanut Butter Sauce together in a bowl. Weigh the mixture and divide the weight by four to get the amount needed to fill one serving.

4. Add the blueberries to a bowl with the stevia. Stir and then microwave for 1-2 minutes. The berries should be warm and melted down.

5. Pour the Peanut Butter Sauce over the hot waffles and top with ¼ of the warm blueberries.

PRO TIP: Make a double or triple batch, then freeze the waffles into individual servings. Reheat in the toaster when ready to serve. Add the Peanut Butter Sauce and toppings fresh.

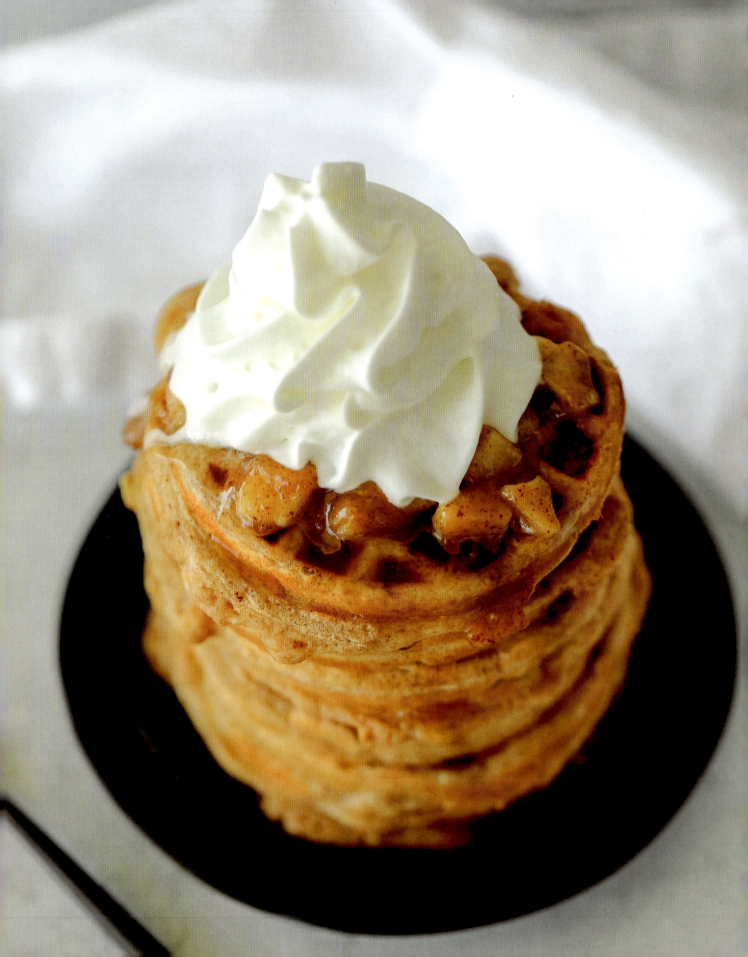

CARAMEL APPLE PIE WAFFLES

Makes 4 servings
350 calories / 11.5F / 39.5C / 24.5P / per serving

Prep: 15 min | **Cook:** 15 min

100g apples
80g CSE Salted Caramel Butter or natural almond butter
1 Tbs. (42g) raw honey
1 ⅓ cups CSE Buttermilk, Gluten-Free Buttermilk,
  or Vanilla Pancake & Waffle Mix
½ cup nonfat, plain Greek yogurt
1 ¼ cups liquid egg whites
1 tsp. cinnamon

Toppings:
8 Tbs. spray whipped cream
2 servings CSE Maple Syrup or other syrup of choice

1. Peel and chop the apples into tiny pieces.

2. Heat a frying pan over low heat. Spray the pan with cooking spray, then add the apples, nut butter and honey. Stir until the apples are well coated. Cook until the apples are soft and the butter and honey are melted. Remove from heat, cover and set aside.

3. Heat a waffle iron.

4. Add the CSE Pancake & Waffle Mix, Greek yogurt, egg whites, and cinnamon to a bowl. Whisk together until smooth. Either fold the caramel apple mixture into the batter or use as a topping once the waffles are cooked. Spray the waffle iron with cooking spray, then add the batter and cook until golden brown. Repeat with the remaining batter.

5. Weigh all the waffles and divide the weight by four to get the amount needed to fill one serving. Top each serving with the caramel apple topping (if applicable), two tablespoons of whipped cream and ½ tablespoon of prepared syrup.

PRO TIP: Make a double or triple batch, then freeze the waffles into individual servings. Reheat in the toaster when ready to serve. Add the toppings fresh.

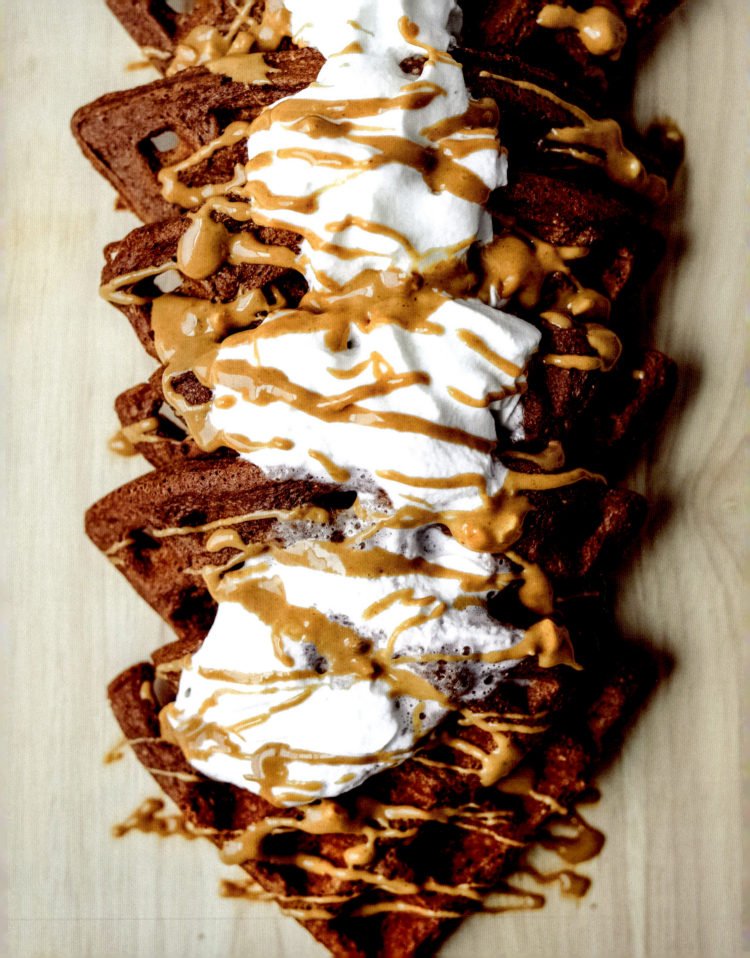

CHOCOLATE WAFFLES
Makes 4 servings
350 calories / 12F / 36C / 25.5P / per serving

Prep: 15 min | **Cook:** 15 min

1 ¾ cups CSE Chocolate Chocolate or Gluten-Free Chocolate Chocolate Pancake & Waffle Mix
1 serving CSE Chocolate Brownie Batter Protein Powder
1 Tbs. cocoa powder
1 ¼ cups water
2 large eggs
40g mashed banana

Toppings per serving:
1 Tbs. CSE Sweet Classic, Buckeye Brownie Peanut Butter or natural peanut butter
2 Tbs. spray whipped cream
CSE Maple Syrup or other syrup of choice (not included in macros)

1. Preheat waffle iron.

2. In a medium-sized bowl, mix together the CSE Pancake & Waffle Mix, protein powder, cocoa powder, water, eggs, and banana. Stir together until well combined.

3. Spray the waffle iron with cooking spray. Pour the batter into the waffle iron. Repeat with the remaining batter. Weigh the waffles and divide the weight by four to get the amount needed to fill one serving.

4. Top each serving with one tablespoon of peanut butter, two tablespoons of whipped cream and syrup. Enjoy!

PRO TIP: Make a double or triple batch, then freeze the waffles into individual servings. Reheat in the toaster when ready to serve. Add the toppings fresh.

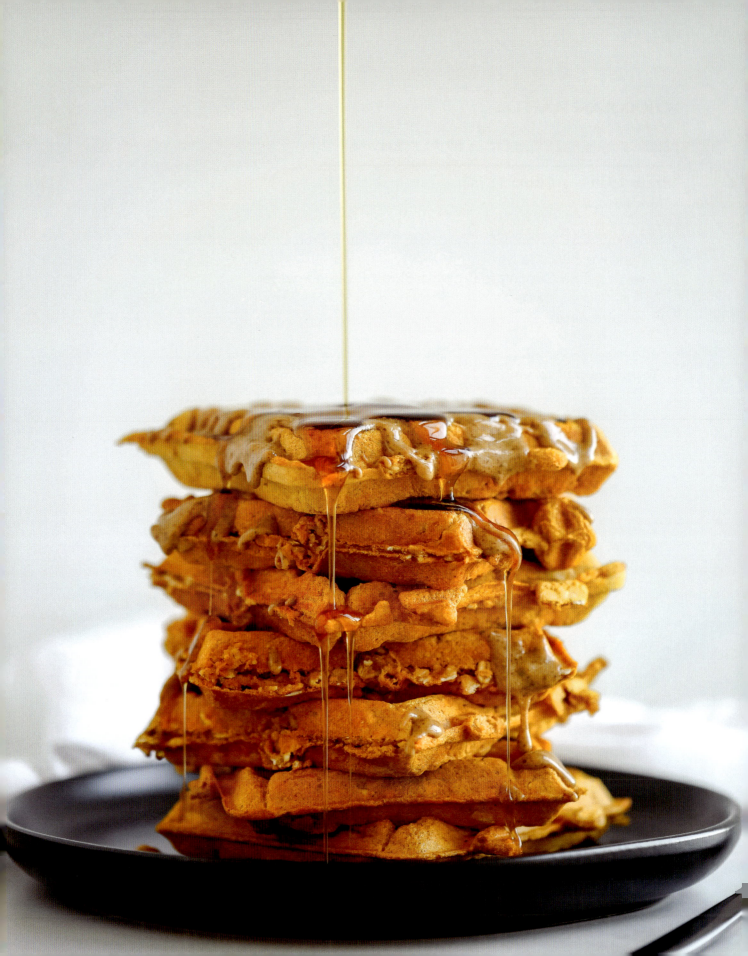

PUMPKIN PROTEIN WAFFLES
Makes 4 servings
350 calories / 12F / 34.5C / 25.5P / per serving

Prep: 15 min | **Cook:** 15 min

1 cup CSE Buttermilk, Gluten-Free Buttermilk, or Vanilla Pancake & Waffle Mix
2 servings (68g) CSE Pumpkin Pie or Simply Vanilla Protein Powder
½ cup canned pumpkin
½ cup unsweetened almond milk
2 large eggs
2 tsp. pumpkin pie spice

Toppings per serving:
1 Tbs. CSE Pumpkin Spice, Salted Caramel Butter
   or natural almond butter
1 serving CSE Maple Syrup or other syrup of choice
2 Tbs. spray whipped cream

1. Heat waffle iron.

2. Add the CSE Pancake & Waffle Mix, protein powder, pumpkin, almond milk, eggs, and pumpkin pie spice to a high-powered blender. Blend until smooth.

3. Pour into the waffle iron and cook for two minutes (these burn easily, so watch closely). Remove from the waffle iron and weigh the waffles, then divide into four servings.

4. Make the CSE Maple Syrup Mix by mixing with water. Drizzle the nut butter and syrup over the waffles and then top with whipped cream.

PRO TIP: Make a double or triple batch, then freeze the waffles into individual servings. Reheat in the toaster when ready to serve. Add the toppings fresh.

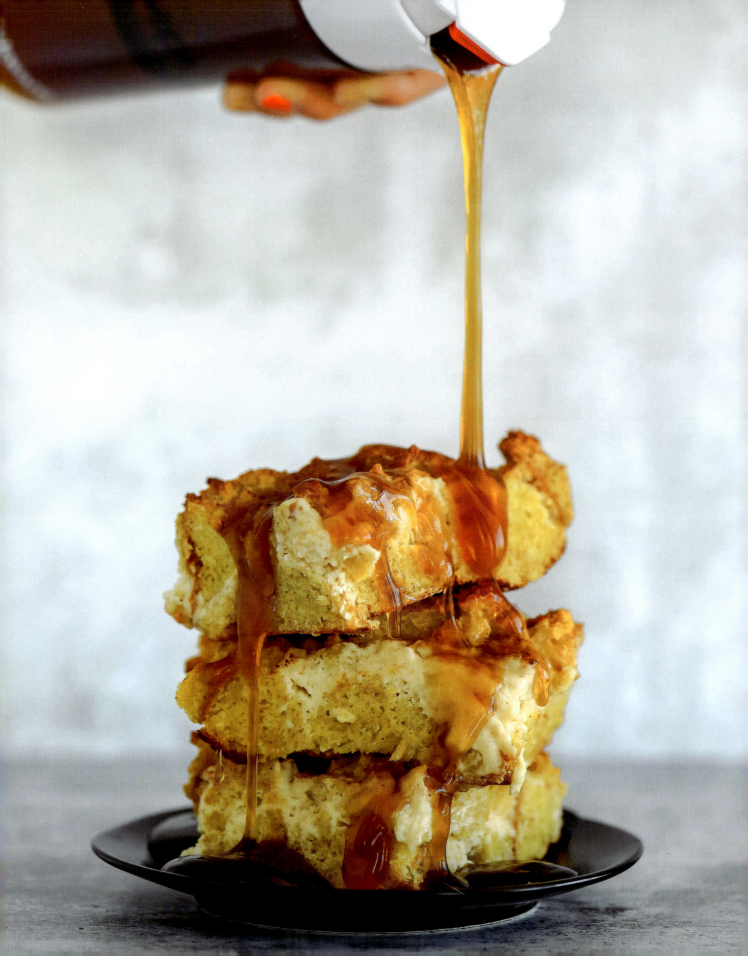

BAKED CINNAMON ROLL FRENCH TOAST
Makes 12 servings
180 calories / 8F / 18.5C / 9P / per serving

Prep: 20 min | **Cook:** 35 min

600g CSE Homemade Honey-Wheat Bread (see page 201 for recipe) or other artisan bread of choice
8 eggs
½ cup fat-free milk or skim milk
1 tsp. vanilla extract
1 tsp. cinnamon (ground)

Cream Cheese Filling:
8 oz. whipped cream cheese
1 serving CSE Cinnamon Roll or Snickerdoodle Protein Powder
¼ cup pure maple syrup
2 Tbs. fat-free milk

1. Preheat oven to 350 degrees. Cube the bread and set aside.

2. Add the eggs, milk, vanilla and cinnamon to a separate mixing bowl. Whisk until well combined. Set aside.

3. In a separate bowl, beat the cream cheese, protein powder, maple syrup and milk together until smooth. Set aside.

4. Add ½ of the bread cubes to a greased 9x13 pan. Pour ½ of the egg mixture over the top. Drizzle the cream cheese mixture over the top. Then top with the remaining bread cubes and egg mixture. Sprinkle with cinnamon.

5. Bake for 30-35 minutes or until the eggs are cooked through and the bread is crispy on the edges. Slice into 12 squares and enjoy warm, topped with your choice of berries, whipped cream, syrup, sweetened Greek yogurt or ice cream (toppings not included in macros).

PRO TIP: Freeze into individual servings and reheat in the microwave or oven when ready to eat. Add the toppings fresh.

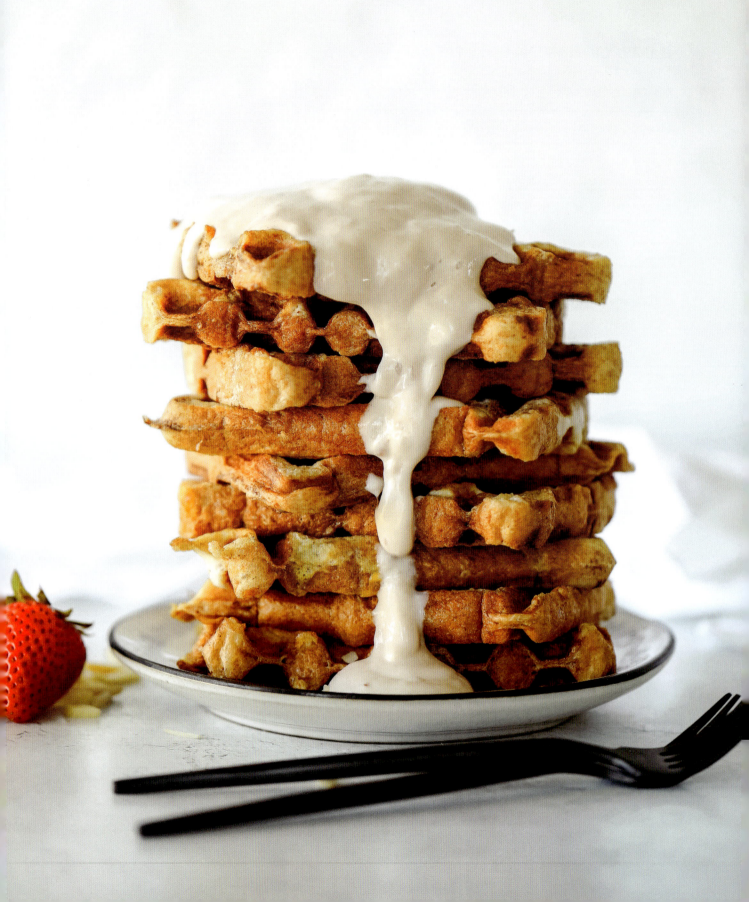

STRAWBERRY CREAM FRENCH TOAST

Makes 4 servings
340 calories / 11F / 34C / 26P / per serving

Prep: 15 min | **Cook:** 20 min

4 large eggs
4 egg whites (½ cup liquid egg whites)
2 Tbs. unsweetened almond milk
Dash cinnamon
6 slices Harper's Bran Bread or Ezekiel Bread

Strawberry Cream Yogurt:
1 ⅓ cups nonfat, plain Greek yogurt
4 Tbs. low-sugar strawberry jam

Toppings:
5 Tbs. sliced almonds
CSE Maple Syrup or other syrup of choice (not included in macros)

1. Heat a griddle or waffle iron over medium heat.

2. Beat eggs, egg whites, almond milk and cinnamon together in a shallow dish. Spray the griddle or waffle iron with cooking spray. Dip both sides of bread into the egg mixture and place on the griddle or waffle iron. Cook until golden brown (about 3 minutes per side), then transfer to a plate and keep warm.

3. Mix the Greek yogurt together with the strawberry jam.

4. Makes 1 ½ slices of French toast per serving. Top each serving with strawberry cream yogurt, almonds and syrup. Enjoy!

PRO TIP: Make ahead and freeze into individual servings. Reheat in the toaster. Prepare the toppings fresh.

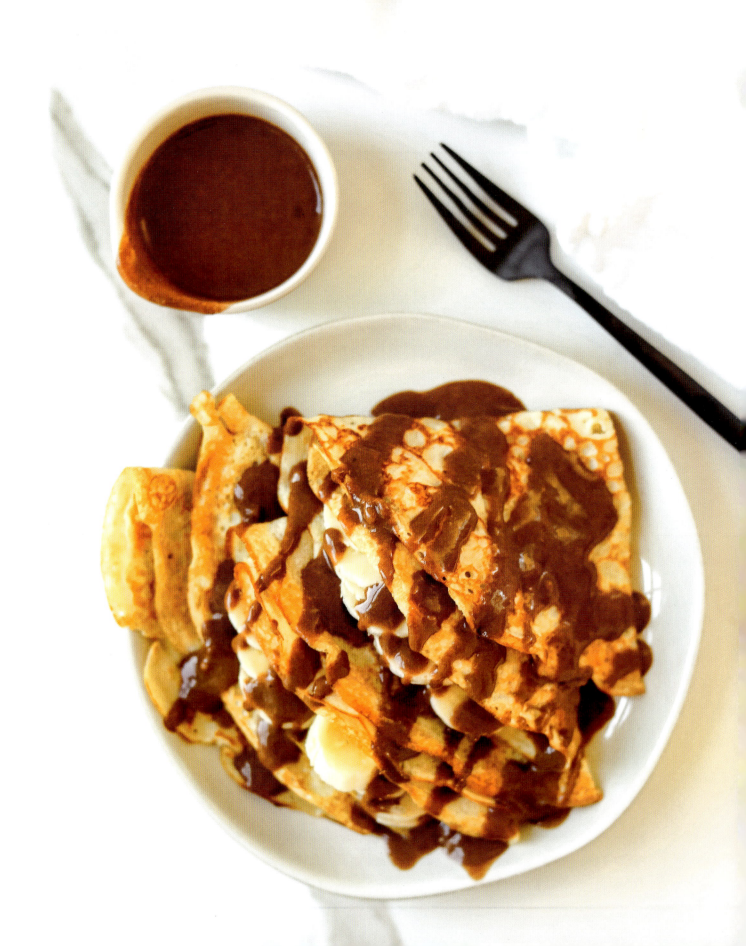

CHOCOLATE GLAZED BANANA CREPES
Makes 4 servings
350 calories / 12.5F / 33C / 26P / per serving

Prep: 15 min | **Cook:** 30 min

8 egg whites (1 cup liquid egg whites)
120g bananas
1 cup CSE Buttermilk, Gluten-Free Buttermilk, or Vanilla Pancake & Waffle Mix
1 cup fat-free milk
Dash sea salt
1 tsp. Stevia in the Raw, optional

Chocolate Glaze:
2 Tbs. CSE Midnight Almond Coconut, Sweet Classic Peanut Butter
   or natural peanut butter
2 Tbs. melted coconut oil
1 serving CSE Chocolate Brownie Batter Protein Powder
1 Tbs. cocoa powder
1 Tbs. raw honey
¼ cup unsweetened almond milk

1. Heat a frying pan over medium heat. Add the egg whites, banana, CSE Pancake & Waffle Mix, milk, sea salt and stevia together in a high-powered blender. Blend on low for 30 seconds, scrape down the sides and blend for another 30 seconds.

2. Spray the pan with cooking spray and pour ¼ cup of the batter into the pan. Swirl the batter around the sides to make a thin crepe. Once the edges start to peel away from the pan, carefully flip the crepe. Cook for one more minute and then transfer to a plate. Repeat with the rest of the batter. It should make about 12 crepes.

3. Whisk together all of the chocolate glaze ingredients. Weigh the glaze and divide the weight by four to get the amount needed to fill one serving.

4. Roll or fold up, then drizzle the chocolate glaze over the top. Enjoy warm.

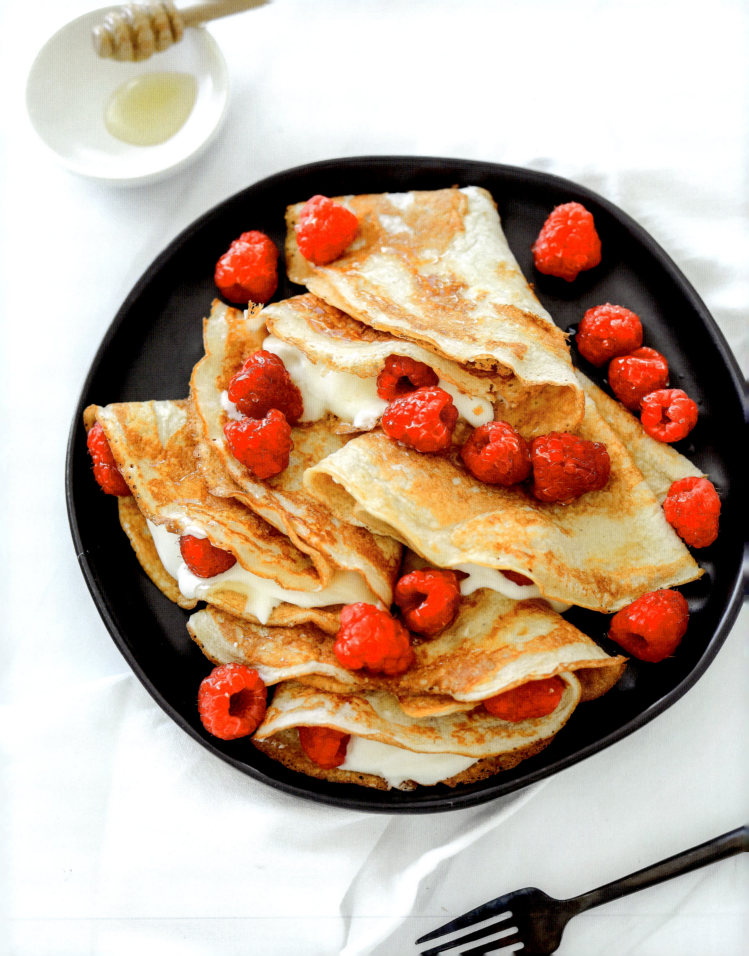

LEMON RASPBERRY FLOURLESS CREPES

Makes 4 servings
340 calories / 12.5F / 32C / 25P / per serving

Prep: 10 min | **Cook:** 30 min

4 large eggs
12 egg whites (1 ½ cups liquid egg whites)
200g bananas
1 serving CSE Simply Vanilla Protein Powder

Toppings per serving:
3 oz. Lemon Noosa Yoghurt
   or 1 Tbs. CSE Lemon Coconut Bliss Butter
½ cup fresh raspberries
1 tsp. raw honey

1. Heat a large frying pan over medium heat.

2. Add the eggs, egg whites, bananas and protein powder to a blender. Blend on high until well combined. Batter will be really thin.

3. Grease the pan well and pour ¼ cup of the mixture into the pan. Twirl the batter around until the pan is coated and the crepe is thin. Once the edges begin to brown and pull away from the sides of the pan, flip carefully. Cook for 30-60 seconds and transfer to a plate. Should make 12 crepes; three per serving.

4. Divide 3 oz. lemon yoghurt or one tablespoon of the Lemon Coconut Bliss Butter, and ½ cup fresh raspberries between three crepes. Drizzle butter or yoghurt in the centers, then add the fresh raspberries. Roll or fold up and then drizzle honey over the top.

SAVORY

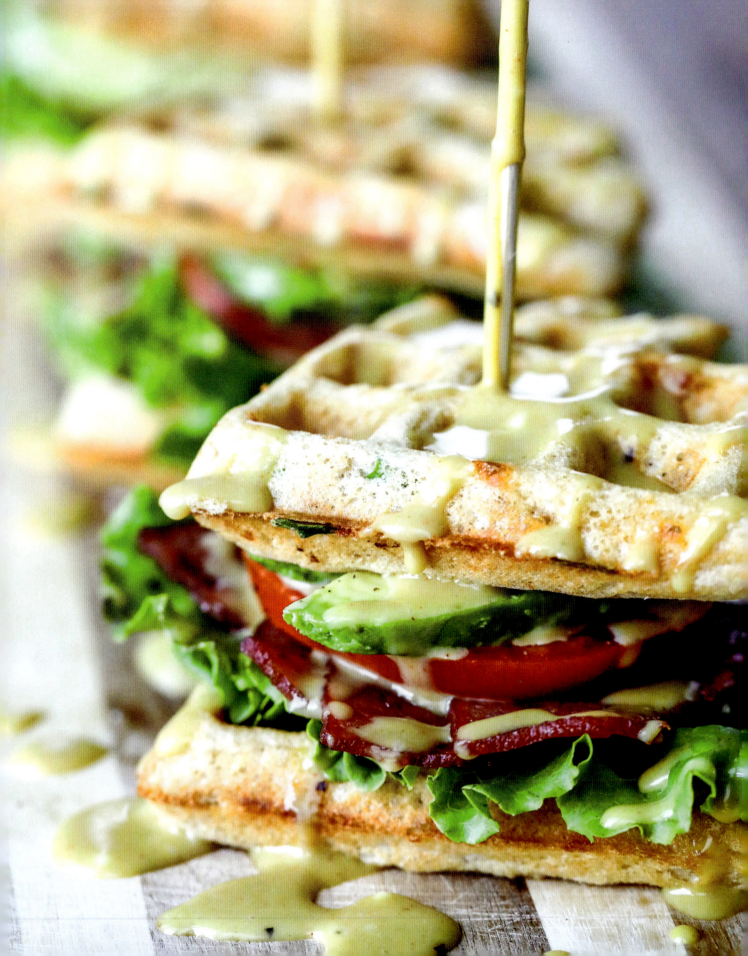

BLTA WAFFLE SANDWICH

Makes 4 servings
350 calories / 12F / 35C / 26P / per serving

Prep: 15 min | **Cook:** 20 min

- 1 ¾ cups CSE Buttermilk or Gluten-Free Buttermilk Pancake & Waffle Mix
- 1 ½ cups water
- ¼ cup low-fat, shredded cheddar cheese
- ¼ cup sliced green onions
- 8 slices turkey bacon
- Green leaf lettuce
- 4 tomato slices
- 80g avocado slices

Honey Mustard Sauce:
- 1 Tbs. olive oil mayo
- 1 Tbs. Dijon mustard
- 1 tsp. yellow mustard
- 1 Tbs. raw honey
- 1 tsp. white wine vinegar
- Dash paprika
- Dash sea salt
- Dash black pepper

1. Whisk all of the Honey Mustard Sauce ingredients together until well combined. Weigh the sauce and divide by four to get the amount needed for one serving. Cover and store in the fridge.

2. Heat a waffle maker. Make waffles by mixing the CSE Pancake & Waffle Mix, water, shredded cheese and green onions together in a bowl. If the batter is too thick, add more water, one tablespoon at a time. Pour the batter onto the greased waffle maker and cook until golden brown. Divide the waffles into four servings and use as a bun.

3. Cook the bacon until crispy.

4. For one serving, sandwich two slices of cooked bacon, lettuce, one tomato slice and 20g avocado in between one serving of the waffle buns. Sprinkle sea salt and pepper on top of the veggies. Use the Honey Mustard Sauce as a dip for the sandwiches. Enjoy warm.

PRO TIP: Make a double or triple batch, then freeze into individual servings. Reheat in the toaster when ready to serve. Add toppings and sauce fresh.

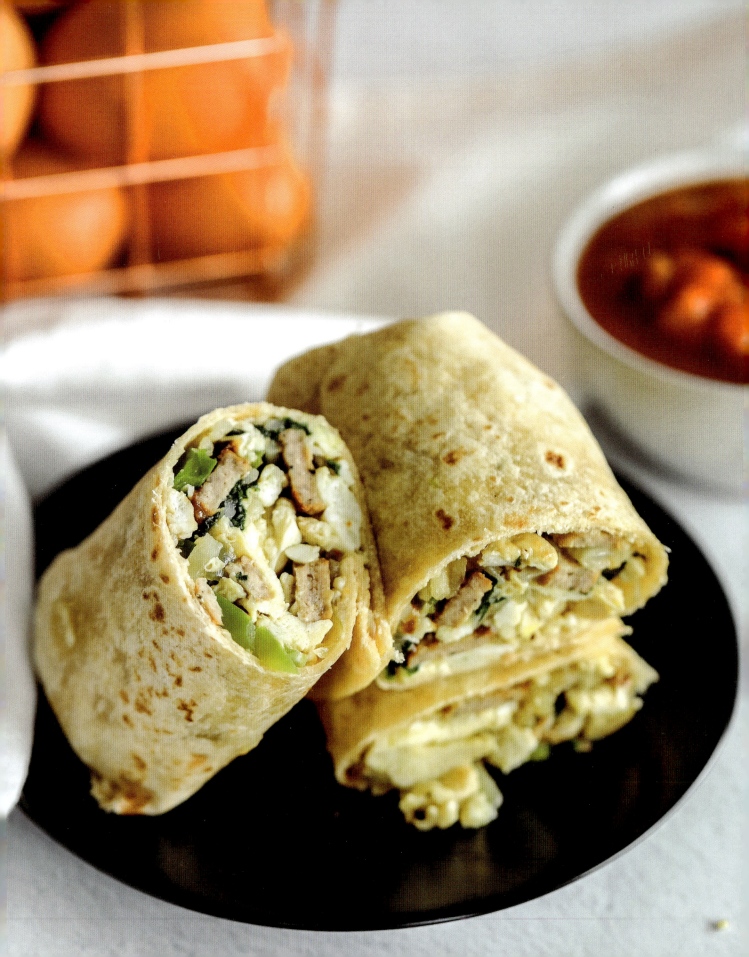

BREAKFAST BURRITOS
Makes 4 servings
340 calories / 11F / 34C / 26P / per serving

Prep: 20 min | **Cook:** 20 min

4 Sugarhouse Maple Chicken Sausages
4 oz. grated red potatoes
½ cup green bell peppers
2 cups chopped spinach
½ cup diced yellow onions
Dash garlic powder
Dash onion powder
Dash sea salt
Dash black pepper
4 large eggs
8 egg whites (1 cup liquid egg whites)
4 large whole grain tortillas (120 calories each)
½ cup low-fat, shredded mozzarella cheese

Topping per serving:
2 Tbs. salsa

1. Heat a skillet to medium heat.

2. Chop chicken sausage and add to the skillet with the grated potatoes, chopped peppers, spinach and diced onions. Sauté until veggies are tender and sausage is browned. Add the eggs, egg whites and seasonings. Cook until eggs are cooked through. Weigh the mixture and divide by four to get the amount needed to fill one serving.

3. Lay out the tortillas and fill them evenly with ¼ of the mixture and two tablespoons of mozzarella cheese. Roll the tortillas up tight and place seam down in pan to seal the edges and melt the cheese. Enjoy warm, dipped in salsa.

PRO TIP: Wrap the extras in foil (spray the foil with nonstick cooking spray when wrapping up the burritos to avoid tortillas from sticking) and store in the fridge or freezer until ready to eat. To reheat from the fridge, place in the oven at 400 degrees for 30 minutes; 50-60 minutes if frozen.

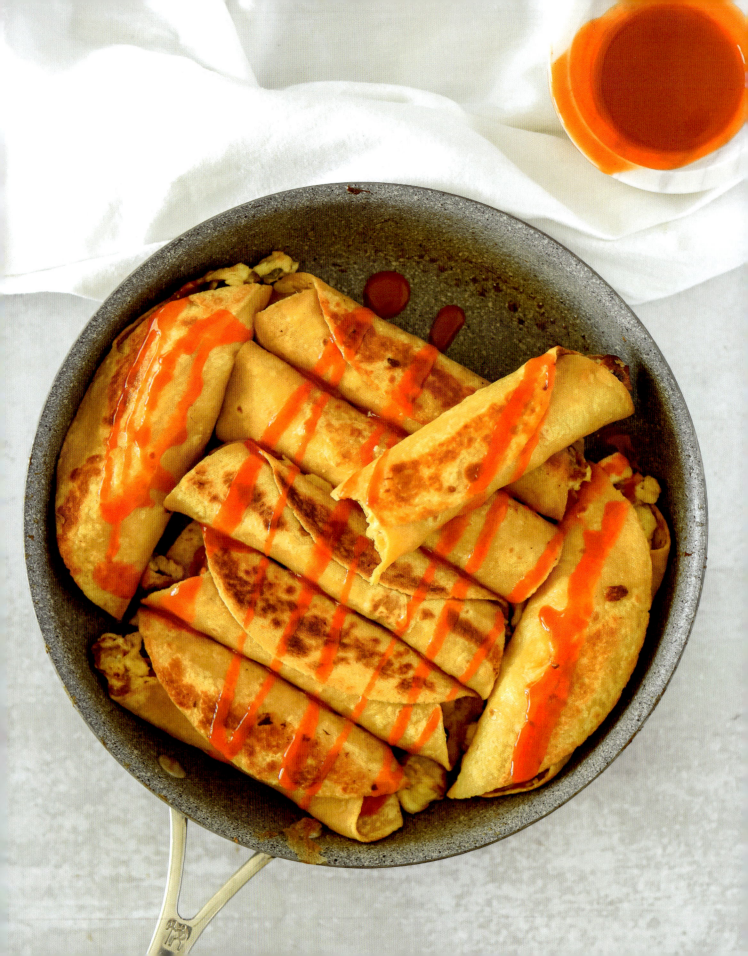

BREAKFAST TAQUITOS

Makes 4 servings
345 calories / 11F / 32.5C / 29P / per serving

Prep: 15 min | **Cook:** 30 min

4 slices turkey bacon
2 Tbs. yellow onions
2 Tbs. green bell peppers
2 Tbs. canned, diced green chiles
2 Tbs. black beans

4 eggs
4 egg whites (½ cup liquid egg whites)
½ cup low-fat, shredded mozzarella cheese
8 yellow corn and wheat blend tortillas
Dash hot sauce

1. Chop the turkey bacon, onions, and bell peppers. Drain the black beans. Add the bacon, onions, peppers, green chiles and black beans to a large, greased frying pan over medium heat. Cook until the bacon is browned and the onions are tender. Remove from the pan.

2. Spray the pan with cooking spray and add the eggs and egg whites. Scramble the eggs over medium heat until the eggs are cooked through. Add the veggies, bacon, beans and cheese to the eggs. Stir until well combined. Remove from the heat and weigh the mixture. Divide the weight by eight to get the amount needed to fill each tortilla.

3. Fill each tortilla with ⅛ of the egg mixture and roll up as tight as you can. Place the seam side down in a large, greased frying pan over medium heat. Let cook until the bottoms are brown, crispy and the seam of the tortilla is sealed down, about 3-5 minutes. Spray the tops of the tortillas with cooking spray and gently flip each taquito over. Brown and crisp the other side for about 3-5 minutes.

4. Enjoy two taquitos per serving with hot sauce, if desired.

PRO TIPS: Wrap the extras in foil (spray the foil with nonstick cooking spray when wrapping up the taquitos to avoid tortillas from sticking) and store in the fridge or freezer until ready to eat. Reheat in the air fryer at 350 degrees for 5 minutes.

Look for tortillas with a combination of yellow corn and wheat flour. They should be around 80 calories each, but macros may vary slightly by brand. All corn tortillas will work, but will be more difficult to roll without cracking.

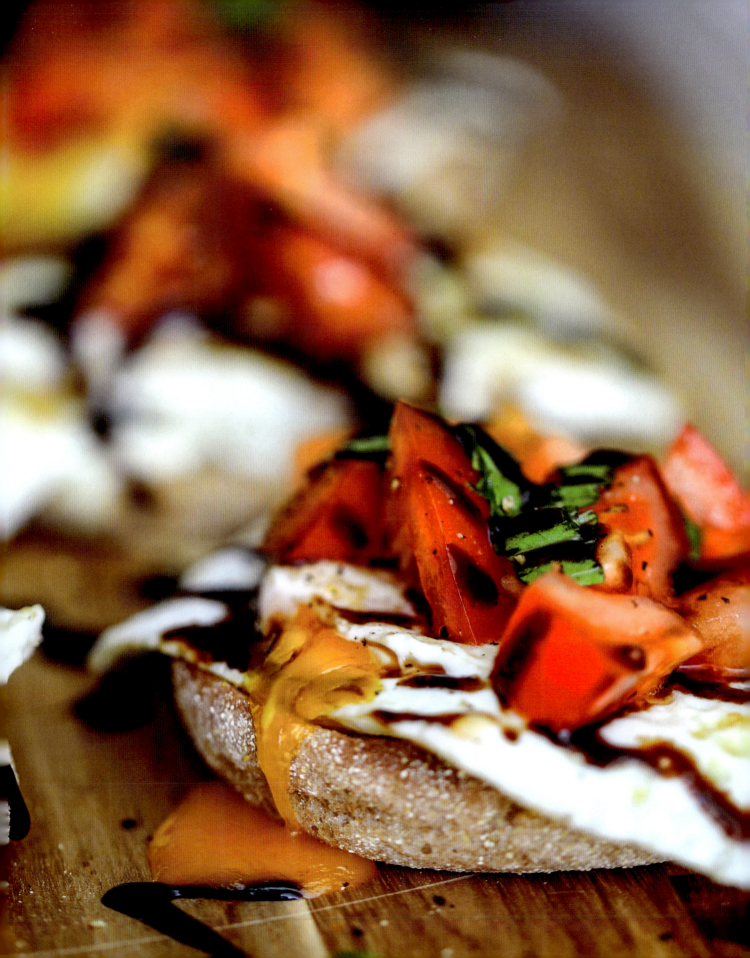

BREKKIE BRUSCHETTA

Makes 4 servings
350 calories / 11.5F / 37C / 25P / per serving

Prep: 10 min | **Cook:** 15 min

2 vine tomatoes
1 Tbs. olive oil
Dash sea salt
Dash black pepper
2 Tbs. fresh basil, chopped
12 egg whites (1 ½ cups liquid egg whites)
½ cup low-fat shredded mozzarella cheese
4 large eggs
4 multigrain English muffins
4 tsp. balsamic glaze

1. Chop tomatoes and place in a bowl. Add the olive oil to the bowl with sea salt, pepper, and chopped basil; set aside.

2. Heat a large frying pan to medium heat. Spray with cooking spray and add the egg whites. Cover and cook until browned on one side. Slice into fourths and flip the egg whites over; cook until browned on the other side. Top with mozzarella cheese, remove from pan and cover to keep warm.

3. Spray the pan again and add the eggs. Cover and cook over-easy or until you reach desired doneness. Toast the English muffins in the toaster while the eggs are cooking.

4. Place one serving of egg whites on one muffin half and one over-easy cooked egg to the other. Evenly distribute ¼ of the bruschetta mixture between each half of the toasted, open-faced muffins and drizzle with one teaspoon of the balsamic glaze per serving. Enjoy!

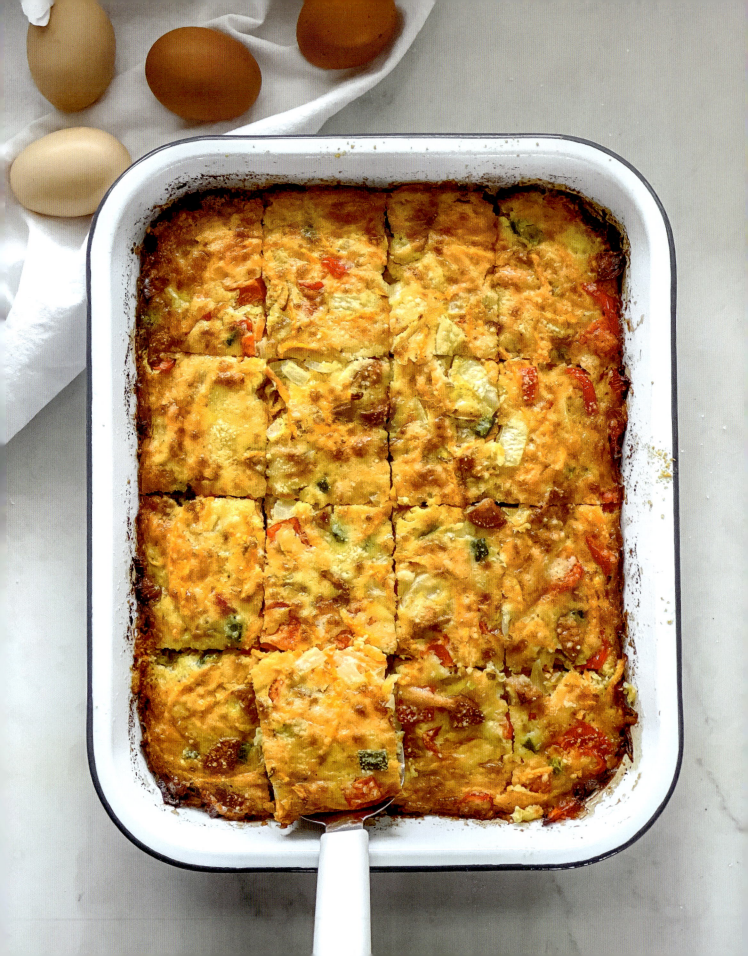

CHEESY SAUSAGE EGG BAKE

Makes 16 servings
130 calories / 7.5F / 5C / 10P / per serving

Prep: 30 min | **Cook:** 35 min

12 eggs
1 cup red bell peppers
1 cup yellow onions
2 cups sweet potatoes
1 jalapeño pepper
2 apple chicken sausage links
1 cup shredded gouda cheese
1 tsp. sea salt
¼ tsp. black pepper
½ cup finely grated Parmesan cheese

1. Preheat the oven to 400 degrees. Add all the eggs to a large mixing bowl. Beat well.

2. Chop the bell peppers, onions, seeded jalapeños and chicken sausage. Grate the sweet potatoes. Add all the veggies, gouda, sea salt and black pepper to the bowl of eggs. Mix until well combined.

3. Pour the egg mixture into a greased 9x13 baking dish. Spread out evenly in the pan and sprinkle Parmesan cheese over the top. Bake for 30-35 minutes. Slice and enjoy!

PRO TIP: Freeze into individual servings, thaw in the fridge and reheat in the oven or microwave.

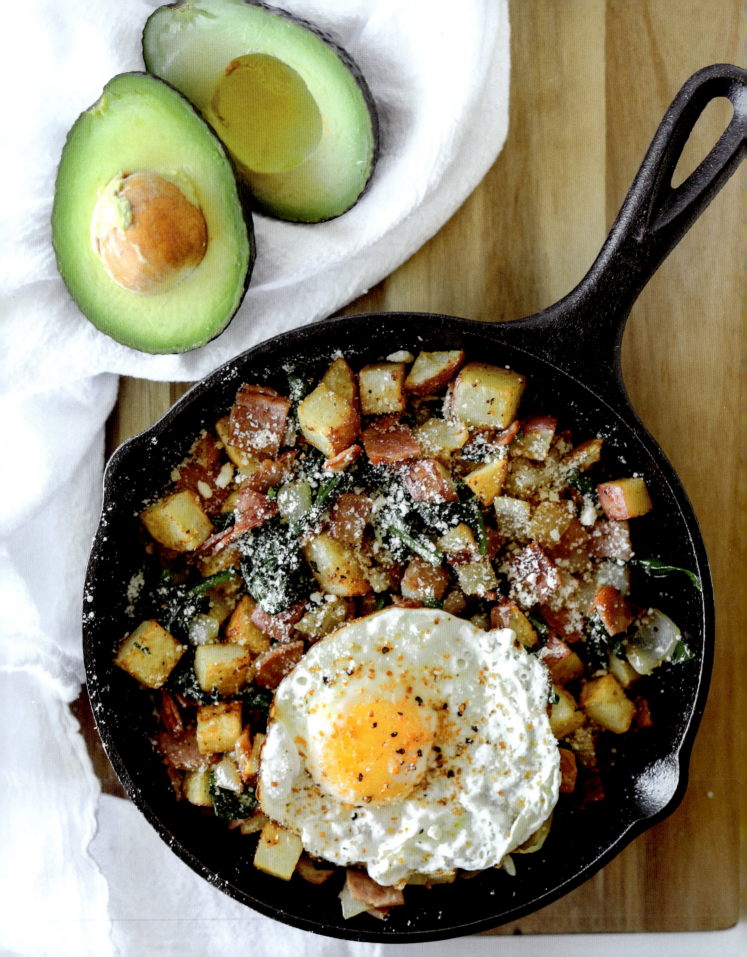

COUNTRY BREAKFAST SKILLET

Makes 4 servings
350 calories / 12F / 35C / 26P / per serving

Prep: 15 min | **Cook:** 50 min

24 oz. baby red potatoes
10 slices turkey bacon
200g chopped yellow onions
2 cups spinach
4 large eggs
80g avocado
2 Tbs. grated Parmesan cheese
Sea salt
Black pepper

1. Preheat the oven to 400 degrees. Move the oven rack to the center of your oven. Wash and cube or cut potatoes into bite-sized pieces or fries with a sharp knife. Spread out in a single layer onto a baking sheet lined with parchment paper. Spray the tops with cooking spray and sprinkle tops with sea salt and other seasonings of choice. Bake for 20 minutes, flip and bake another 15 minutes. Potatoes should be fork-tender.

2. Heat a frying pan over medium-high heat. Chop the turkey bacon. Spray the pan with cooking spray and add the bacon, onions, spinach and roasted potatoes. Sprinkle it with sea salt and black pepper. Cook until the onions are tender and bacon is crispy. Remove from the pan. Weigh the hash and divide the total weight by four to get the amount needed to fill one serving.

3. Spray the pan again and crack the eggs into it. Cook the eggs over-easy or to your liking. Top one serving of the hash with one egg, 20g avocado and ½ tablespoon of Parmesan cheese.

PRO TIP: Cook the potatoes in advance and store in the fridge or freezer. This will make the meal come together in a snap.

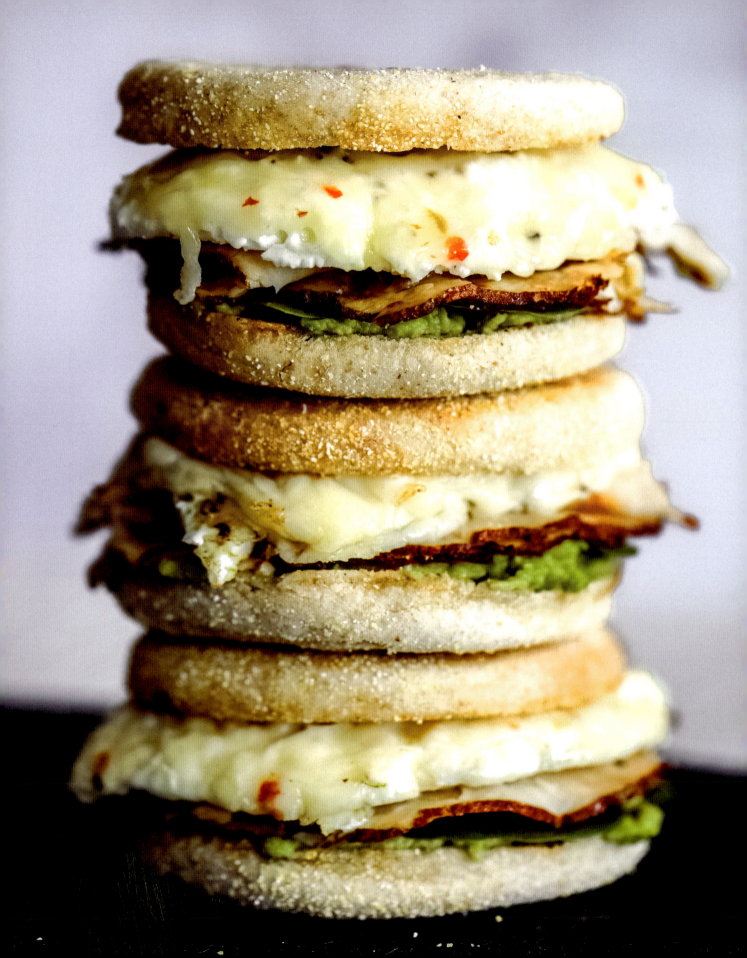

EGG WHITE, PEPPER JACK & AVOCADO SANDWICH

Makes 1 serving
345 calories / 11F / 34.5C / 26.5P

Prep: 5 min | **Cook:** 20 min

3 egg whites (6 Tbs. liquid egg whites)
1 oz. pepper jack cheese
1 oz. deli-sliced chicken breast
1 multigrain English muffin
15g smashed avocado
Handful of spinach
Dash sea salt
Dash black pepper

1. Heat a frying pan over medium-high heat. Spray the pan with cooking spray. Add the egg whites and season with salt and pepper. Cover with a lid and heat until fully cooked through. Fold in half and then in half again. Top with cheese and then transfer to a plate.

2. Add the deli meat to the pan and brown on both sides; remove from heat.

3. Slice muffin in half and toast in the toaster. Once toasted, smash the avocado onto the bottom of the muffin and sandwich the spinach, egg whites, cheese and chicken in the middle.

PRO TIP: Make the sandwich without the avocado and spinach. Wrap each one in foil and freeze. Thaw in the fridge overnight before eating. Reheat in the oven at 400 degrees for 30-45 minutes. Add avocado and spinach fresh.

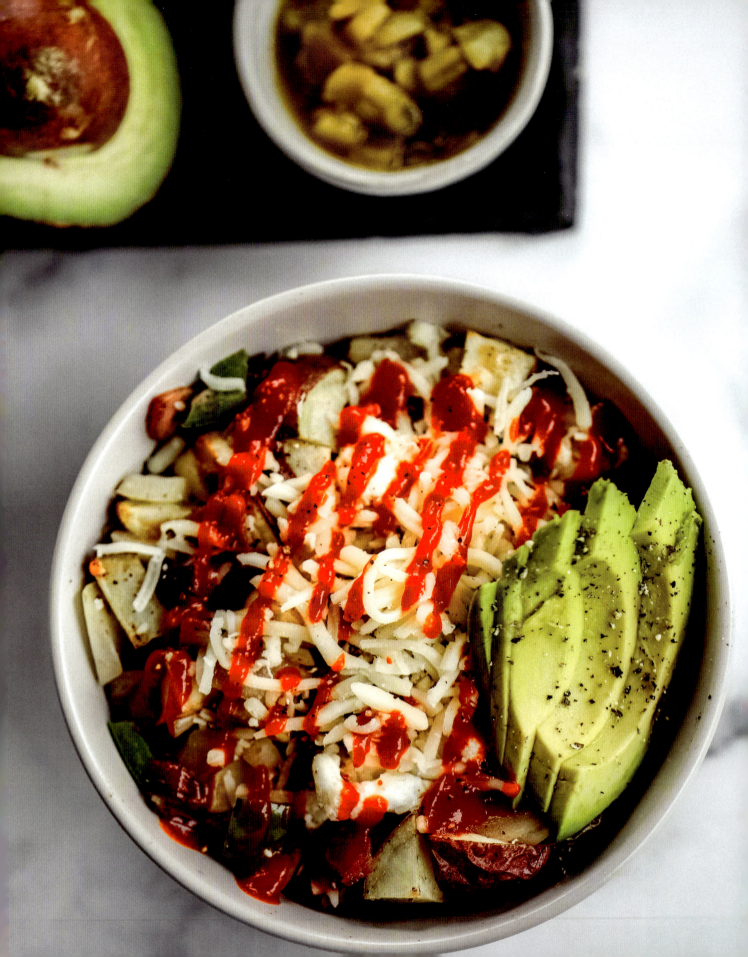

LOADED BREAKFAST BURRITO BOWL

Makes 1 serving
350 calories / 12F / 34C / 27P

Prep: 20 min | **Cook:** 40 min

3 oz. baby red potatoes
Dash sea salt
Dash paprika
Dash black pepper
Dash garlic powder
¼ cup green bell peppers
¼ cup yellow onions
1 slice chopped turkey bacon
3 egg whites (6 Tbs. liquid egg whites)
¼ cup black beans, drained and rinsed
1 Tbs. low-fat, shredded mozzarella cheese
40g sliced avocado
1 Tbs. canned green chilies
1 Tbs. salsa
Dash hot sauce, optional

1. Heat oven to 400 degrees.

2. Place the potatoes on a baking sheet lined with parchment paper. Spray tops with cooking spray and sprinkle with sea salt, paprika, pepper and garlic powder. Bake for 20 minutes. Flip potatoes and add sliced peppers and onions to the pan. Bake for another 20 minutes.

3. While baking, add the chopped bacon to a frying pan. Cook until crispy. Remove from the pan. Spray the pan with cooking spray and add the egg whites. Scramble and season with sea salt and pepper, to taste. Add the bacon and beans to the pan and cook until heated through.

4. Place the potatoes, peppers, onions, egg whites, beans and turkey bacon in a bowl. Top with cheese, avocado, green chilies, salsa and hot sauce. Enjoy!

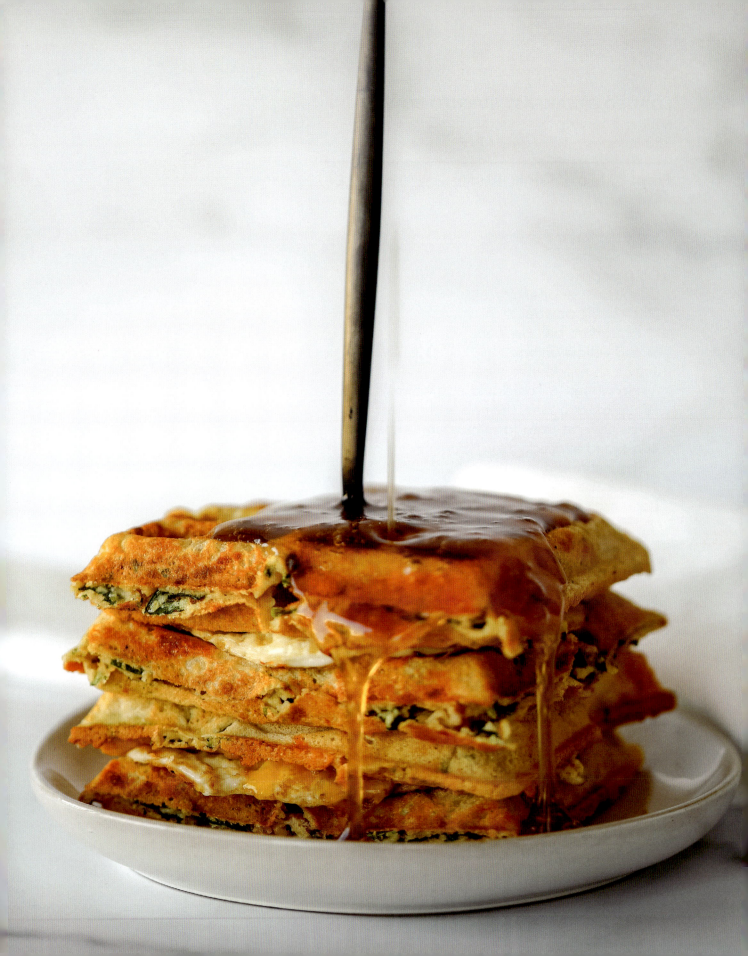

SAVORY STUFFED WAFFLES
Makes 4 servings
335 calories / 10F / 31C / 29.5P / per serving

Prep: 10 min | **Cook:** 20 min

2 slices turkey bacon
2 cups CSE Buttermilk or Gluten-Free Buttermilk Pancake & Waffle Mix
1 ½ cups water
2 cups chopped spinach
½ cup low-fat, shredded mozzarella cheese
2 Tbs. chopped, fresh chives
¼ cup zero calorie syrup of choice
4 large eggs

1. Heat a waffle iron. Chop the bacon and cook in a frying pan over medium-high heat until crispy. Remove from the pan.

2. Whisk the CSE Pancake & Waffle Mix and water together in a bowl until well combined. Fold in the chopped spinach, cheese, chives and ¼ cup syrup. Spray the waffle iron with cooking spray and add the batter. Cook until golden brown. Repeat with the remaining batter. Weigh the waffles and divide the weight by four to get the amount needed to fill one serving and use as a bun.

3. While the waffles are cooking, heat the frying pan over medium heat and cook the eggs and bacon to your liking. Sandwich one egg and a ½ slice of bacon in between the waffle bun. Use extra syrup for a dip, if desired.

PRO TIP: Make a double or triple batch and freeze waffles in individual servings. Reheat in the toaster when ready to serve. Add egg and bacon fresh.

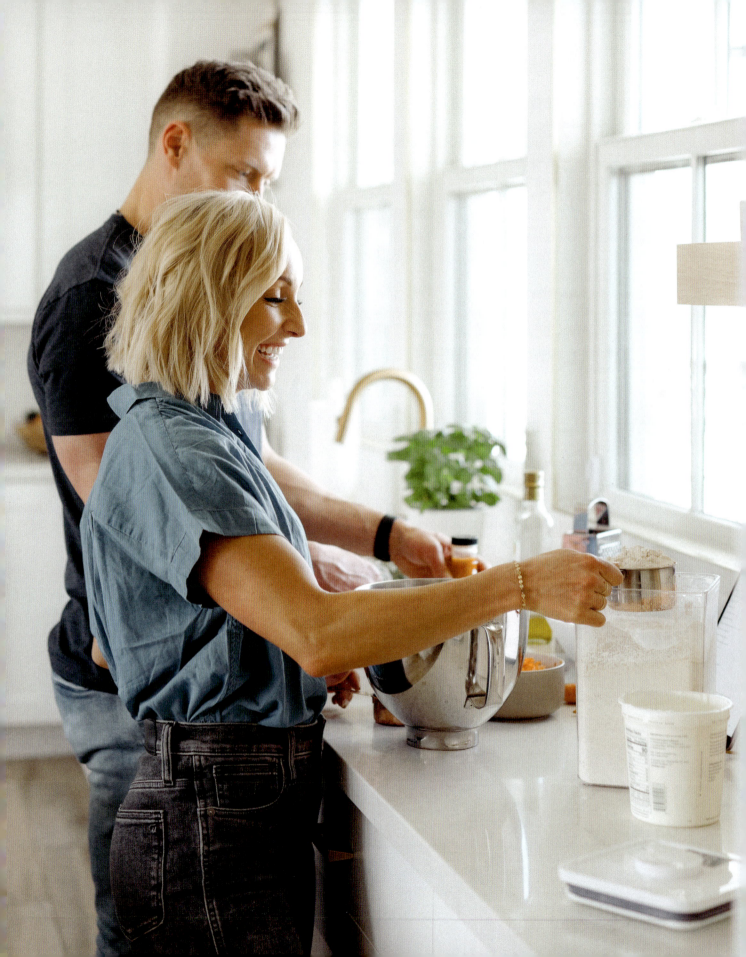

SNACKS

The perfect snack starts with a great recipe, simple ingredients and lots of flavor. Take your snack game to the next level with our **Crunchy & Savory** snacks like the Kickin' Avo Toast or Chips & Cheesy Chile Dip! Whip up a **Parfait or Fruit Dip** if you're craving a sweet little something-something! And of course we can't forget our must-have-in-the-fridge-at-all-times snacks, **Muffins** and **Power Bites**! I recommend always making a double batch because they will go fast! Your future self will thank you as you pop one (or two) on-the-go!

CRUNCHY, SAVORY

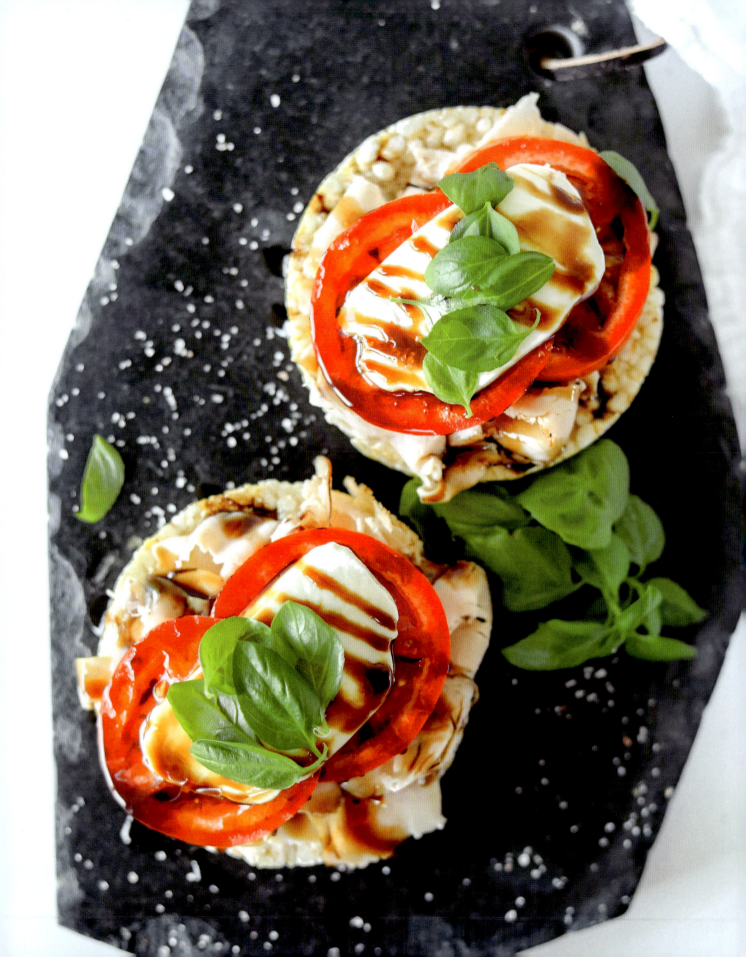

CAPRESE CRUNCH SNACK

Makes 1 serving
230 calories / 8F / 21C / 18P

Prep: 5 min

2 white cheddar rice cakes
2 oz. nitrate-free deli turkey
1 oz. fresh mozzarella slices
2 tomato slices
1 tsp. balsamic glaze
Fresh basil

1. Top the rice cakes with turkey, mozzarella and tomato slices.

2. Drizzle the balsamic glaze over the top and garnish with fresh basil.

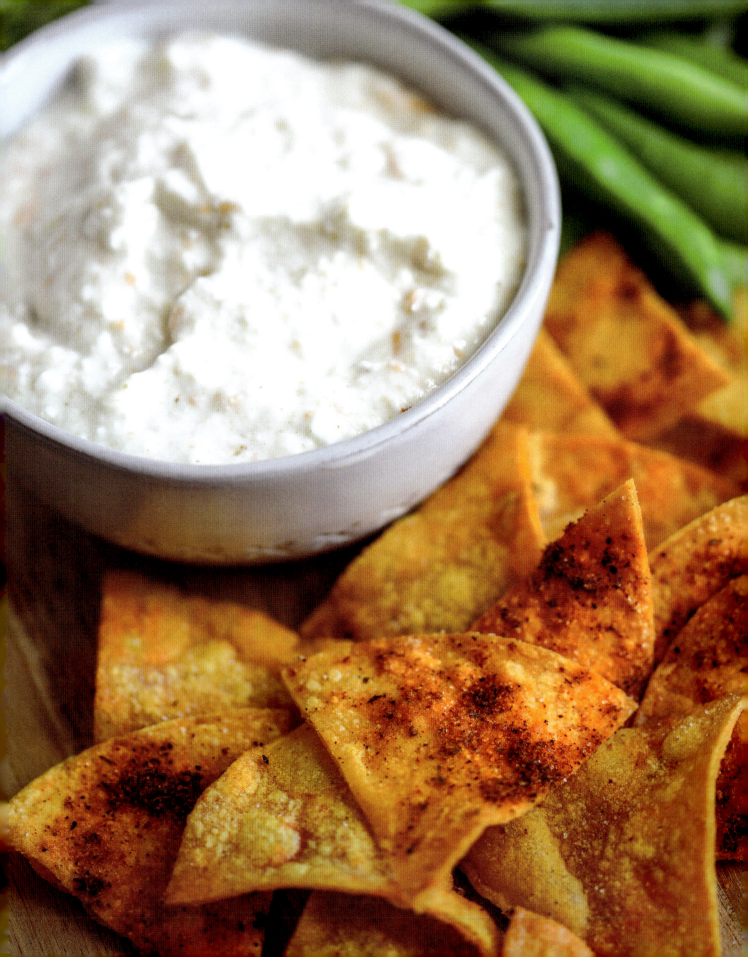

CHIPS & CHEESY CHILE DIP

Makes 2 servings
230 calories / 5.5F / 24.5C / 18.5P / per serving

Prep: 10 min | **Cook:** 20 min

3 corn tortillas
Dash chili-lime seasoning
Dash sea salt
¾ cup low-fat cottage cheese
¼ cup shredded cheddar cheese
1-2 Tbs. chopped green chiles
Dash garlic powder
Dash onion powder
Dash cumin
2 cups sugar snap peas

1. Heat oven to 350 degrees.

2. Place corn tortillas on a cutting board. Spray both sides of each tortilla with cooking spray and sprinkle with chili-lime seasoning and sea salt. Slice into triangles, six per tortilla. Lay out in a single layer on a baking sheet lined with parchment paper. Bake for 10 minutes. Flip the chips, then bake for another 5-10 minutes or until golden brown and crispy.

3. While the chips are baking, add the cottage cheese, cheddar cheese, green chiles, garlic powder, onion powder and cumin to a food processor or blender. Pulse until broken up and smooth. Evenly distribute into two separate serving bowls.

4. Serve nine chips and one cup of sugar snap peas with the dip. Enjoy cold or heat the dip in the microwave for 10-20 seconds before dipping.

PRO TIP: Use the air fryer for a quicker method. Place in the air fryer and spread out evenly. Heat at 400 degrees for 3 minutes, toss the chips around and heat for another 3 minutes. Transfer chips to a plate and start dipping.

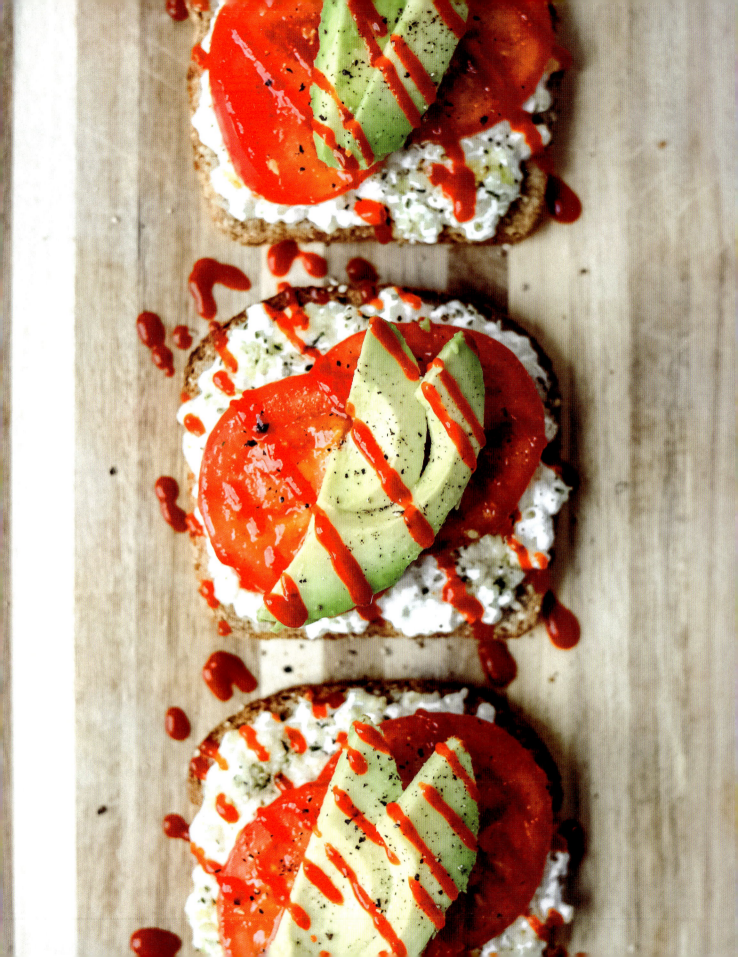

KICKIN' AVO TOAST
Makes 1 serving
220 calories / 9F / 22C / 15P

Prep: 10 min │ **Cook:** 10 min

1 slice Ezekiel Bread, Harper's Bran Bread or Dave's Killer Thin-Sliced Bread
⅓ cup low-fat cottage cheese
2 tomato slices
Dash sea salt
½ tsp. olive oil
20g avocado
1 tsp. hemp hearts
Sriracha sauce or hot sauce, optional

1. Preheat the oven to 375 degrees.

2. Place one piece of bread onto a baking sheet. Spray the top with cooking spray and toast in the oven for 5 minutes.

3. Remove from the oven and top with cottage cheese, tomato slices, a dash of sea salt and a drizzle of olive oil. Bake for another 5 minutes.

4. Remove from the oven and top with sliced avocado, hemp hearts and a drizzle of hot sauce. Enjoy!

PRO TIP: Use the air fryer for a quicker method. Spray the bread with cooking spray and air fry for 2 minutes at 375 degrees. Add the cottage cheese, tomato slices, sea salt and olive oil. Air fry for another 2 minutes or until you reach your desired doneness.

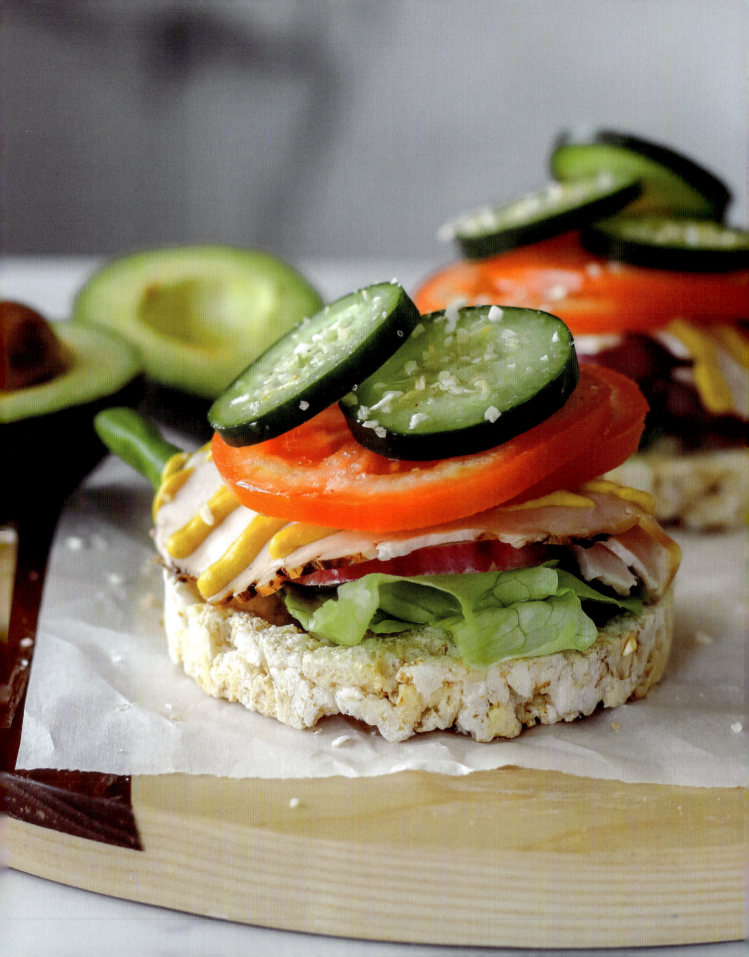

OPEN-FACED TURKEY & VEGGIE SANDWICH
Makes 1 serving
225 calories / 6F / 26C / 16P

Prep: 5 min

2 rice cakes (any flavor)
2 lettuce leaves
2 red onion slices
2 oz. nitrate-free deli turkey
2 Tbs. yellow mustard
4 tomato slices
4 cucumber slices
30g avocado
Dash dried, minced onion
Dash sea salt
Dash black pepper

1. On each rice cake, layer a lettuce leaf, slice of red onion, 1 oz. turkey, one tablespoon of mustard, two slices of tomato, two slices of cucumbers, and 15g of avocado. Sprinkle the minced onion, salt, and pepper over the top. Enjoy!

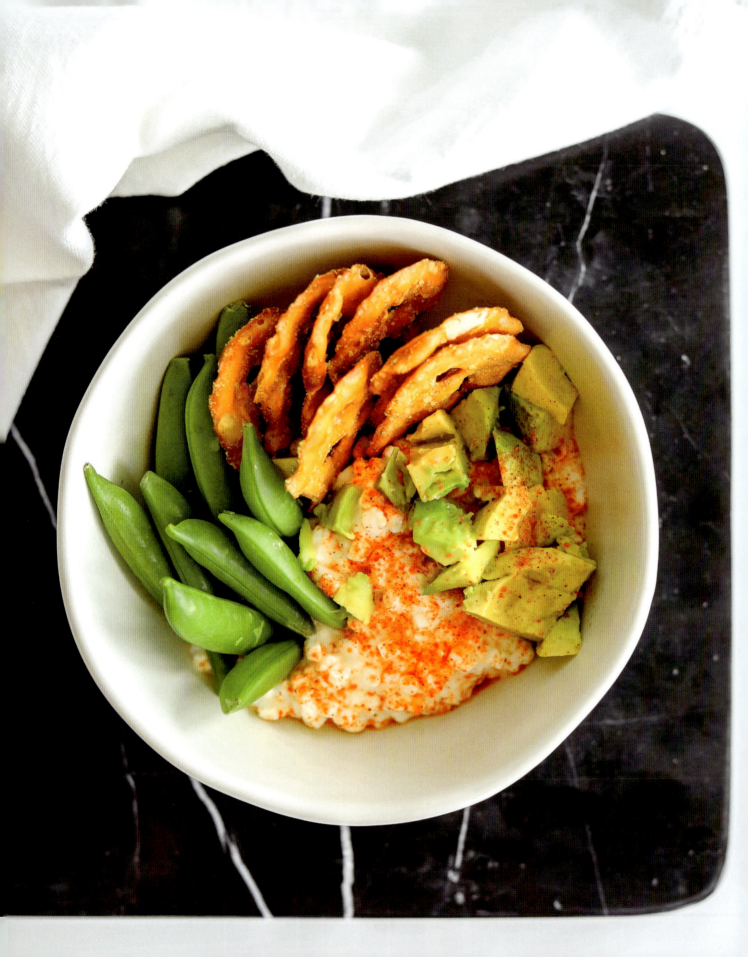

PRETZEL SNAP DIP
Makes 1 serving
240 calories / 8F / 26C / 17P

Prep: 5 min

½ cup low-fat cottage cheese
30g avocados
1 dash Traeger Chicken Rub seasoning
20g Pretzel Crisps Sea Salt & Cracked Pepper
50g sugar snap peas

1. Add the cottage cheese and chopped avocado to a bowl. Sprinkle with seasoning. Use it as a dip for the pretzels and sugar snap peas. Enjoy!

PARFAITS & FRUIT DIPS

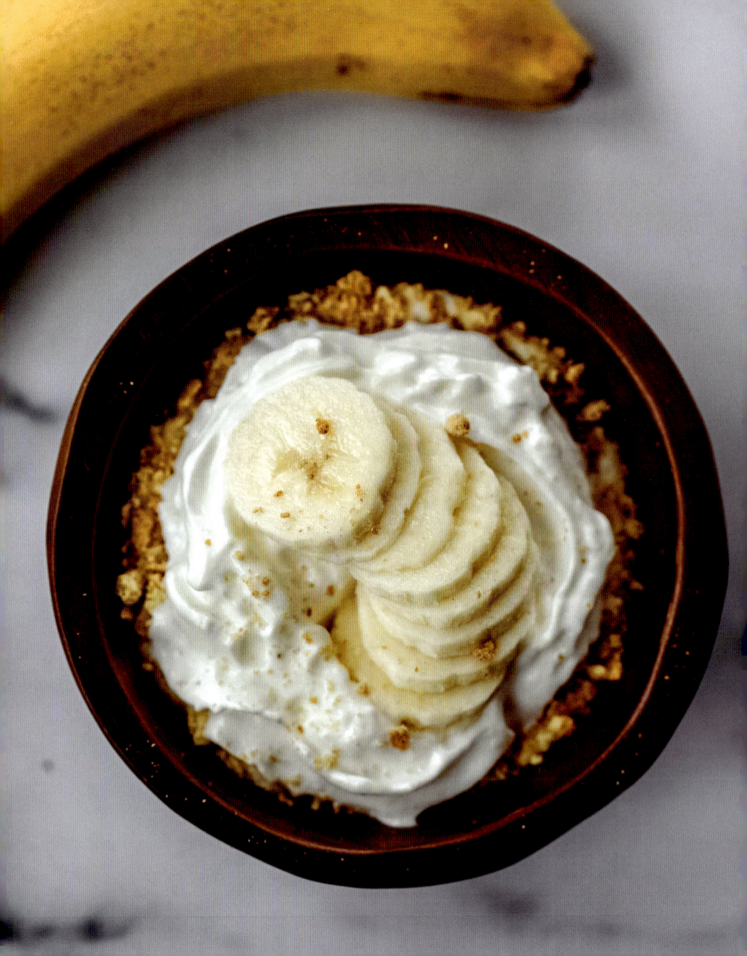

BANANA CREAM PIE PARFAIT

Makes 1 serving
210 calories / 5F / 23.5C / 18P

Prep: 10 min

½ cup nonfat, plain Greek yogurt
Vanilla stevia drops, optional for sweetness
¼ serving (8g) CSE Simply Vanilla or Bananas Foster Protein Powder
½ cup spray whipped cream
8g graham cracker crumbs
30g banana slices

1. Add the yogurt, stevia and protein powder to a small bowl; mix until smooth.

2. Top with whipped cream, graham cracker crumbs and banana slices.

PRO TIP: Try with other protein powder flavors for a new variation.

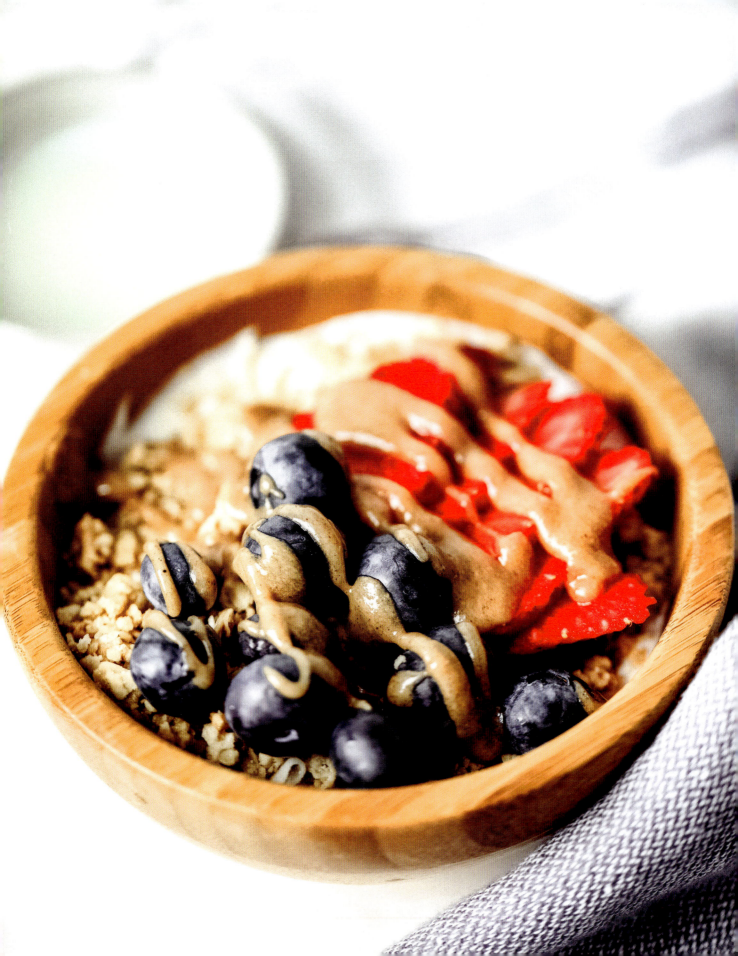

BIRCHGROVE MUESLI

Makes 1 serving
235 calories / 7.5F / 26.5C / 16.5P

Prep: 10 min

½ cup nonfat, plain Greek yogurt
Vanilla stevia drops, to taste
¼ cup Nature's Path Coconut & Cashew Butter Granola
2 Tbs. sliced strawberries
2 Tbs. fresh blueberries
2 Tbs. fat-free milk
1 tsp. CSE Cinnamon Bun, Salted Caramel, Aloha Butter,
   or natural almond butter
½ tsp. raw honey

1. Place the Greek yogurt and stevia together in a bowl. Mix together until you reach your desired sweetness.

2. Add the granola, strawberries and blueberries to the yogurt. Pour milk over the top and finish with a drizzle of nut butter and honey.

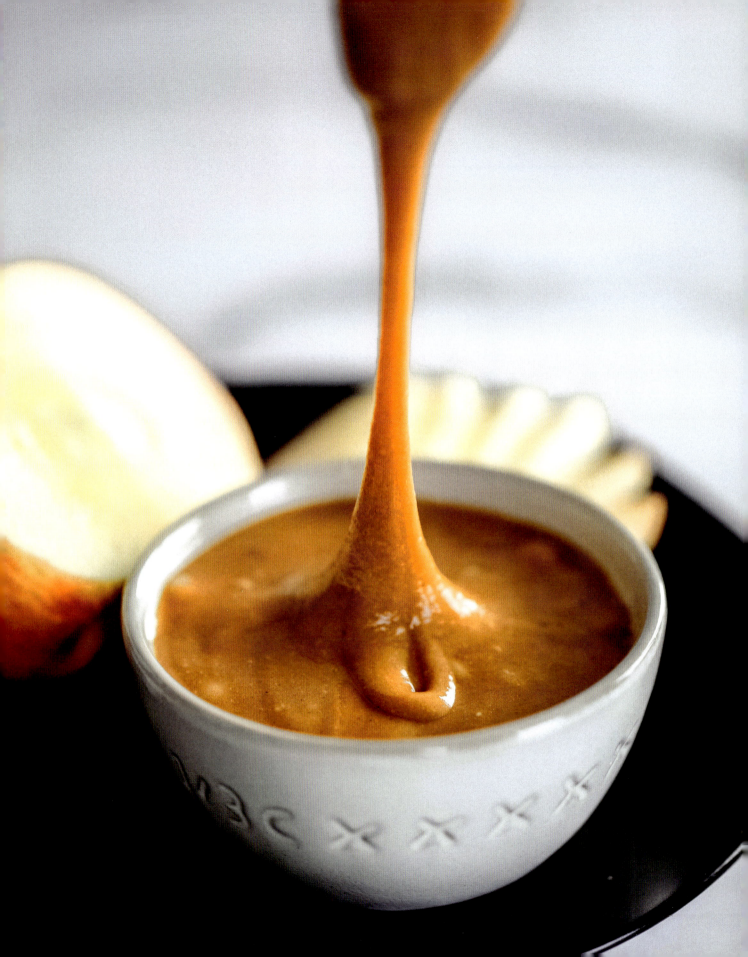

CARAMEL APPLE DIP

Makes 1 serving
235 calories / 7.5F / 26C / 16P

Prep: 10 min

3 Tbs. CSE Powdered Peanut Butter
2 Tbs. CSE Caramel Toffee or Simply Vanilla Protein Powder
2 Tbs. water
1 tsp. raw honey
½ Tbs. CSE Salted Caramel, Sweet Classic Peanut Butter,
   or natural peanut butter
Dash cinnamon
1 tsp. mini chocolate chips
70g apple slices

1. Stir the powdered peanut butter, protein powder and water together in a small bowl. Add the honey, nut butter and cinnamon. Stir until well combined.

2. Top with mini chocolate chips and use as a dip for the apple slices.

PRO TIP: Try with other protein powder or nut butter flavors for a new variation.

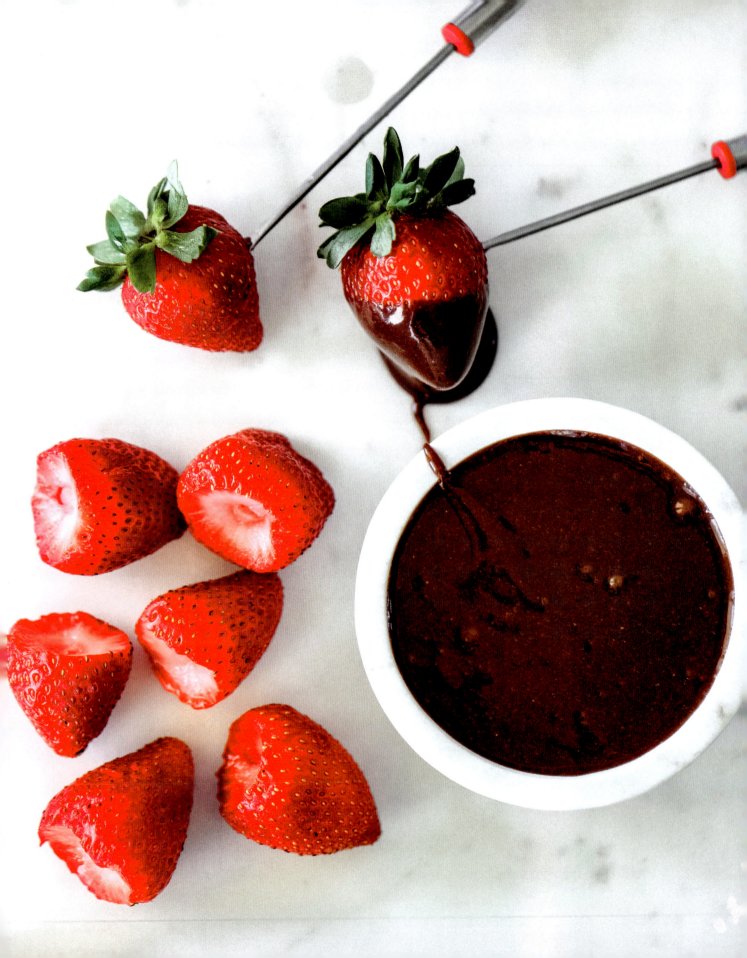

CHOCOLATE FONDUE POWER DIP

Makes 1 serving
230 calories / 6F / 28C / 16P

Prep: 10 min

140g strawberries
2 Tbs. CSE Powdered Peanut Butter
2 Tbs. water
2 Tbs. (8g) CSE Chocolate Brownie Batter
   or Chocolate Peanut Butter Protein Powder
1 Tbs. CSE Buckeye Brownie Peanut Butter
   or 14g melted chocolate chips
1 tsp. raw honey

1. Mix all the ingredients, except the fruit, together in a bowl.

2. Warm in the microwave for 10 seconds and stir. Use as a fondue dip for the fruit. Enjoy!

PRO TIP: Swap the strawberries for 50g banana or 85g apple slices for a new variation.

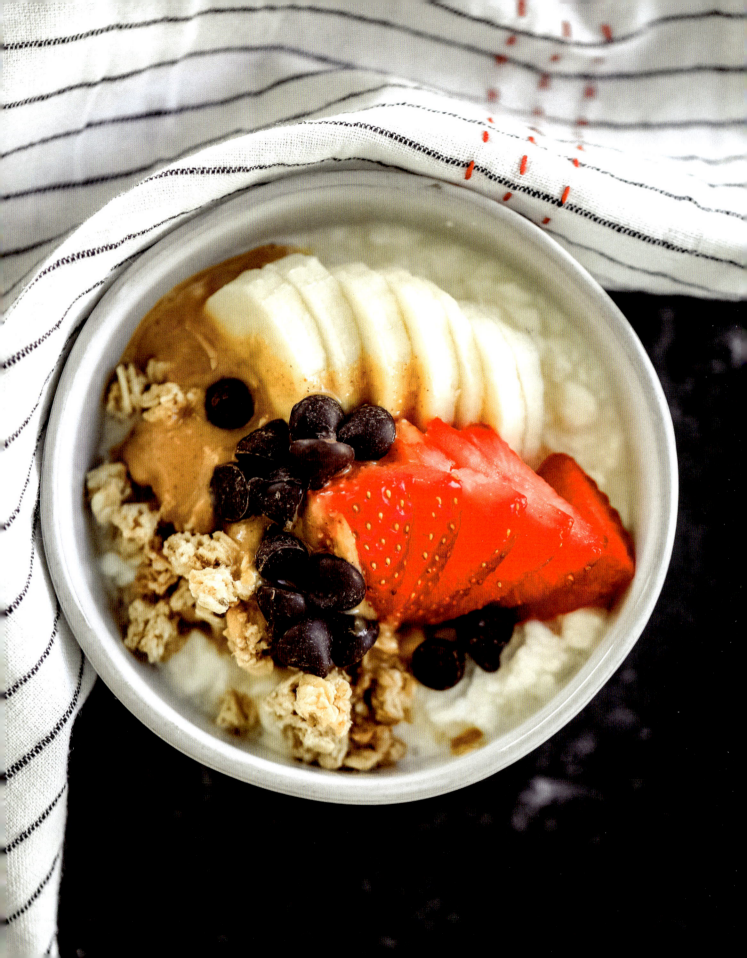

CHUNKY MONKEY BOWL

Makes 1 serving
250 calories / 10F / 23C / 17P

Prep: 5 min

½ cup low-fat cottage cheese
Vanilla stevia drops
30g banana slices
1 large strawberry, sliced
2 Tbs. Nature's Path Pumpkin Seed & Flax Granola
½ Tbs. CSE Sweet Classic or Monkey Business Butter
   or natural peanut butter
8 (4g) dark chocolate chips

1. Combine the cottage cheese and stevia in a bowl.

2. Top with bananas, strawberries, granola, peanut butter and chocolate chips.

PRO TIP: Swap nonfat, plain Greek yogurt in place of cottage cheese.

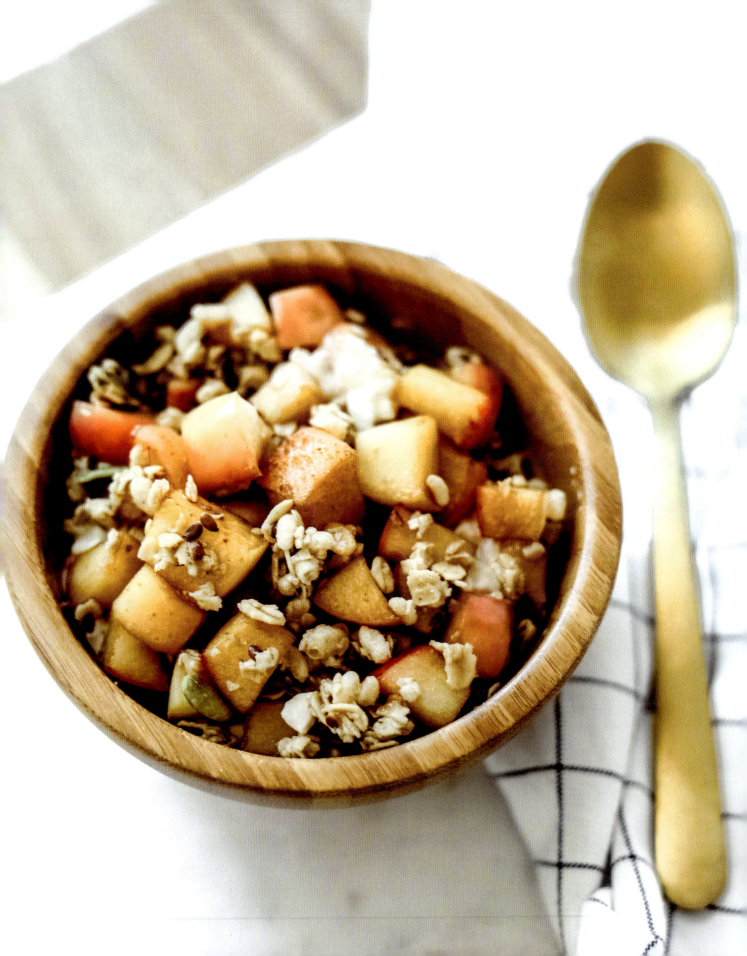

CREAMY CINNAMON SUGAR APPLE BOWL

Makes 1 serving
240 calories / 9F / 25C / 15P

Prep: 5 min | **Cook:** 5 min

½ cup low-fat cottage cheese
Vanilla stevia drops
75g chopped apple
1 tsp. coconut oil
1 tsp. coconut sugar
1 tsp. ground cinnamon
2 Tbs. Nature's Path Pumpkin Seed & Flax Granola

1. Combine the cottage cheese and stevia drops in a bowl; set aside.

2. In a frying pan over medium heat, sauté the apples in coconut oil, coconut sugar and cinnamon. Cook until fragrant.

3. Pour the apples over the cottage cheese and sprinkle granola over the top.

PRO TIP: Swap nonfat, plain Greek yogurt in place of cottage cheese.

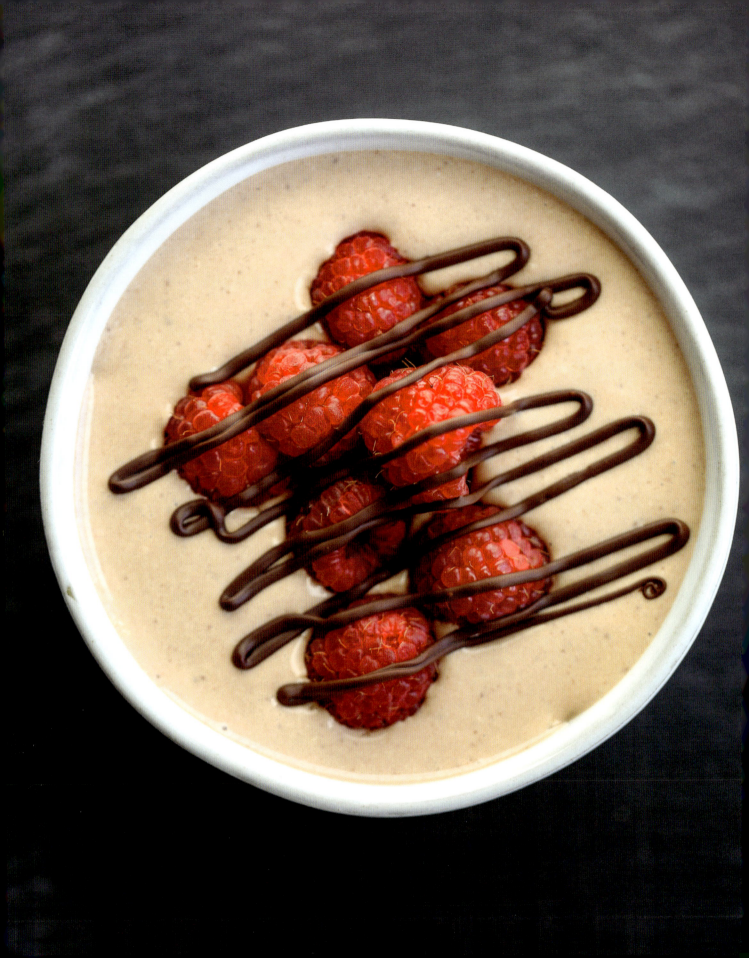

DARK CHOCOLATE MOUSSE
Makes 1 serving
250 calories / 8F / 28C / 17P

Prep: 10 min | **Cook:** 1 min

⅔ cup nonfat, plain Greek yogurt
1 Tbs. cocoa powder
1 tsp. raw honey
Vanilla stevia drops, optional
¼ cup fresh raspberries
15g dark chocolate chips, melted
2 Tbs. spray whipped cream

1. Stir the Greek yogurt, cocoa powder, honey and stevia together in a bowl. Add the fresh raspberries.

2. Optional step: Place the chocolate chips in a bowl and heat in the microwave for 30 seconds at a time until melted and smooth; stirring in between.

3. Drizzle the chocolate over the raspberries and top with whipped cream.

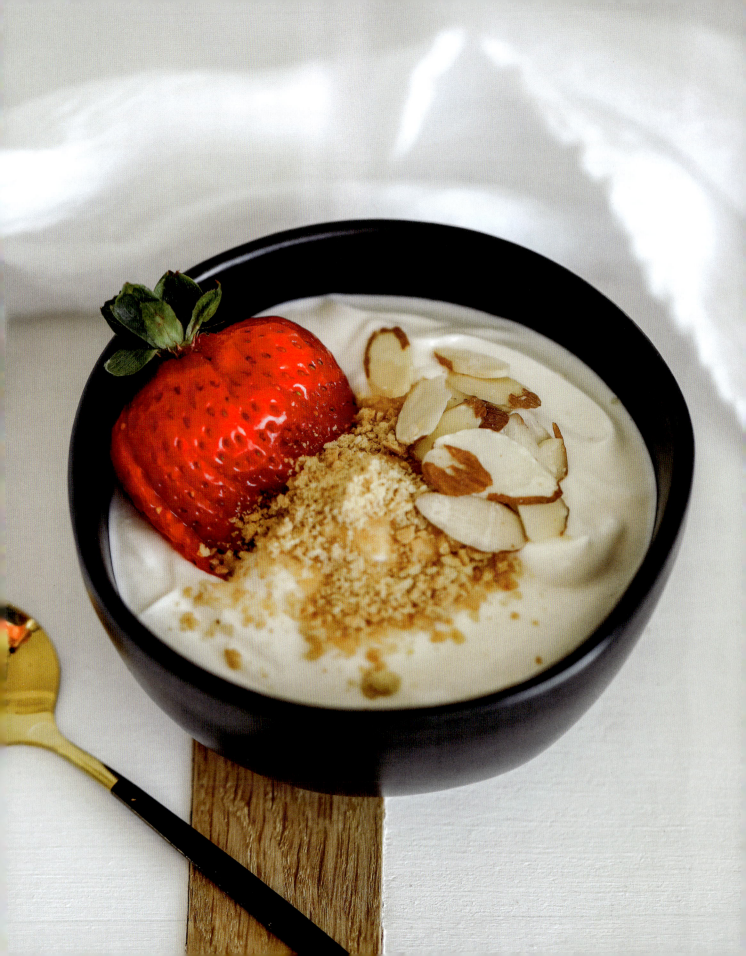

STRAWBERRY CHEESECAKE BOWL
Makes 1 serving
240 calories / 6F / 25C / 22P

Prep: 10 min

⅔ cup nonfat, plain Greek yogurt
2 Tbs. unsweetened almond milk
4g CSE Strawberry Cheesecake Protein Powder
150g sliced strawberries
8g graham cracker crumbs
1 Tbs. sliced almonds

1. Add the Greek yogurt, almond milk and protein powder to a bowl. Stir until well combined.

2. Top with fresh strawberries, graham cracker crumbs and sliced almonds.

PRO TIP: Sprinkle a little sugar-free Cheesecake Jello Pudding Mix into the yogurt to make it extra yummy.

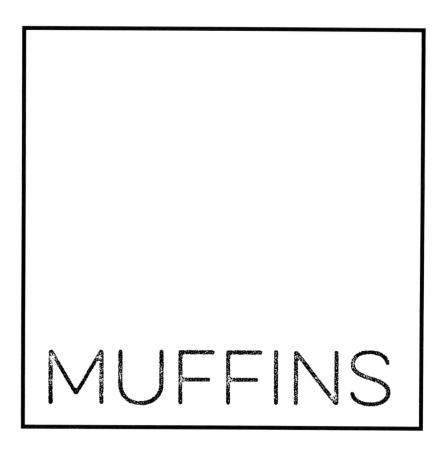

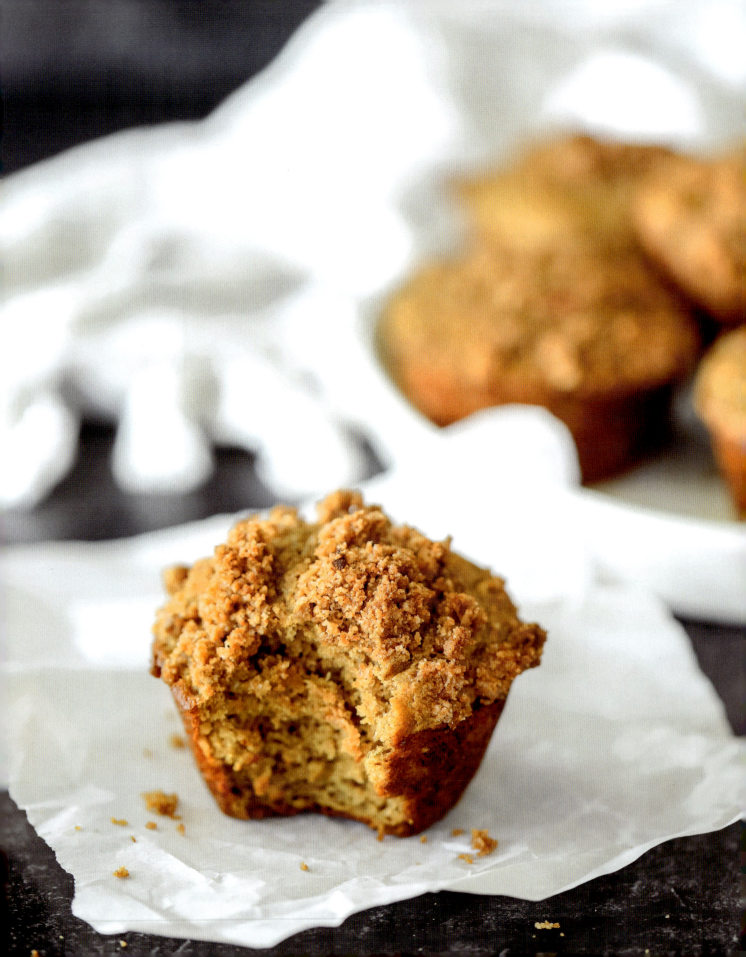

APPLE CRUMB MUFFINS

Makes 14 muffins
140 calories / 3F / 23.5C / 6P / per muffin

Prep: 15 min | **Cook:** 15 min

Crumb Topping:
¼ cup CSE Buttermilk, Gluten-Free Buttermilk, or Vanilla Pancake & Waffle Mix
¼ cup coconut palm sugar
2 Tbs. melted coconut oil or butter
½ tsp. cinnamon
Dash sea salt

Muffins:
½ cup unsweetened almond milk
½ tsp. white wine vinegar
½ cup unsweetened applesauce
½ cup coconut palm sugar
2 large eggs
½ Tbs. vanilla extract
2 cups CSE Buttermilk, Gluten-Free Buttermilk, or Vanilla Pancake & Waffle Mix
1 tsp. baking powder
1 tsp. baking soda
1 tsp. cinnamon
½ tsp. sea salt
75g peeled and grated apples

1. Heat the oven to 375 degrees. Make the crumb topping first by mixing the CSE Pancake & Waffle Mix, coconut sugar, cinnamon, and sea salt together in a bowl. Stir in the melted coconut oil or butter and store in the fridge.

2. In a small bowl, combine the almond milk and vinegar. Set aside. Beat the applesauce, coconut sugar, and almond milk mixture in a large bowl. Add the eggs and vanilla. Mix until well combined.

3. In a separate bowl, combine the CSE Pancake & Waffle Mix, baking powder, baking soda, cinnamon and sea salt. Mix until well combined. Add the dry ingredients to the wet ingredients and mix until just combined. Fold in the grated apples.

4. Add muffin liners to a muffin tin and spray the liners with cooking spray. Add ¼ cup of the batter to each muffin cup. Sprinkle ½ tablespoon of the crumb mixture over each muffin. Bake in the oven for 14-15 minutes.

PRO TIP: Pour batter into a greased 9x13 pan instead of baking in a muffin tin. Cook for the same amount of time. Let cool and cut into squares.

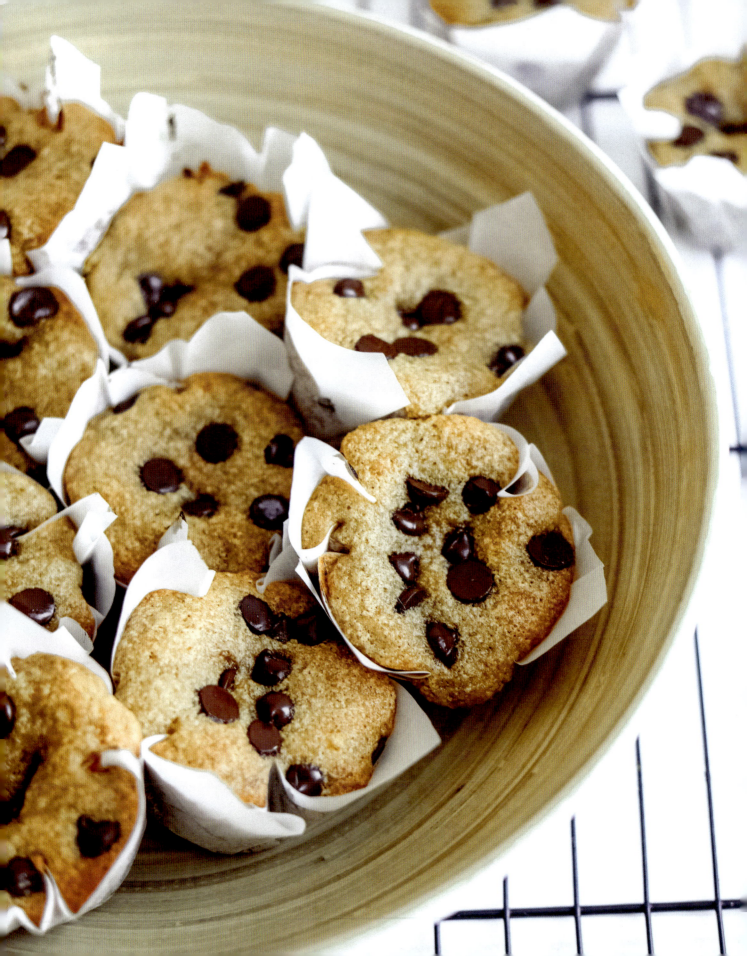

BANANA CHOCOLATE CHIP MUFFINS

Makes 13 muffins
180 calories / 6.5F / 26C / 6.5P / per muffin

Prep: 15 min | **Cook:** 15 min

2 (240g) ripe bananas
½ cup raw honey
3 Tbs. melted coconut oil
½ cup unsweetened applesauce
1 large egg
1 tsp. vanilla extract
1 ½ cups CSE Buttermilk, Gluten-Free Buttermilk,
  or Vanilla Pancake & Waffle Mix
1 serving CSE Simply Vanilla Protein Powder
2 Tbs. flaxseed meal
1 tsp. baking soda
1 tsp. baking powder
¼ tsp. sea salt

Topping per muffin:
10 dark chocolate chips (5 grams per muffin)

1. Preheat the oven to 350 degrees.

2. Mash the bananas in a large mixing bowl. Beat in the honey and coconut oil. Add in the applesauce, egg and vanilla; mix well and set aside.

3. In a separate bowl, combine the CSE Pancake & Waffle Mix, protein powder, flaxseed meal, baking soda, baking powder and sea salt. Add the wet ingredients to the dry ingredients and whisk together until just combined.

4. Line a muffin tin with liners. Scoop about ¼ cup of the batter into each muffin cup and top with chocolate chips. Bake for 15-16 minutes. Transfer from the pan to the cooling rack.

PRO TIP: Make an extra batch and freeze! Allow muffins to cool completely and store in a freezer bag. Thaw (or microwave) before serving and enjoy!

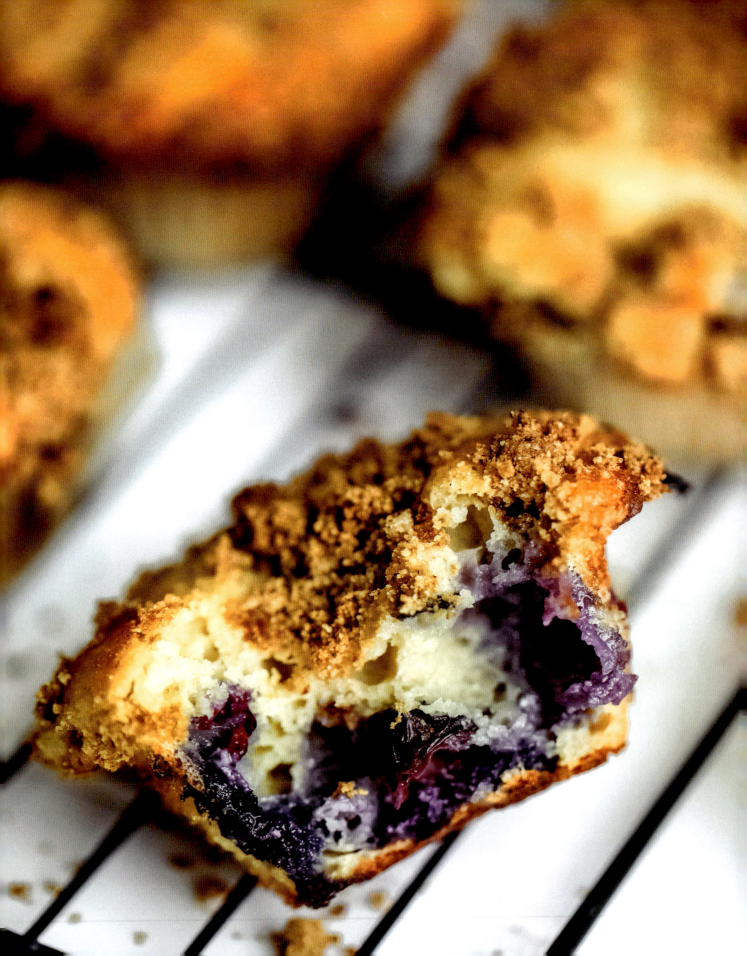

BLUEBERRY MUFFINS
Makes 12 muffins
150 calories / 5F / 21C / 7P / per muffin

Prep: 15 min | **Cook:** 15 min

Crumb Topping:
⅓ cup coconut sugar
⅓ cup CSE Buttermilk, Gluten-Free Buttermilk, or Vanilla Pancake & Waffle Mix
2 Tbs. melted grass-fed butter or coconut oil
1 tsp. ground cinnamon

Muffin Mix:
1 ½ cups CSE Buttermilk, Gluten-Free Buttermilk, or Vanilla Pancake & Waffle Mix
1 serving CSE Simply Vanilla or Coconut Cream Protein Powder
½ cup xylitol sweetener
½ tsp. sea salt
2 tsp. baking powder
1 large egg
⅓ cup unsweetened applesauce
⅓ cup unsweetened almond milk
2 Tbs. melted coconut oil
1 cup fresh blueberries

1. Heat the oven to 400 degrees.

2. Make the topping by adding the coconut sugar, CSE Pancake & Waffle Mix, melted butter/coconut oil and cinnamon to a bowl. Mix with a fork until well combined; set aside.

3. Place the CSE Pancake & Waffle Mix, protein powder, xylitol, sea salt and baking powder in a bowl. Stir until combined.

4. In a separate bowl, beat the egg, applesauce, almond milk and melted coconut oil. Add the wet ingredients to the dry ingredients; mix until just combined. Fold in the blueberries.

5. Add muffin liners to a muffin pan. Spray the liners with cooking spray. Add the batter to the liners until they are ¾ full; about ¼ cup in each. Add one tablespoon of the crumble topping to each muffin. Bake for 13-15 minutes or until golden and cooked through.

PRO TIP: Pour batter into a greased 9x13 pan instead of baking in a muffin tin. Cook for the same amount of time. Let cool and cut into squares.

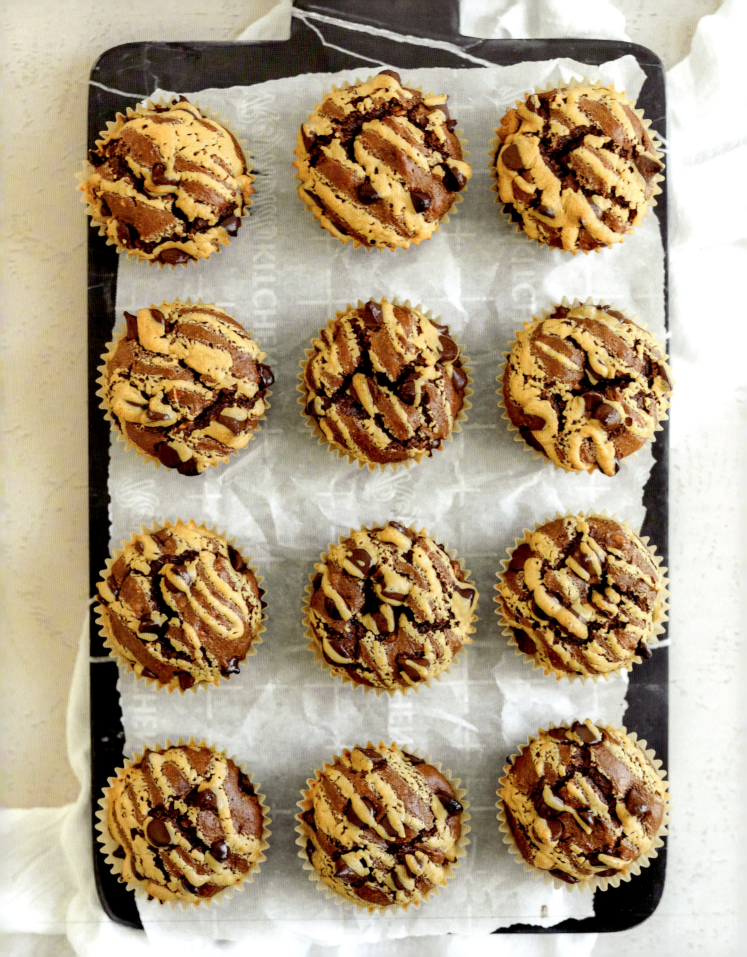

CHOCOLATE PB SWIRL MUFFINS
Makes 16 muffins
175 calories / 8F / 20C / 6P / per muffin

Prep: 15 min | **Cook:** 12 min

¾ cup bananas
¼ cup raw honey
¼ cup organic cane sugar
2 eggs
½ cup CSE Sweet Classic Peanut Butter or natural peanut butter
1 tsp. vanilla extract
½ cup old-fashioned rolled oats
½ cup white whole wheat flour
¼ cup cocoa powder
1 serving CSE Chocolate Brownie Batter or Chocolate Peanut Butter Protein Powder
1 tsp. baking powder
½ tsp. baking soda
½ tsp. sea salt
½ cup dark chocolate chips

Topping:
16 tsp. CSE Sweet Classic Peanut Butter or natural peanut butter

1. Preheat the oven to 350 degrees.

2. Mash the banana. Add the mashed bananas, honey, sugar, eggs, peanut butter and vanilla extract into a large mixing bowl. Beat until smooth. Set aside.

3. In a separate bowl, mix the oats, flour, cocoa powder, protein powder, baking powder, baking soda and sea salt together. Add to the wet ingredients and mix until just combined. Fold in the chocolate chips.

4. Add muffin liners to a muffin tin. Fill each muffin liner ¾ full with the batter. Drizzle about one teaspoon of peanut butter over the top of each muffin. Place in the oven and bake for 10-12 minutes.

5. Let cool for a couple minutes and then remove each muffin from the muffin tin. Store leftovers in the fridge.

PRO TIP: Make an extra batch and freeze! Allow muffins to cool completely and store in a freezer bag. Thaw (or microwave) before serving and enjoy!

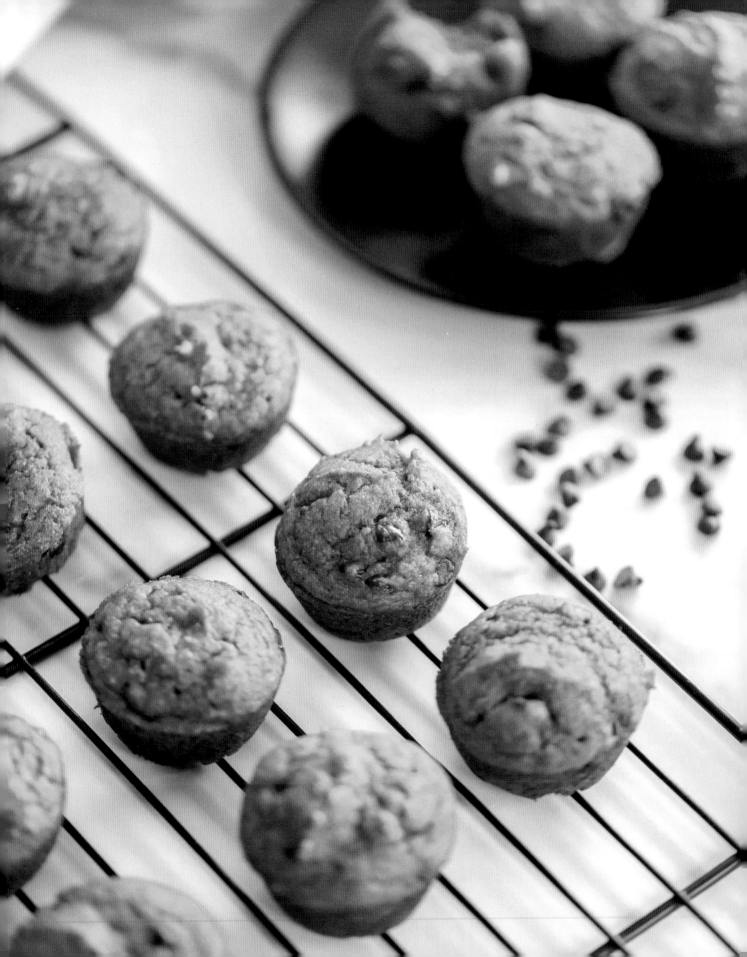

MINI PUMPKIN CHOCOLATE CHIP MUFFINS

Makes 46 muffins
40 calories / 1.5F / 5.5C / 1.5P / per muffin

Prep: 15 min | **Cook:** 12 min

1 serving CSE Pumpkin Pie Protein Powder
1 ½ cups Kodiak Cakes Pumpkin Flax Mix
1 tsp. baking soda
1 tsp. baking powder
½ tsp. sea salt
½ tsp. ground cinnamon
2 eggs
1 cup canned pumpkin
1 tsp. vanilla extract
½ cup coconut sugar
¼ cup nonfat, plain Greek yogurt
¼ cup unsalted, grass-fed butter
⅓ cup fat-free milk or skim milk
½ cup chocolate chips mini

1. Preheat the oven to 350 degrees. Grease a mini muffin tin. No liners needed. Melt the butter.

2. Add the protein powder, Kodiak Cakes Mix, baking soda, baking powder, sea salt and cinnamon to a large bowl. Stir until combined; set aside.

3. In a separate bowl, whisk the eggs, pumpkin, vanilla, coconut sugar, Greek yogurt, melted butter and milk together until well combined. Add the wet ingredients to the dry ingredients and whisk until just combined. Fold in the chocolate chips.

4. Spoon about one tablespoon of the batter into each muffin cup, filling about ¾ of the way full. Bake for 12 minutes. Let cool for a couple minutes. Transfer to a cooling rack.

PRO TIP: Make an extra batch and freeze! Allow muffins to cool completely and store in a freezer bag. Thaw (or microwave) before serving and enjoy!

POWER BITES

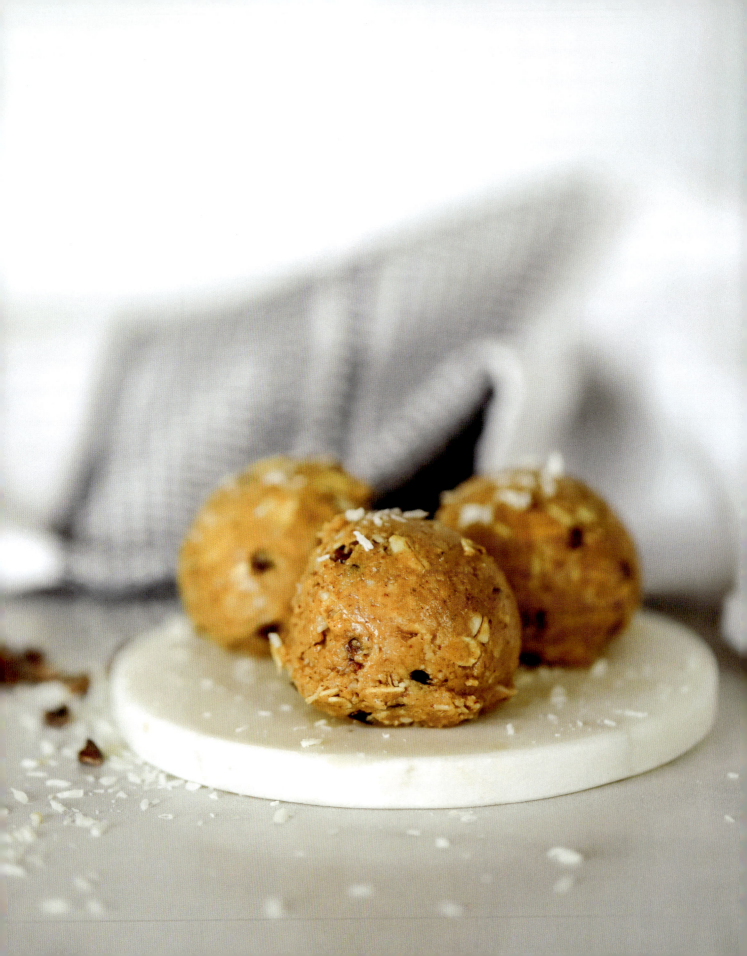

ALMOND JOY COOKIE DOUGH BITES

Makes 32 servings
100 calories / 5F / 11C / 3P / per bite

Prep: 15 min

- ½ cup CSE Midnight Almond Coconut Butter or natural almond butter
- ½ cup CSE Sweet Classic Peanut Butter or natural peanut butter
- ½ cup raw honey
- 1 serving CSE Simply Vanilla or Coconut Cream Protein Powder
- ½ cup unsweetened shredded coconut
- ¼ cup flaxseed meal
- 2 Tbs. cocoa nibs or mini chocolate chips
- 1 cup old-fashioned rolled oats

1. Mix all of the ingredients together, adding the oats last.

2. Using a small cookie scoop, scoop into balls and store in the fridge or freezer. Enjoy!

PRO TIPS: Easily prepared in a Kitchen Aid Mixer.

Bites stay fresh for up to two weeks in the fridge and up to three months in the freezer. We encourage you to make a double batch!

Try swapping in CSE Chocolate Brownie Batter Protein Powder in for a chocolatey treat!

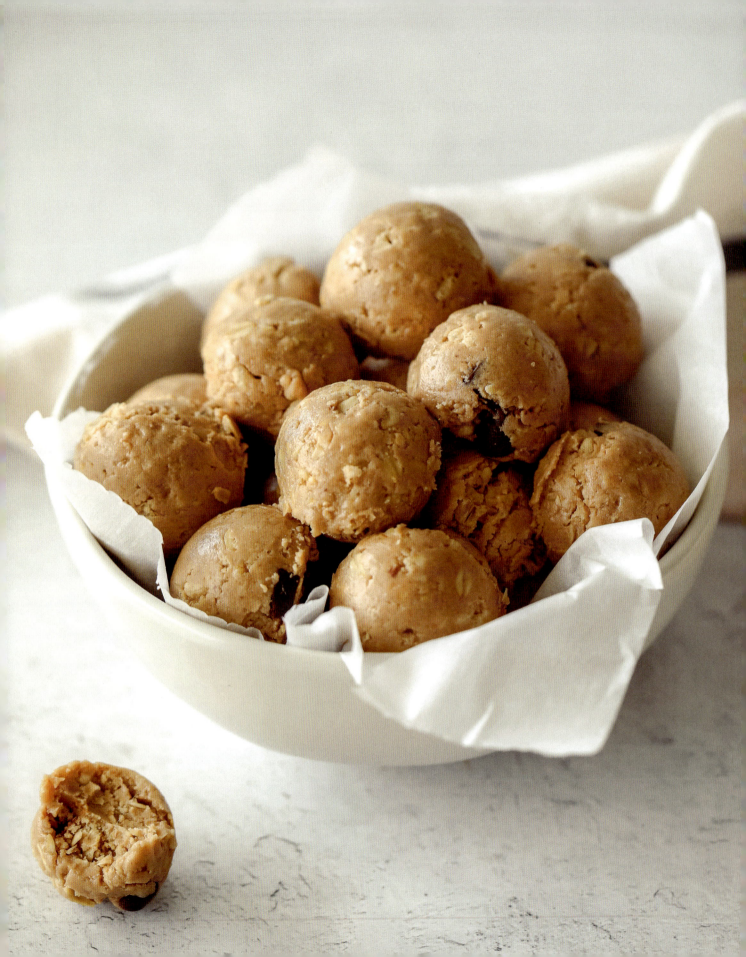

CRISPY CHOCOLATE PB BITES

Makes 25 servings
100 calories / 5F / 10C / 4P / per bite

Prep: 15 min

1 cup CSE Sweet Classic Peanut Butter or natural peanut butter
½ cup raw honey
2 servings CSE Chocolate Peanut Butter Protein Powder
Dash sea salt
1 tsp. vanilla extract
1 cup old-fashioned rolled oats
1 cup Nature's Path Crispy Rice Cereal
2 Tbs. mini chocolate chips

1. Add the peanut butter, honey, protein powder, salt and vanilla to a large mixing bowl. Mix until well combined.

2. Add in the remaining ingredients and mix well.

3. Using a small cookie scoop, scoop into balls and store in the fridge or freezer. Enjoy!

PRO TIP: Bites stay fresh for up to two weeks in the fridge and up to three months in the freezer. We encourage you to make a double batch!

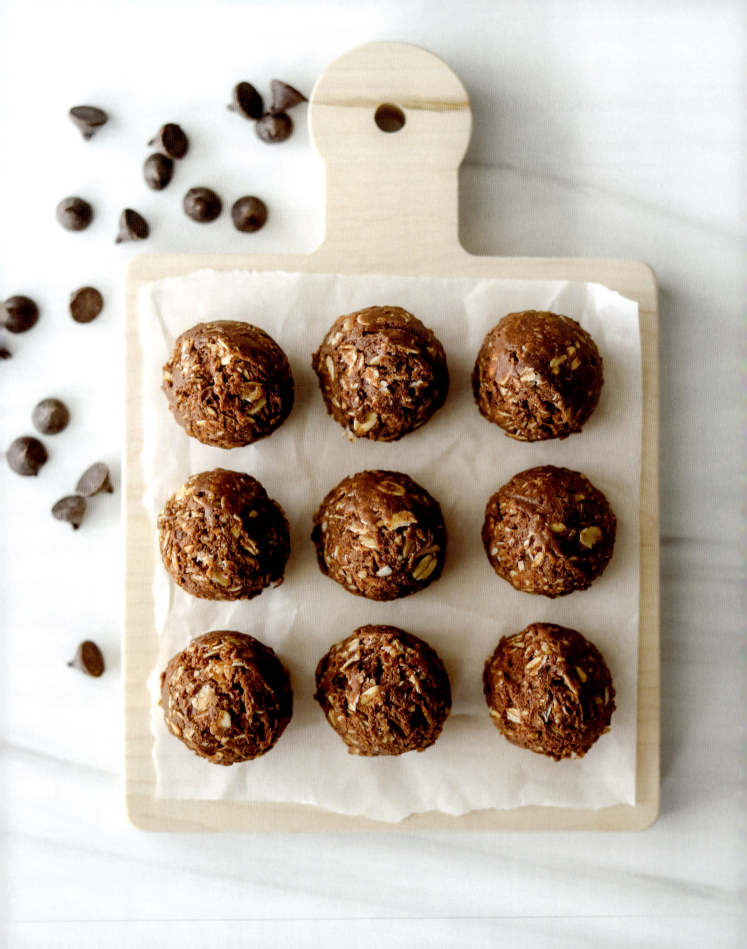

DARK CHOCOLATE PEANUT BUTTER BITES

Makes 26 servings
110 calories / 5.5F / 11.5C / 4P / per bite

Prep: 15 min

1 cup CSE Sweet Classic Peanut Butter, Buckeye Brownie Peanut Butter or natural peanut butter
½ cup raw honey
1 serving CSE Chocolate Brownie Batter or Chocolate Peanut Butter Protein Powder
1 ½ cups old-fashioned rolled oats
2 Tbs. cocoa powder
30 extra dark chocolate chips

1. Add all the ingredients to a large bowl and mix until well combined.

2. Using a small cookie scoop, scoop into balls and store in the fridge or freezer. Enjoy!

PRO TIP: Bites stay fresh for up to two weeks in the fridge and up to three months in the freezer. We encourage you to make a double batch!

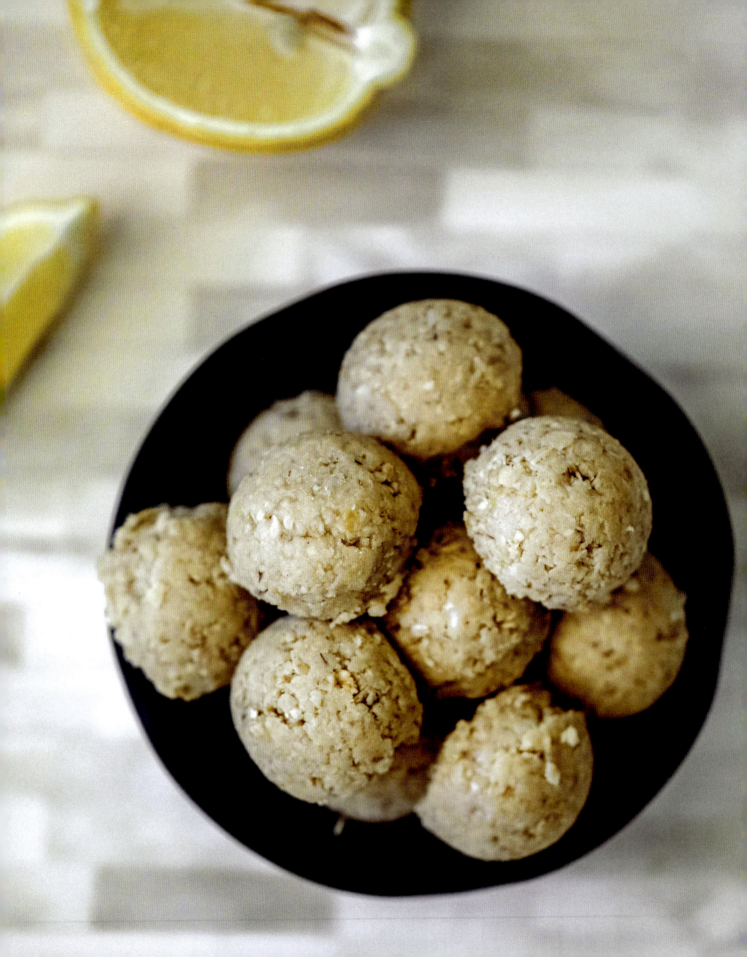

LEMON COCONUT BLISS BITES

Makes 32 servings
100 calories / 6F / 10C / 2.5P / per bite

Prep: 15 min

1 cup CSE Lemon Coconut Bliss Butter or coconut butter, softened
½ cup raw honey
1 serving CSE Simply Vanilla or Coconut Cream Protein Powder
¼ cup unsweetened shredded coconut
2 Tbs. lemon zest
2 tsp. fresh lemon juice
1 tsp. vanilla extract
Dash sea salt
1 ½ cups old-fashioned rolled oats

1. Place the coconut butter in the microwave for 30 seconds to soften. Make sure the foil liner is completely removed from the jar.

2. Add all of the ingredients into a mixing bowl and stir together until well combined.

3. Using a small cookie scoop, scoop into balls and store in the fridge or freezer. Enjoy!

PRO TIPS: Easily prepared in a Kitchen Aid Mixer.

Bites stay fresh for up to two weeks in the fridge and up to three months in the freezer. We encourage you to make a double batch!

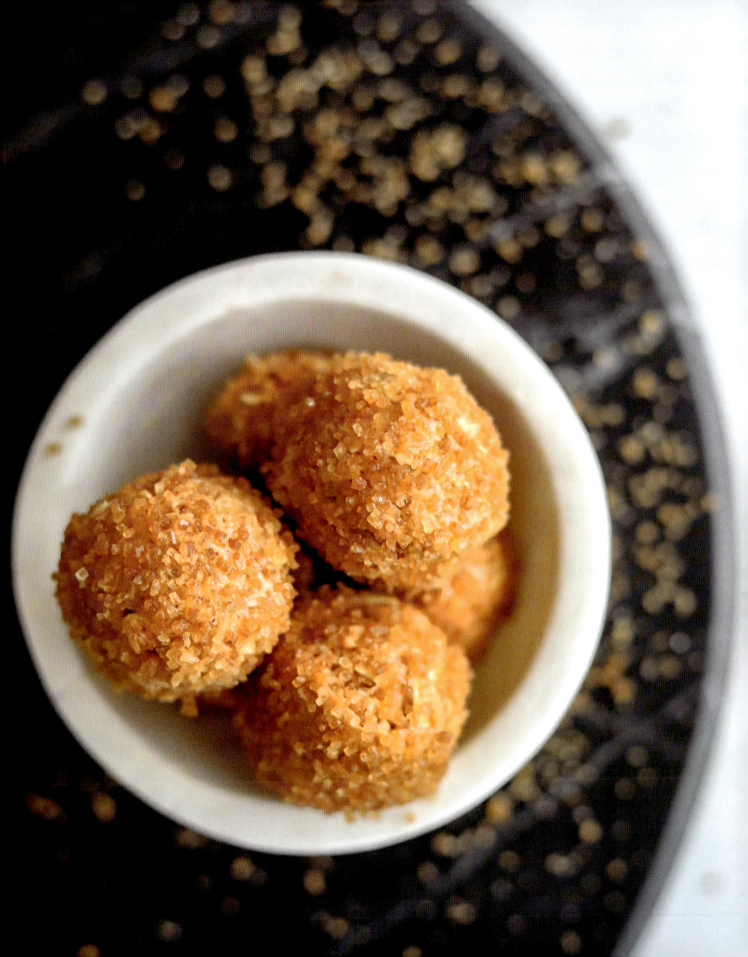

SALTED CARAMEL BITES

Makes 26 servings
100 calories / 5F / 12C / 4P / per bite

Prep: 15 min

- 1 cup CSE Salted Caramel Butter or natural almond butter
- ½ cup raw honey
- 1 serving CSE Simply Vanilla or Caramel Toffee Protein Powder
- 1 ½ cups old-fashioned rolled oats
- ¼ cup turbinado sugar

1. Add the nut butter to a bowl with the honey, protein powder and rolled oats. Mix until well combined.

2. Using a small cookie scoop, scoop into balls.

3. Place the sugar in a bowl and roll each ball into the sugar. Place all of the balls into a container. Store in the fridge or freezer. Enjoy!

PRO TIPS: Easily prepared in a Kitchen Aid Mixer.

Bites stay fresh for up to two weeks in the fridge and up to three months in the freezer. We encourage you to make a double batch!

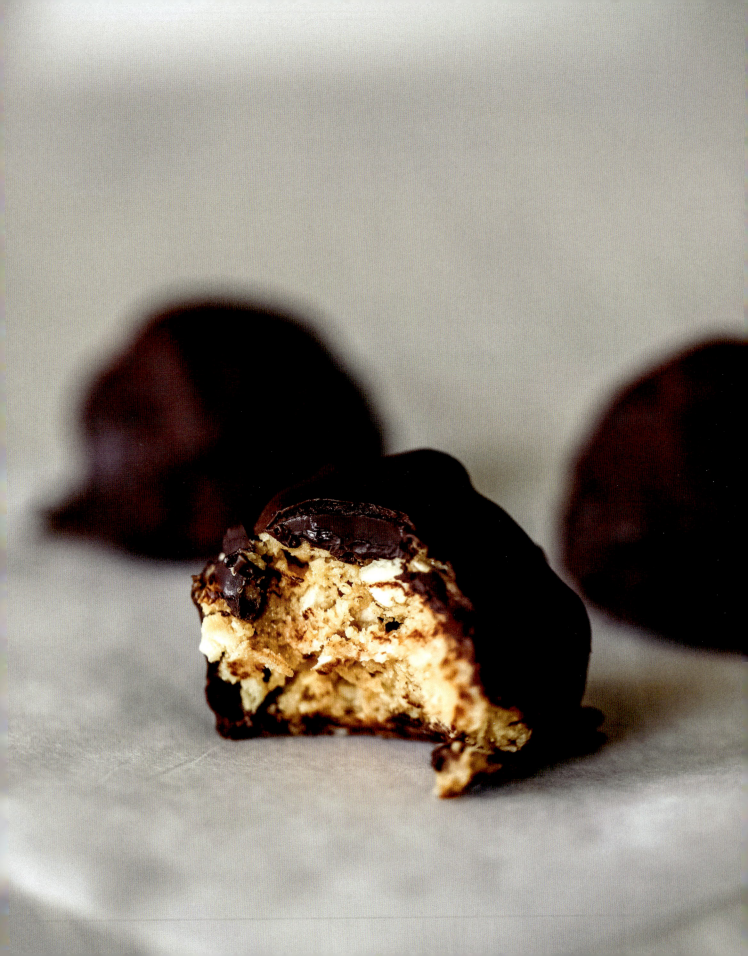

SNICKERS POWER BITES

Makes 28 servings
Macros with the cocoa dusting:
   100 calories / 5F / 10.5C / 4P / per bite
Macros with the chocolate coating:
   110 calories / 5.5F / 11C / 4P / per bite

Prep: 25 min

1 cup CSE Candy Bar, Sweet Classic Peanut Butter
   or natural peanut butter
½ cup raw honey
1 serving CSE Caramel Toffee or Simply Vanilla Protein Powder
½ tsp. vanilla extract
Dash sea salt
1 ½ cups old-fashioned rolled oats
Cocoa Dusting:
¼ cup cocoa powder
Chocolate Coating:
120g dark chocolate chips

1. Add all the ingredients to a large bowl and mix until well combined.

2. Using a small cookie scoop, scoop into balls.

3A. If using the Cocoa Dusting method: Add the cocoa powder to a bowl and roll each ball into it. Place in a container and store in the fridge or freezer.

3B. If using the Chocolate Coating method: Add the chocolate chips to a microwave-safe bowl. Microwave in 30-second increments, stirring after each one, until melted and smooth. Place the balls on a baking sheet lined with parchment paper. Drizzle the melted chocolate evenly over each one. Place in the fridge or freezer to allow the chocolate coating to set. Transfer to a container and store in the fridge or freezer. Enjoy!

PRO TIPS: Easily prepared in a Kitchen Aid Mixer.

Bites stay fresh for up to two weeks in the fridge and up to three months in the freezer. We encourage you to make a double batch!

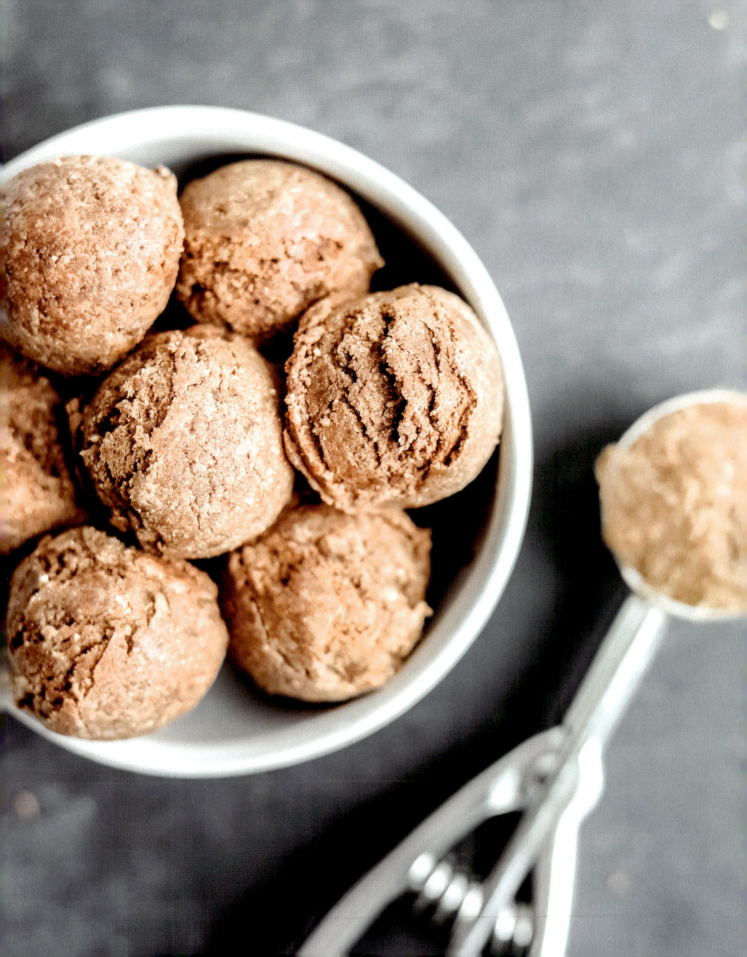

THIN MINT COOKIE BITES

Makes 34 servings
95 calories / 3.5F / 12.5C / 4P / per bite

Prep: 15 min

- 12 oz. CSE Mint Chocolate Chip Cookie Butter or natural chocolate almond butter
- ½ cup raw honey
- 2 servings CSE Mint Chocolate Cookie or Chocolate Brownie Batter Protein Powder
- 1 ½ cups oat flour
- Dash vanilla extract
- Dash sea salt

1. Place all ingredients into a mixing bowl and stir together until well combined.

2. Scoop into balls using a small cookie scoop. Store in the fridge or freezer. Enjoy!

PRO TIPS: Easily prepared in a Kitchen Aid Mixer.

Drizzle melted chocolate over the top to take these to the next level!

Bites stay fresh for up to two weeks in the fridge and up to three months in the freezer. We encourage you to make a double batch!

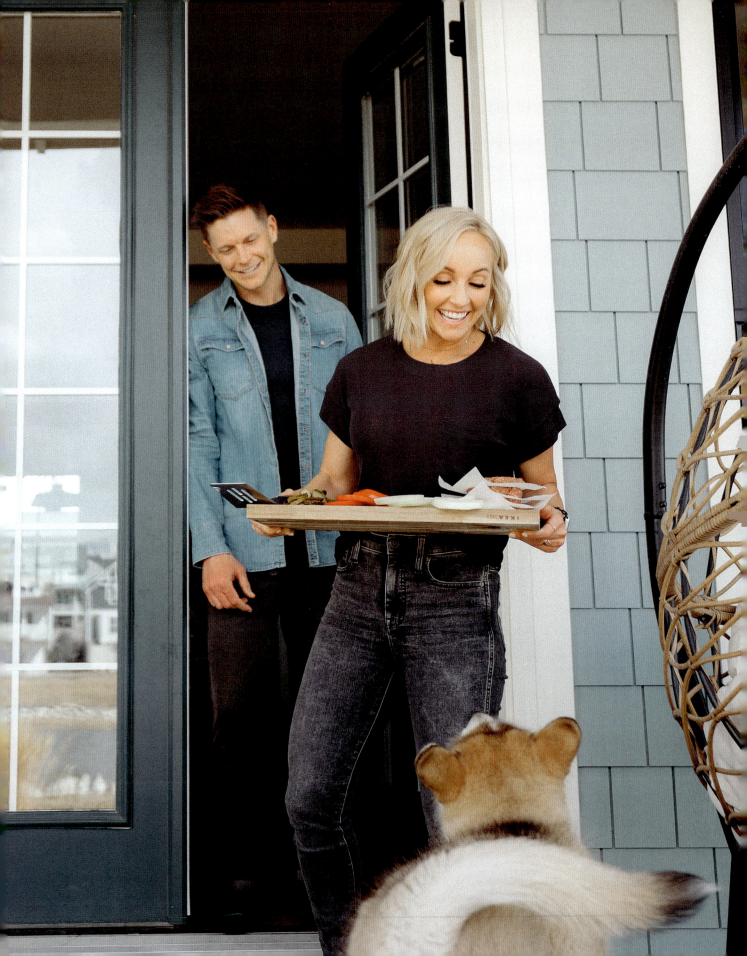

ENTREES

We can't pick a favorite meal, so don't even ask! We went and did one better though by including ALL of our favorites — **Soups, Salads, & Sandwiches**, **Tex-Mex**, **Pizza & Pasta**, and good old-fashioned **Comfort Food** classics! We share lots of quick and easy weeknight meals (we're talking 25 minutes or less), dinners your kids will actually eat (hello, homemade chicken nuggets), and meals to please a crowd. At our house, we believe that food should be enjoyed and celebrated! Because there's nothing better than a big bowl of pasta or a warm bowl of soup on a cold day, there's a lot more to pizza than just plain cheese, and tacos aren't just for Tuesday. These meals are sure to fill hungry bellies and bring families back to the dinner table.

SOUPS, SALADS & SANDWICHES

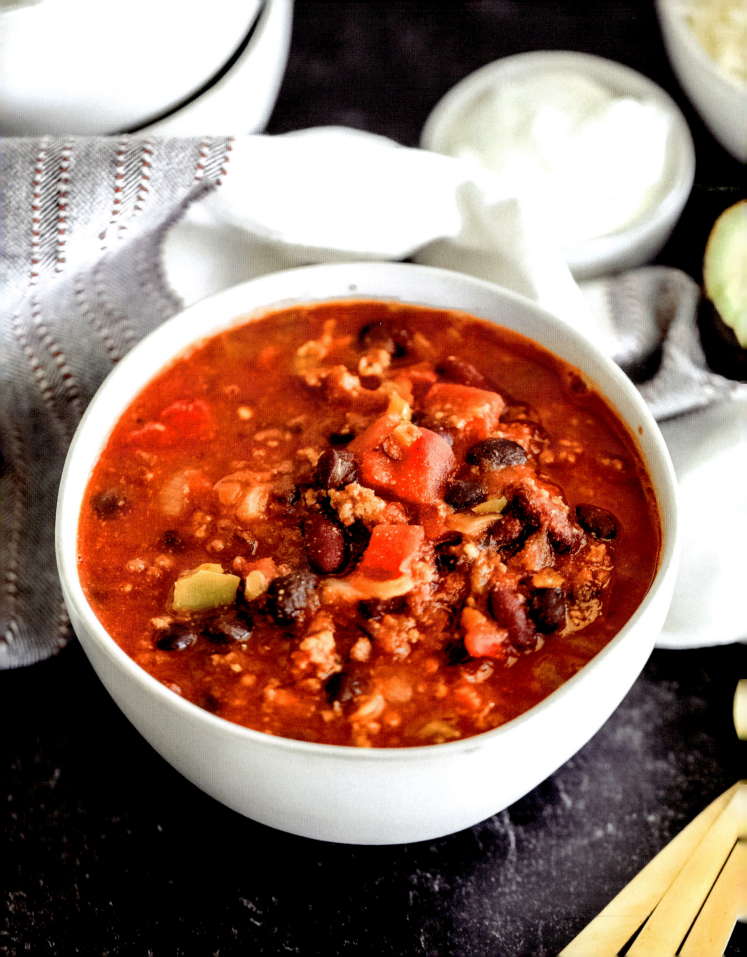

BEST EVER CHILI

Makes 4 servings
350 calories / 12F / 36C / 24P / per serving

Prep: 30 min | **Cook:** 1-4 hrs

8 oz. lean ground beef
1 cup fresh, minced yellow onion
2 cups minced green bell pepper
1 tsp. fresh, minced garlic
2 Tbs. chopped flat-leaf parsley
1 chopped jalapeño pepper, optional
2 tsp. ground chili powder
1 tsp. ground cumin
½ tsp. dried oregano
½ tsp. sea salt
½ tsp. black pepper
1 cup tomato sauce
2 cups diced tomatoes
1 cup black beans, drained and rinsed
1 cup kidney beans, drained and rinsed

Toppings per serving:
1 Tbs. low-fat, shredded mozzarella cheese
1 Tbs. nonfat, plain Greek yogurt
30g chopped avocado

1. In a skillet, brown the ground beef until no longer pink. Transfer to a crockpot.

2. Spray the skillet with cooking spray and add the onions, bell peppers, garlic, parsley and jalapeño peppers. Cook over medium heat for about five minutes or until veggies are tender and fragrant. Remove from heat and add all the seasonings.

3. Add all ingredients, except for the toppings, to the crockpot. Cook on low for 3-4 hours (or simmer in a pot on the stovetop for 1 hour).

4. Weigh the entire recipe and divide the weight by four to get the amount needed for one serving. Serve warm topped with cheese, Greek yogurt and avocado.

PRO TIPS: To cut down on cook time, make this recipe in a large pot, cooking the meat first, then simmering for 30 minutes.

To make this a freezer meal, make and freeze without toppings. To thaw, place in a crockpot on high for 4-6 hours. Add toppings fresh.

My kids love eating this with Frito Scoops or toasted french bread.

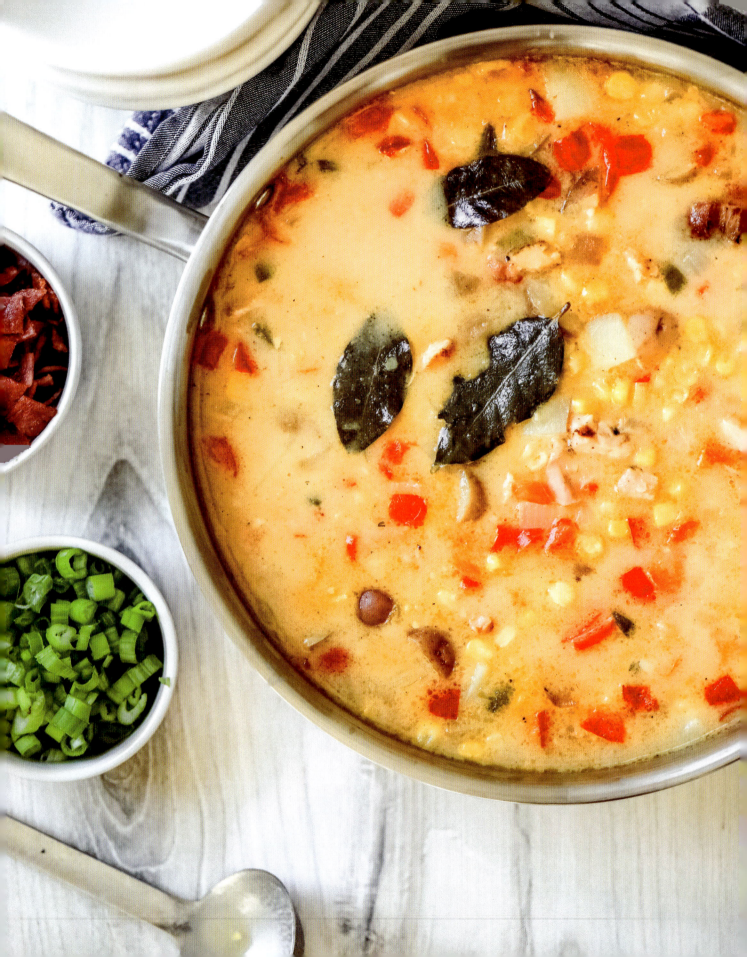

CREAMY CHICKEN CORN CHOWDER

Makes 4 servings
350 calories / 12F / 34C / 26P / per serving

Prep: 30 min | **Cook:** 45 min

- 4 oz. cooked, shredded chicken breast (5.2 oz. raw)
- 2 Tbs. grass-fed butter
- 1 cup diced red bell pepper
- ½ cup diced yellow onion
- 1 jalapeño, seeded and finely chopped
- 2 garlic cloves, minced
- 2 Tbs. CSE Buttermilk or Gluten-Free Buttermilk Pancake & Waffle Mix
- 2 cups low-sodium chicken broth
- 8 oz. raw, diced red potatoes
- 2 bay leaves
- Dash sea salt
- Dash black pepper
- 2 cups fresh or frozen corn
- ½ cup plain, nonfat Greek yogurt

Toppings per serving:
- 2 Tbs. low-fat, shredded mozzarella cheese
- 1 slice cooked, chopped turkey bacon
- Green onions, chopped

1. Cook or grill the chicken over medium heat until all sides are golden and the chicken is cooked through, about 5-7 minutes per side or until internal temperature reaches 160 degrees. Cook the bacon according to the directions on the package.

2. In a large pot, melt the butter over medium heat. Add the red bell peppers, onions and jalapeños; sauté until tender, about three minutes. Add the garlic and cook until fragrant. Stir in the CSE Pancake & Waffle Mix and then slowly whisk in the chicken broth until well blended.

3. Add the potatoes, bay leaves, salt and pepper to taste. Bring mixture to a boil, stirring constantly. Reduce heat to medium-low and cook uncovered, about 10 minutes or until the potatoes are tender.

4. Add in the cooked chicken, corn and Greek yogurt. Simmer uncovered for 10-15 minutes, stirring occasionally. Weigh the entire recipe and divide the weight by four to get the amount needed to fill one serving. Serve warm topped with cheese, bacon and green onions.

PRO TIPS: Make and freeze without toppings. To thaw, place in a crockpot on high for 4-6 hours. Add toppings fresh.

Use pre-cooked rotisserie chicken to cut down on your cook time.

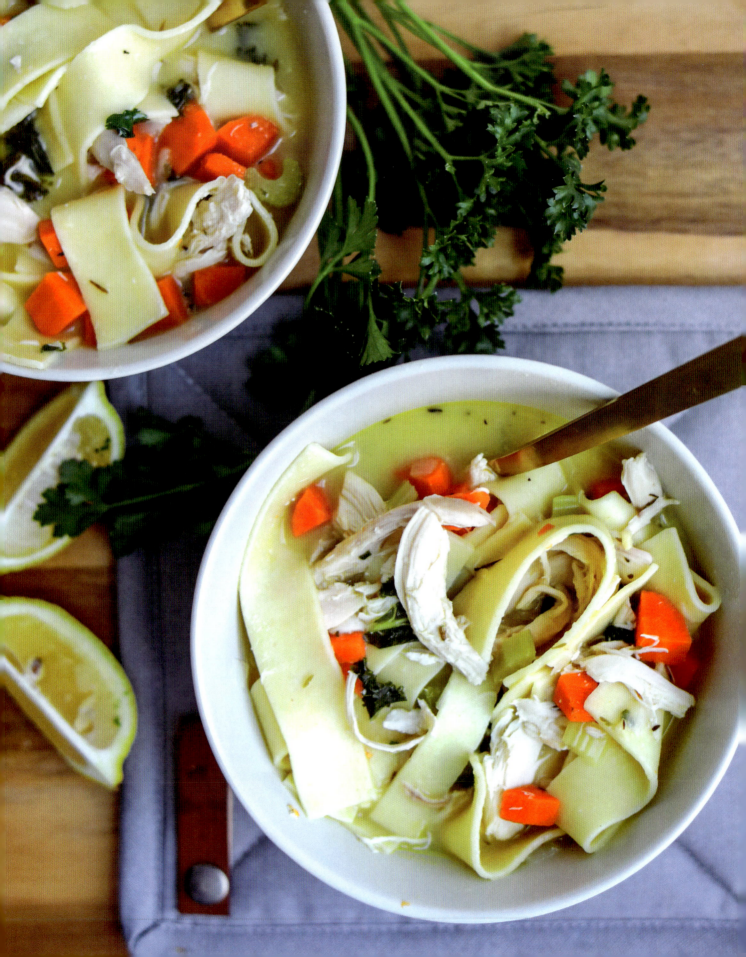

CREAMY CHICKEN NOODLE SOUP

Makes 4 servings
350 calories / 12F / 33C / 27P / per serving

Prep: 25 min | **Cook:** 35 min

- 1 Tbs. olive oil
- ½ cup diced yellow onion
- 3 cups chicken broth
- 2 cups water
- 1 bay leaf
- 1 tsp. fresh minced garlic
- ½ tsp. dried thyme
- ½ tsp. sea salt
- 1 ½ cups chopped carrots
- 1 cup chopped celery
- 1 cup chopped kale
- 4 oz. uncooked egg noodles
- 1 Tbs. grass-fed butter
- 2 Tbs. CSE Buttermilk or Gluten-Free Buttermilk Pancake & Waffle Mix
- ¼ cup canned, lite coconut milk
- 11 oz. rotisserie chicken breast, shredded
- ½ of a lemon, juice of
- 2 Tbs. fresh chopped parsley

1. Add the olive oil and diced onion to a large pot over medium heat. Sauté for about 3 minutes or until fragrant and tender. Stir in the chicken broth and water. Add the bay leaf, minced garlic, thyme and sea salt. Bring to a boil and then reduce heat and let simmer for 20 minutes.

2. Add in the carrots, celery and kale. Let cook for about five minutes and then add the uncooked egg noodles. Cook the noodles al dente according to the directions on the package.

3. Add the butter to a large frying pan over low heat. Once melted, stir in the CSE Pancake & Waffle Mix. Add one cup of broth from the soup to the pan, then slowly whisk it in along with the coconut milk. Bring to a boil; stirring constantly. Remove from heat and add to the pot of soup once the noodles are done cooking.

4. Add the shredded chicken last and simmer until the chicken is warm. Squeeze lemon juice over the soup and it is ready to serve. Weigh the entire soup and divide the weight by four to get the amount needed for one serving. Garnish each bowl with fresh parsley.

PRO TIP: Make and freeze without toppings. To thaw, place in a crockpot on high for 4-6 hours. Add toppings fresh.

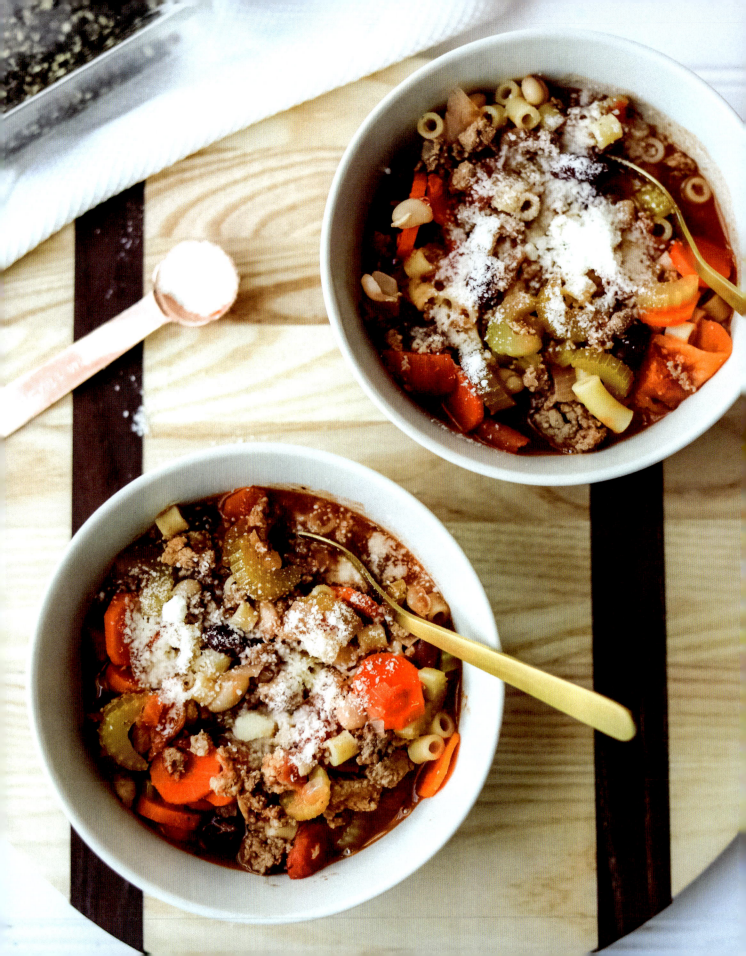

PASTA E FAGIOLI

Makes 4 servings
355 calories / 12F / 36C / 25P / per serving

Prep: 10 min | **Cook:** 50 min

- 12 oz. lean ground beef
- ½ cup diced yellow onion
- 1 tsp. minced garlic
- 2 chopped celery sticks
- 2 sliced, medium-sized carrots
- 2 cups canned diced tomatoes
- ½ cup red kidney beans, drained
- ½ cup great northern beans, drained
- 1 cup tomato sauce
- ½ cup vegetable broth
- 2 tsp. white wine vinegar
- ½ tsp. dried basil
- ½ tsp. dried oregano
- ½ tsp. sea salt
- ¼ tsp. dried thyme
- ¼ tsp. black pepper
- 2 oz. uncooked ditalini or macaroni pasta

Topping per serving:
- 1 tsp. grated Parmesan cheese

1. Brown the ground beef in a large pot over medium heat. Add the onions, garlic, celery and carrots. Sauté for about 10 minutes. Add the remaining ingredients, except for the pasta, and simmer for 30 minutes.

2. Cook the pasta al dente according to the directions on the package; drain.

3. Add the pasta to the pot of soup and then simmer for five minutes. Weigh the entire soup and divide the weight by four to get the amount needed to fill one serving. Serve warm topped with Parmesan cheese.

PRO TIP: Make and freeze without toppings. To thaw, place in a crockpot on high for 4-6 hours. Add toppings fresh.

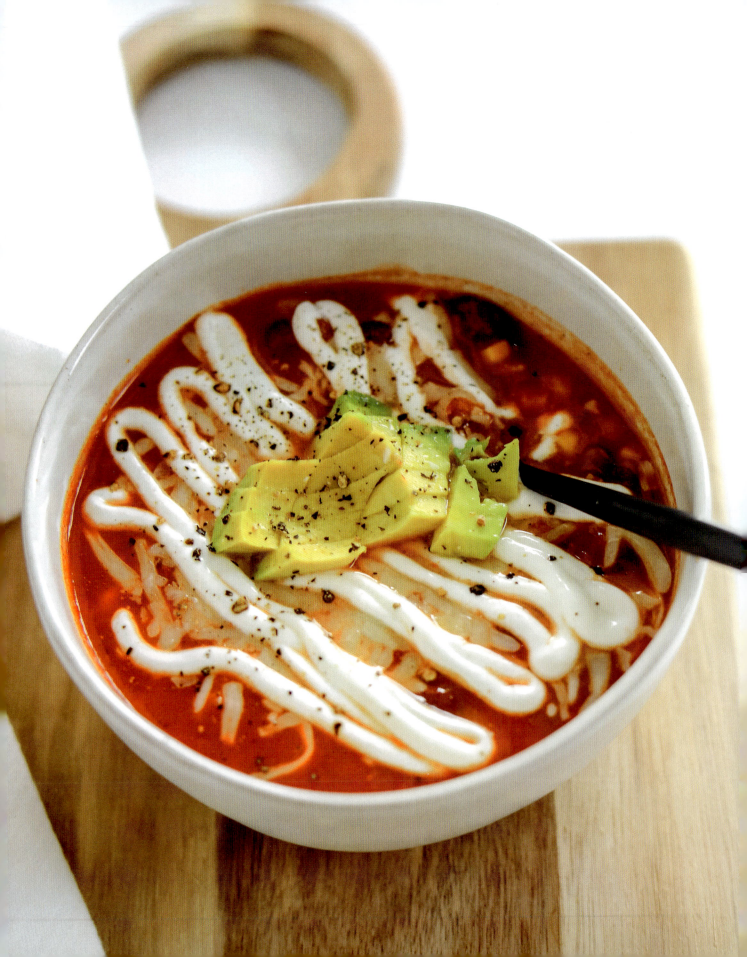

TACO SOUP

Makes 4 servings
340 calories / 12F / 33C / 26P / per serving

Prep: 10 min | **Cook:** 40 min

8 oz. lean ground turkey
½ cup chopped yellow onion
2 cups crushed tomatoes
1 cup frozen yellow corn
1 cup black beans or kidney beans
2 Tbs. taco seasoning
Toppings per serving:
2 Tbs. mozzarella cheese
1 Tbs. nonfat, plain Greek yogurt
25g avocado
Dash sea salt
Dash black pepper

1. In a large soup pot, brown the ground turkey with the chopped yellow onion over medium-high heat. Once browned, add the crushed tomatoes, corn, beans and taco seasoning. Let simmer for 30 minutes.

2. Weigh the entire recipe and divide the weight by four to get the amount needed to fill one serving. Top each serving with two tablespoons of shredded mozzarella cheese, one tablespoon of plain Greek yogurt, 25g avocado, salt and pepper to taste.

PRO TIPS: Make and freeze without toppings. To thaw, place in a crockpot on high for 4-6 hours. Add toppings fresh.

My kids love eating this soup with Frito Scoops.

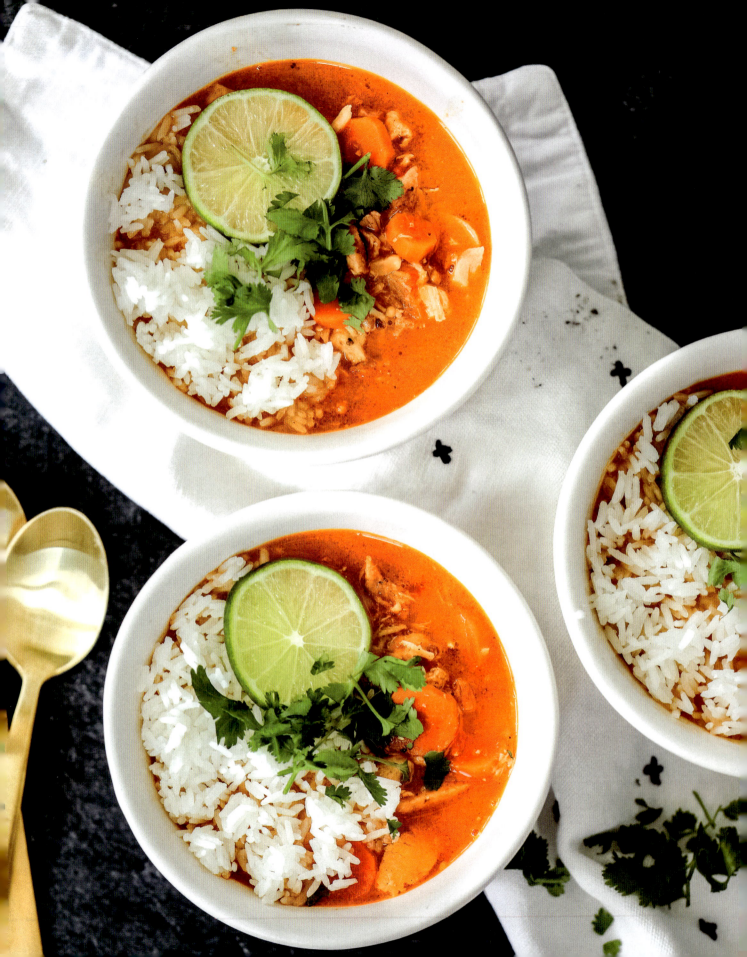

THAI CHICKEN SOUP

Makes 4 servings
345 calories / 10F / 35C / 28P / per serving

Prep: 15 min | **Cook:** 4-6 hrs

1 Tbs. red curry paste
1 ½ cups light, canned coconut milk
1 cup low-sodium chicken broth
1 Tbs. fish sauce
1 Tbs. raw honey
2 Tbs. CSE Sweet Classic Peanut Butter
  or natural peanut butter
14 oz. raw chicken breast
1 cup sliced red bell pepper
½ cup thin sliced yellow onion
1 cup peeled, chopped carrots
2 tsp. fresh, grated ginger
½ cup uncooked white or brown jasmine rice
Toppings per serving:
Lime wedge
Cilantro, for garnish

1. In a crockpot, whisk together the curry paste, coconut milk, chicken stock, fish sauce, honey and peanut butter. Cut the chicken into slices. Add in the chicken, uncooked rice, red bell peppers, onions, carrots and ginger. Cover and cook on low for 6 hours or on high for 4 hours.

2. Weigh the entire soup and divide by four to get the amount needed to fill one serving. Spoon into bowls. Top each serving with lime juice and cilantro. Enjoy warm.

PRO TIP: To cut down on cook time, make this recipe in a large pot, cooking the meat first, then simmering for 30 minutes.

Use pre-cooked rotisserie chicken to cut down on cook time.

Use microwavable rice pouches to cut down on cook time.

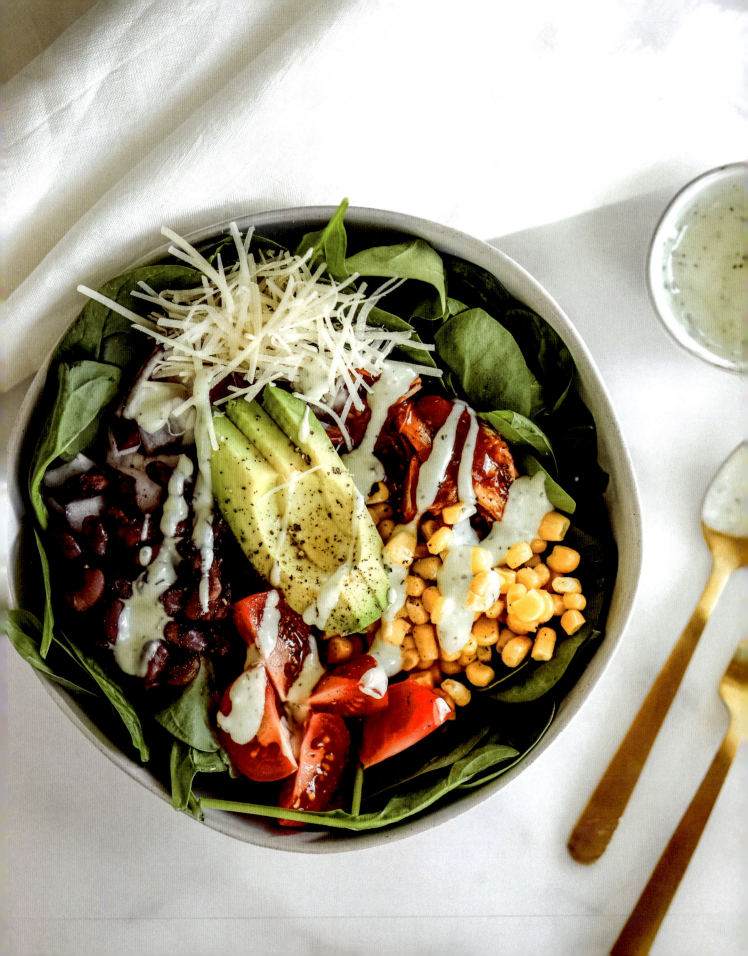

BBQ CHICKEN CHOPPED SALAD
Makes 4 servings
345 calories / 12F / 33C / 24P / per serving

Prep: 10 min | **Cook:** 15 min

8 oz. cooked chicken breast (10.6 oz. raw)
½ cup Stubb's BBQ Sauce
8 cups chopped spinach or romaine lettuce
1 cup black beans, drained and rinsed
1 cup frozen corn, thawed
2 diced vine tomatoes
½ cup diced red onion
Toppings per serving:
30 grams chopped avocado
2 Tbs. Bolthouse Farms Cilantro Avocado or Classic Ranch Dressing
1 Tbs. grated Parmesan or mozzarella cheese

1. Cook or grill the chicken over medium heat until all sides are golden and the chicken is cooked through, about 5-7 minutes per side or until internal temperature reaches 160 degrees.

2. Cube or shred the chicken and mix together with the BBQ sauce.

3. For one serving, layer two cups of chopped spinach, ¼ of the BBQ chicken mixture, ¼ cup of the black beans, ¼ cup of the corn, ½ of a tomato, two tablespoons of diced red onion, 30g avocado, two tablespoons of dressing and one tablespoon cheese.

PRO TIPS: Prep your salad in advance and store in a 32 oz. wide mouth mason jar. Prepare each salad individually. Layer in this order: tomatoes, red onion, corn, beans, chicken and spinach/lettuce on the top. Store in the fridge. When ready to eat, dump the salad out onto a plate and add the toppings and dressing fresh.

Use pre-cooked rotisserie chicken to cut down on your cook time.

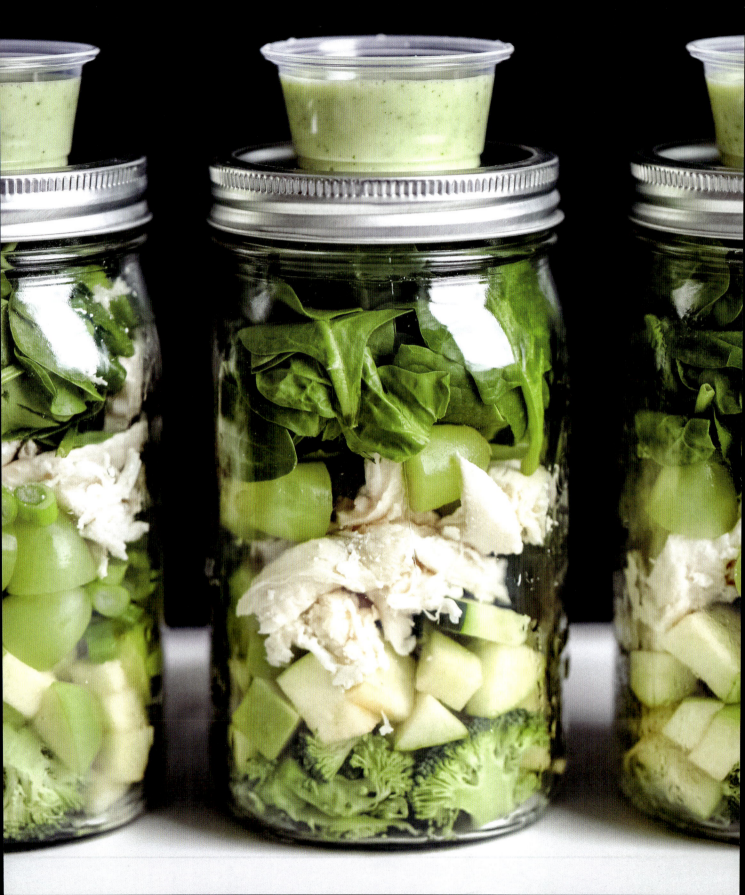

GREEN GODDESS SALAD

Makes 4 servings
350 calories / 11F / 35.5C / 27P / per serving

Prep: 10 min | **Cook:** 15 min

11 oz. cooked chicken breast
  (14.8 oz. raw)
4 cups spinach
2 cups broccoli
160g green grapes
160g green apples
1 cup cucumber
4 Tbs. green onion
160g avocados

Green Goddess Dressing:
⅓ cup olive oil mayo
2 Tbs. raw honey
1 tsp. apple cider vinegar
2 tsp. lemon juice
Pinch fresh cilantro
Dash sea salt
Dash black pepper

1. Cook or grill the chicken over medium heat until all sides are golden and the chicken is cooked through, about 5-7 minutes per side or until internal temperature reaches 160 degrees. Let cool after cooking.

2. Chop the spinach, broccoli, grapes, apples, cucumber and green onion.

3. Make the dressing by placing all of the ingredients into a blender. Blend on high until smooth. Weigh the entire dressing and divide the weight by four to get the amount needed to fill one serving.

4. Add one cup chopped spinach, ½ cup chopped broccoli, 40g sliced grapes, 40g chopped apples, ¼ cup chopped cucumber, 2.75 oz. grilled chicken, one tablespoon of green onions and 40g sliced avocado. Top with one serving of dressing. Enjoy!

PRO TIPS: Prep your salad in advance and store in a 32 oz. wide-mouth mason jar. Prepare each salad individually. Layer in this order: broccoli, green apples, cucumbers, chicken, green grapes, green onions and spinach. Seal the lid and store in the fridge. When ready to eat, dump the salad out onto a plate. Top with dressing and avocado.

Use pre-cooked rotisserie chicken to cut down on your cook time.

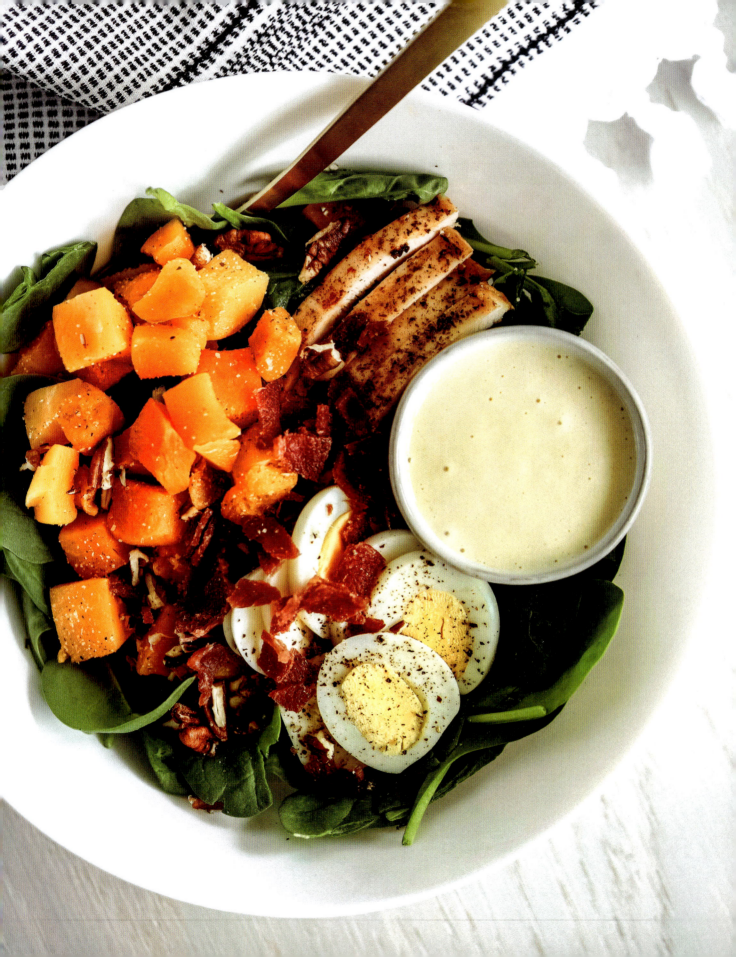

HARVEST COBB SALAD

Makes 4 servings
350 calories / 14F / 30C / 25P / per serving

Prep: 20 min | **Cook:** 50 min

- 4 oz. grilled chicken breast (6 oz. raw)
- 4 hard-boiled eggs, sliced
- 4 cups cubed and roasted butternut squash
- 4 slices turkey bacon
- 8 cups chopped spinach
- 4 Tbs. chopped pecans
- Dash sea salt
- Dash black pepper

Honey Mustard Dressing:
- ½ cup low-fat mayo
- 2 Tbs. lemon juice
- 2 Tbs. raw honey
- 2 Tbs. Dijon mustard
- 1 tsp. dry mustard

1. Cook or grill the chicken over medium heat until all sides are golden and the chicken is cooked through, about 5-7 minutes per side or until internal temperature reaches 160 degrees. Place eggs in a pot with water. Bring to a boil for 2 minutes, then remove from heat; keep covered and allow to keep cooking in the pot for 10 minutes. Drain and place eggs in a bowl of ice. Cook the bacon until crispy.

2. Place butternut squash in a single layer on a large baking sheet lined with parchment paper. Spray the tops with cooking spray and sprinkle with sea salt. Roast for 50-60 minutes, flipping halfway.

3. For one serving, layer two cups of chopped spinach, one sliced hard-boiled egg, 1 oz. grilled chicken breast, one slice cooked and chopped bacon, one cup of roasted butternut squash and one tablespoon chopped pecans.

4. Blend all the dressing ingredients together in a blender until smooth. Weigh the dressing and divide by four to get the amount needed to fill one serving. Drizzle one portion over each salad. Top with sea salt and black pepper.

PRO TIPS: Bulk prep the chicken, eggs, butternut squash and dressing in advance and store in the fridge. When it comes time to eat, this meal will come together in a snap!

Use pre-cubed butternut squash, pre-cooked rotisserie chicken and pre-cooked hard boiled eggs to cut down on your cook time.

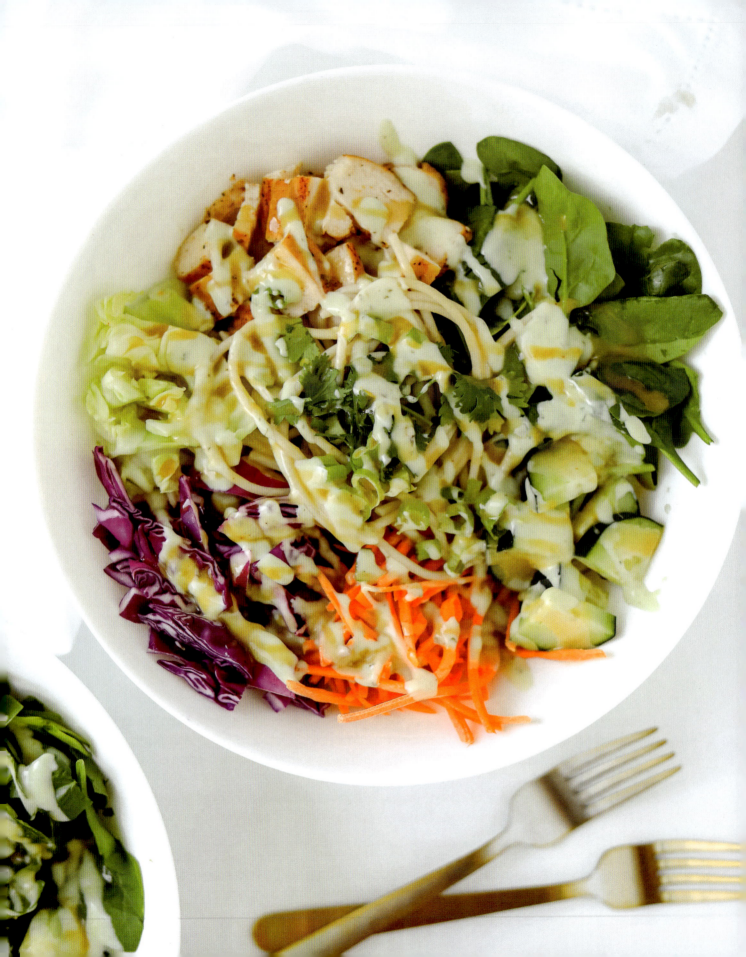

THAI CRUNCH SALAD

Makes 4 servings
340 calories / 13F / 30C / 25P / per serving

Prep: 15 min | **Cook:** 15 min

8 oz. cooked chicken breast
  (10.6 oz. raw)
4 oz. cooked brown rice spaghetti
  (.8 oz. uncooked)
2 cups chopped green cabbage
2 cups chopped red cabbage
2 cups matchstick carrots
1 cup chopped cucumbers
4 cups chopped spinach
1 bunch green onions, sliced
½ cup chopped cilantro
½ cup Bolthouse Farms Classic Ranch
  or Cilantro Avocado Dressing

Thai Peanut Dressing:
2 Tbs. CSE Sweet Classic Peanut Butter
  or natural peanut butter
2 Tbs. raw honey
1 Tbs. olive oil
2 tsp. water
2 tsp. rice vinegar
2 tsp. coconut aminos
Dash sea salt
Dash cayenne pepper

1. Cook or grill the chicken over medium heat until all sides are golden and the chicken is cooked through, about 5-7 minutes per side or until internal temperature reaches 160 degrees. Cook the spaghetti according to the directions on the package.

2. Place all of the Thai Peanut Dressing ingredients into a blender; blend until smooth. Weigh the dressing and divide the weight by four to get the amount needed to fill one serving.

3. For one serving, layer one cup of chopped spinach, ½ cup chopped green cabbage, ½ cup chopped red cabbage, ½ cup matchstick carrots, ¼ cup cucumbers, 2 oz. grilled chicken breast, two tablespoons of cooked spaghetti noodles, two tablespoons of sliced green onions and two tablespoons of chopped cilantro. Drizzle one serving of the dressing over the top. Enjoy!

PRO TIP: Prep your salad in advance and store in a 32 oz. wide-mouth mason jar. Prepare each salad individually. Layer in this order: green cabbage, red cabbage, matchstick carrots, cucumbers, chicken, spaghetti, spinach, green onions and cilantro. Seal lid and store in the fridge. When ready to eat, dump salad out onto a plate. Top with one serving each of the Thai Peanut Dressing and Bolthouse Dressing.

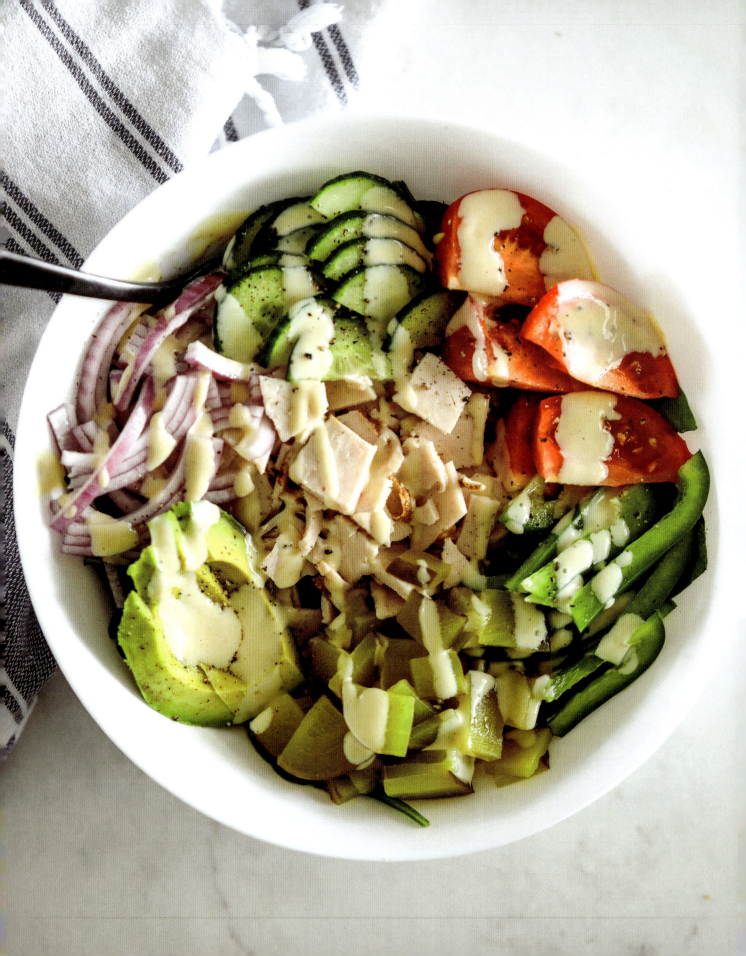

TURKEY SUB SALAD

Makes 4 servings
350 calories / 13F / 33C / 26P / per serving

Prep: 20 min

Honey Mustard Dressing:
½ cup olive oil mayo
2 Tbs. lemon juice
2 Tbs. raw honey
2 Tbs. Dijon or yellow mustard
1 tsp. dry mustard
Salad:
8 cups spinach
16 oz. chopped nitrate-free deli turkey
4 Roma tomatoes
½ of a small red onion, thinly sliced
24 slices cucumber
24 slices pickles
1 green bell pepper, thinly sliced
80g chopped avocado
Side:
400g fresh strawberries

1. Place all the dressing ingredients in a blender. Blend on high until smooth. Weigh the dressing and divide by four to get the amount needed to fill one serving.

2. For one serving, layer two cups of spinach, 4 oz. chopped turkey, one chopped tomato, ¼ cup red onion, six slices of cucumber, six slices of pickles, ¼ of a green bell pepper, 20g avocado and one serving of the dressing. Enjoy 100g strawberries on the side.

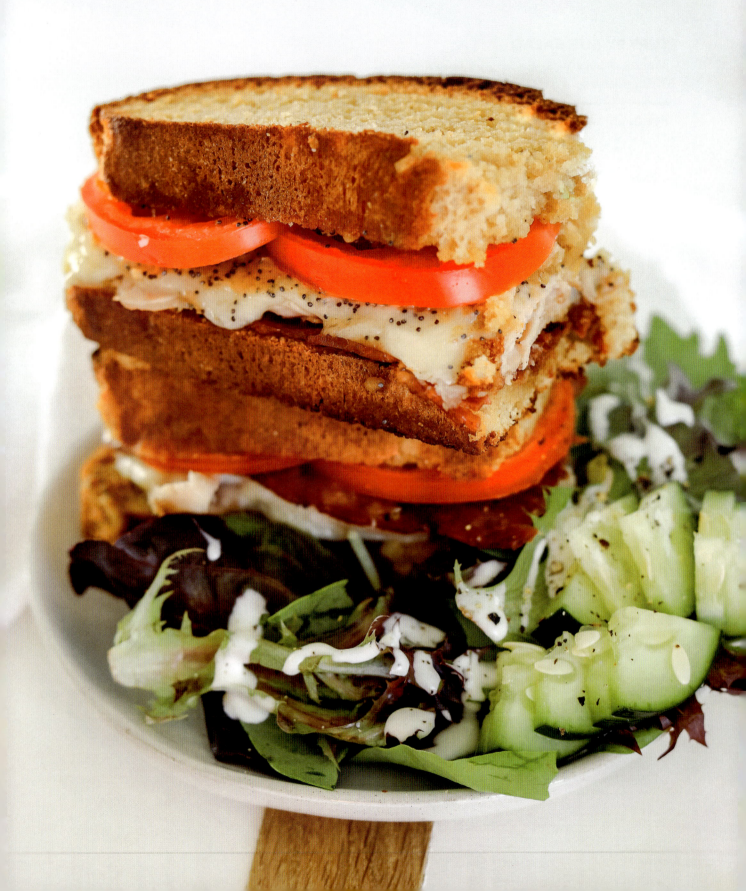

HOT TURKEY & SWISS

Makes 4 servings
360 calories / 14F / 34C / 25P / per serving

Prep: 20 min | **Cook:** 25 min

- 10 oz. CSE Homemade Honey-Wheat Bread (recipe on the next page)
- 4 slices nitrate-free turkey bacon
- 1 ½ Tbs. melted grass-fed butter
- 2 tsp. dried onion
- 2 tsp. Dijon mustard
- 2 tsp. Worcestershire sauce
- 6 oz. nitrate-free deli turkey
- 56g Swiss cheese
- ½ tsp. poppy seeds
- 4 tomato slices

Side salad per serving:
- 1 cup spring salad mix
- ¼ cup matchstick carrots
- ¼ cup sliced cucumbers
- 1 Tbs. Bolthouse Farms Dressing, any variety

1. Make the Homemade Honey-Wheat Bread.

2. Preheat the oven to 400 degrees.

3. Preheat a frying pan to medium heat. Add the turkey bacon to the pan and cook until crispy.

4. In a small bowl, combine the melted butter, dried onion, Dijon mustard and Worcestershire sauce. Whisk until smooth.

5. Make sandwiches by layering a 2.5 oz. slice of the wheat bread, ½ of the sauce, 3 oz. deli turkey, 28g Swiss cheese, ¼ tsp. poppy seeds, two slices of turkey bacon and top with another 2.5 oz. slice wheat bread. Cut the sandwich in half and spray tops with nonstick cooking spray. Repeat for a second sandwich.

6. Grease an 8x8 baking dish. Place the sandwiches in the baking dish. Cover with foil and bake for 20 minutes. Remove foil and bake for an additional 5 minutes or until the bread is golden brown and crispy on the top. Add two tomato slices and a dash of sea salt and pepper to each sandwich. Serve ½ of a sandwich warm with a salad on the side.

PRO TIP: For a quicker method, cook the sandwiches in a panini press.

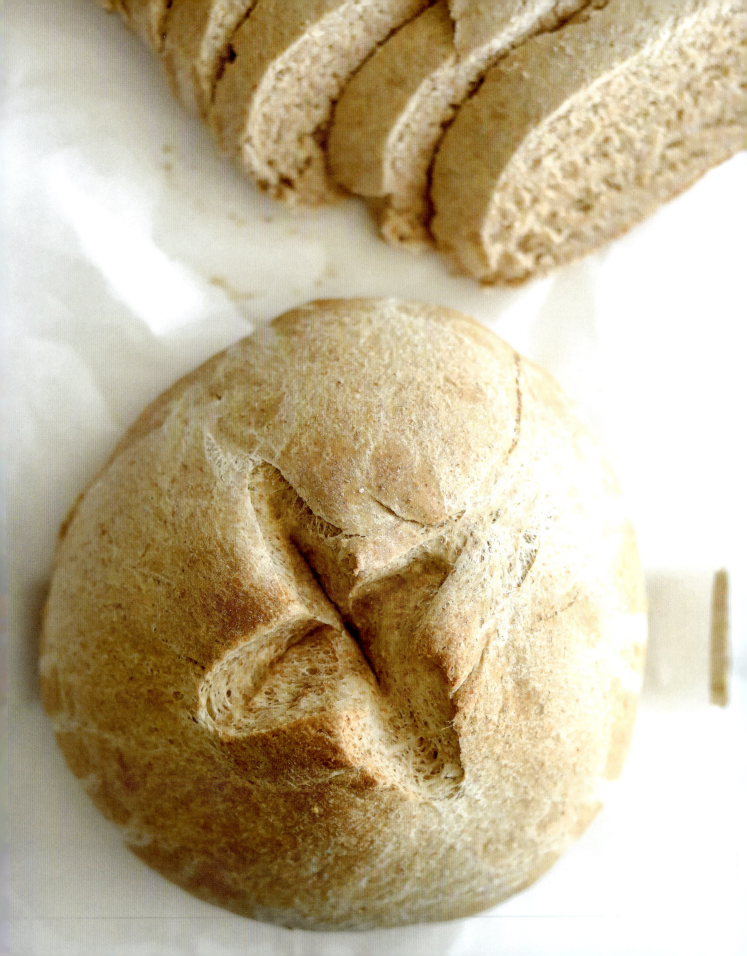

HOMEMADE HONEY-WHEAT BREAD

Makes 24 servings
105 calories 1.5F / 22C / 4P / per serving

Prep: 40 min | **Cook:** 25 min

4 cups (715g) white whole wheat flour
1 ½ Tbs. quick rise yeast
1 ½ Tbs. sea salt
2 cups warm water (100-115 degrees)
4 Tbs. raw honey
1 ½ Tbs. olive oil

1. Stir dry ingredients together in a bowl. Add the wet ingredients and mix for one minute. Dough should be slightly sticky. If dry, add more water. If too sticky to handle, add more flour.

2. Knead for 5 minutes using a bread mixer, Kitchen Aid Mixer, or your hands.

3. Form dough into two balls. Place on a baking sheet lined with parchment paper. Cover with a dish towel and let rise for 25 minutes. Preheat oven to 350 degrees.

4. Score the top of each loaf with a sharp knife. Bake for 22-25 minutes or until golden brown. Remove from the oven and cool on a wire rack.

5. Weigh the bread and divide the weight by 24 to get the amount needed for one serving.

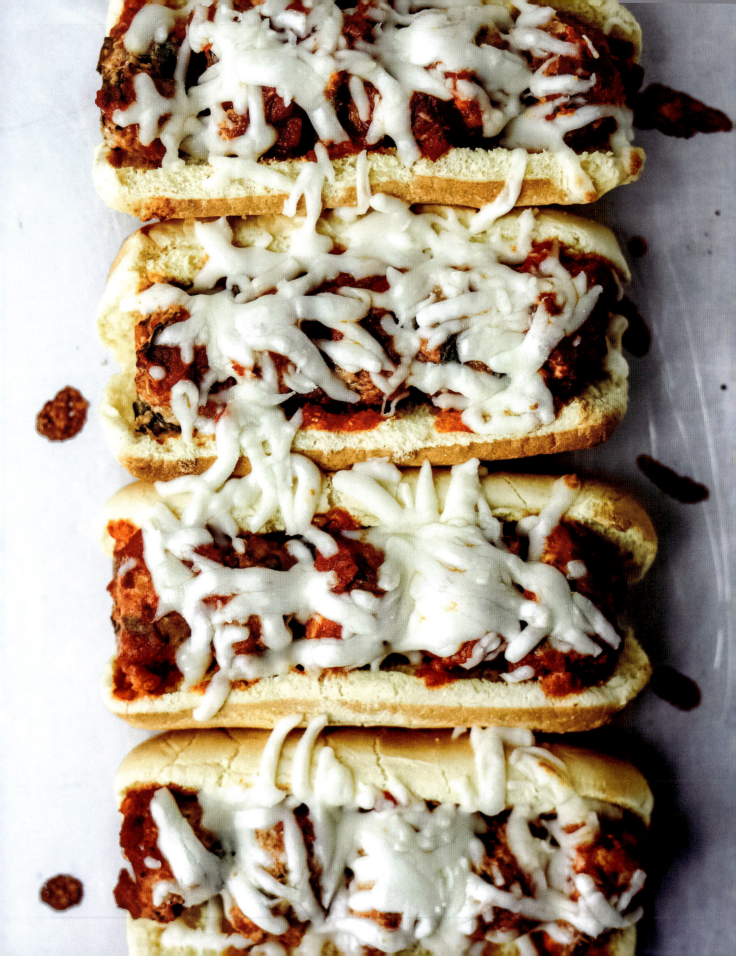

MEATBALL SUBS

Makes 4 servings
350 calories / 11.5F / 33C / 28.5P / per serving

Prep: 30 min | **Cook:** 30 min

- 1 slice Ezekiel bread
- 10 oz. raw lean ground turkey
- 1 large egg
- 1 cup finely chopped spinach
- ½ cup finely chopped red bell peppers
- 1 Tbs. dried minced onion
- 1 Tbs. tomato paste
- 1 tsp. fresh, minced garlic
- 1 tsp. all-purpose seasoning
- ¼ tsp. sea salt
- Dash black pepper
- 1 cup marinara sauce
- ½ cup low-fat, shredded mozzarella cheese
- 4 whole wheat or potato hot dog buns

1. Preheat the oven to 400 degrees.

2. Toast the bread in a toaster until browned and crispy. Break up into pieces and place in a blender. Pulse into crumbs; set aside.

3. Add the ground turkey, egg, homemade bread crumbs, spinach, bell peppers, onion, tomato paste, garlic and seasonings to a bowl. Mix with hands until well combined. Using a cookie scoop, scoop into 20, 1-inch meatballs and place in a greased 9x13 baking dish. Cover with marinara sauce and bake for 15-20 minutes or until cooked through.

4. Place the hotdog buns on a baking sheet lined with parchment paper. Open the buns and spray the inside lightly with cooking spray. Place in the oven at 350 degrees for 5 minutes to toast the inside.

5. Distribute the meatballs evenly between the four hot dog buns. Top each sub sandwich with two tablespoons of mozzarella cheese and return to the oven for 3-5 minutes, or until the cheese is melted and the subs are heated through.

PRO TIPS: Only make the subs that you are going to eat immediately. The buns will get soggy if the meatballs are left on them too long.

Make and freeze the meatballs. Let thaw overnight and then bake to reheat by following the recipe.

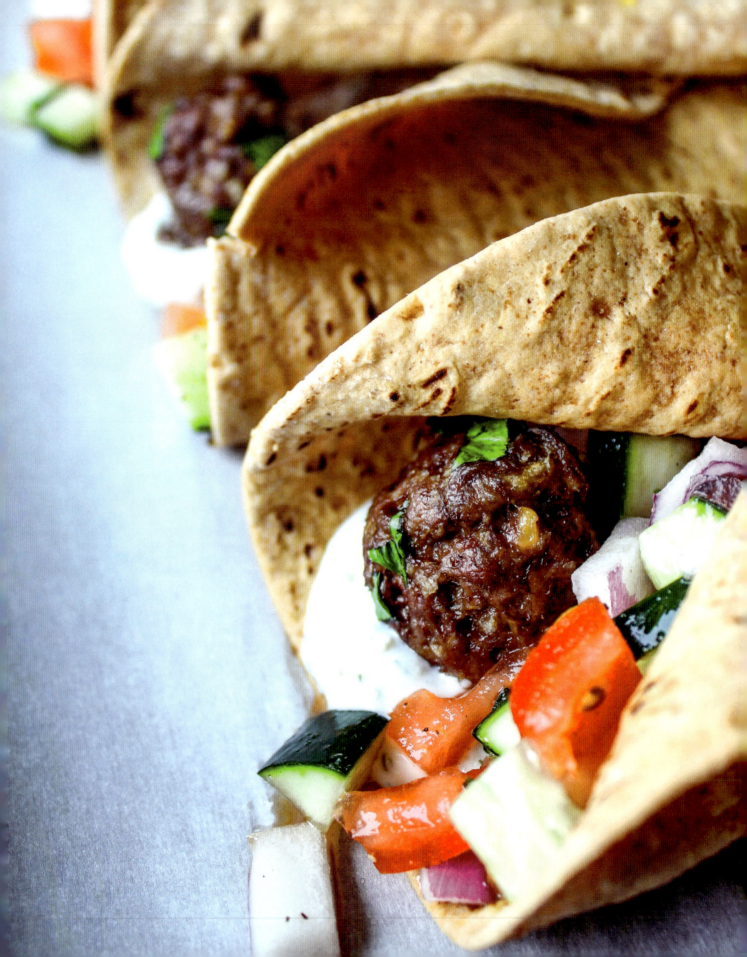

MEDITERRANEAN MEATBALL GYRO

Makes 4 servings
345 calories / 11F / 35C / 26P / per serving

Prep: 35 min | **Cook:** 12 min

Tzatziki Sauce:
- ¼ cup plain Greek yogurt
- ¼ tsp. minced garlic
- ¼ tsp. olive oil
- ½ tsp. fresh dill
- Dash sea salt
- Dash black pepper
- 1 tsp. fresh lemon juice

Meatballs:
- 8 oz. lean ground beef
- 2 Tbs. breadcrumbs
- 2 egg whites
- 2 tsp. flat-leaf Italian parsley, chopped
- 1 tsp. minced garlic
- ¼ tsp. cumin
- ¼ tsp. sea salt
- Dash black pepper

Side Per Serving:
- 100g pineapple

Tomato & Cucumber Salad:
- ½ cup tomatoes, diced
- ½ cup cucumber, diced
- ¼ cup red onion, diced
- 1 tsp. parsley, chopped
- Dash sea salt
- Dash black pepper
- 4 Flatout flatbread wraps

1. Combine all sauce ingredients together in a bowl and store in the fridge until ready to use. Weigh the sauce and divide by four to get the amount needed to fill one serving.

2. Preheat the oven to 425 degrees.

3. Combine all the meatball ingredients together in a large bowl. Mix well and form into meatballs about one to two tablespoons in size. Place on a baking sheet lined with parchment paper. Bake for 10-12 minutes or until they are fully cooked through.

4. Dice up all the veggies for the Tomato & Cucumber Salad and combine in a bowl.

5. Distribute the meatballs, Tzatziki sauce and salad evenly between the flatbread wraps. Roll up and enjoy! Serve pineapple on the side.

PRO TIP: Bake and freeze meatballs. To reheat, bake at 350 degrees for 20-25 minutes. Make and freeze Tzatziki Sauce into individual servings. Make the Tomato & Cucumber Salad fresh.

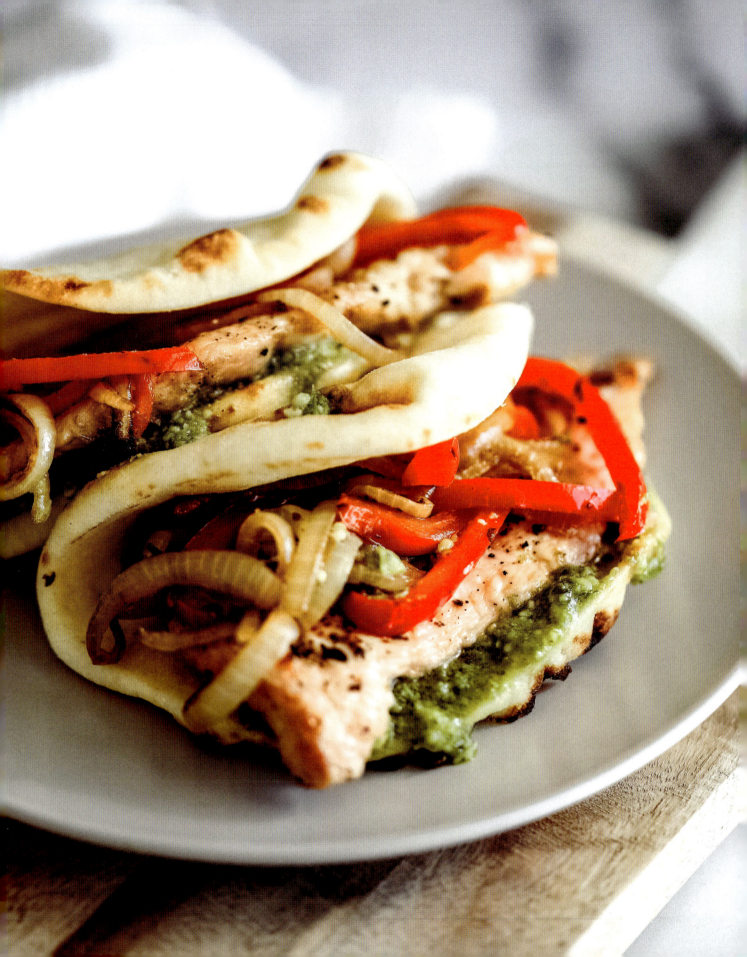

PESTO CHICKEN PANINI
Makes 4 servings
345 calories / 11F / 33C / 28P / per serving

Prep: 10 min | **Cook:** 25 min

9 oz. grilled chicken breast (12 oz. raw)
1 yellow onion, thinly sliced into rings
1 red bell pepper, thinly sliced
3 Tbs. pesto sauce
2 wedges Light Laughing Cow Cheese
4 pieces (about 50g each) Mini Stonefire Naan Bread

1. Cook or grill the chicken over medium heat until all sides are golden and the chicken is cooked through, about 5-7 minutes per side or until internal temperature reaches 160 degrees.

2. Brown the onions and peppers in a greased frying pan until tender and fragrant.

3. Spread 1 ½ tablespoons of pesto sauce on two pieces of the mini naan bread and one cheese wedge on the other two. Add 4.5 oz. chicken, ½ the onions and ½ the peppers to each pesto naan bread. Then sandwich it all together with the cheese naan bread on top.

4. Place in a preheated panini maker or frying pan and cover. Cook and press until lightly browned. Enjoy ½ of a sandwich per serving, hot or cold.

PRO TIP: Use pre-cooked rotisserie chicken to cut down on your cook time.

TEX-MEX

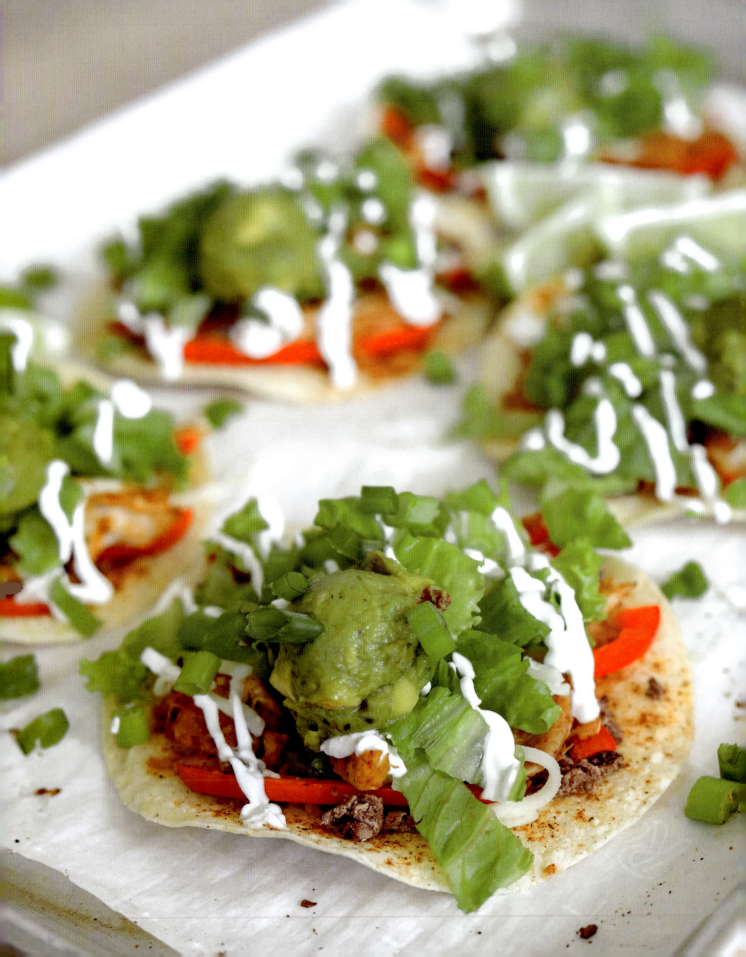

BLACK BEAN TOSTADAS

Makes 4 servings
350 calories / 12F / 34C / 27P / per serving

Prep: 15 min | **Cook:** 30 min

8 corn tortillas
⅔ cup black or refried beans
4 tsp. taco seasoning
1 red bell pepper
8 oz. grilled chicken breast
 (10.6 oz. raw)
2 green onions, chopped
8 Tbs. low-fat, shredded mozzarella cheese

Toppings:
Shredded lettuce
8 oz. guacamole
4 Tbs. nonfat, plain Greek yogurt
4 Tbs. salsa
1 lime, juice of

1. Cook or grill the chicken over medium heat until all sides are golden and the chicken is cooked through, about 5-7 minutes per side or until internal temperature reaches 160 degrees.

2. Preheat the oven to 375 degrees.

3. Line a baking sheet with foil. Spray foil with cooking spray. Lay tortillas in a single layer on foil and spray tops with cooking spray. Sprinkle tops of tortillas with taco seasoning. Bake for 8 minutes.

4. Drain and rinse the beans. Place on a plate and microwave for 30-45 seconds. Mash with a fork, then spread a rounded tablespoon onto each warm tortilla. Slice the bell peppers, grilled chicken and green onions. Layer the bell peppers evenly on tortillas and top each one with 1 oz. grilled chicken, one tablespoon of shredded cheese and green onions.

5. Return to the oven for another 8 minutes. Enjoy two tostadas per serving. Serve warm with shredded lettuce, 2 oz. guacamole, one tablespoon of plain Greek yogurt, one tablespoon of salsa and a squirt of lime juice.

PRO TIP: Use pre-cooked rotisserie chicken to cut down on your cook time.

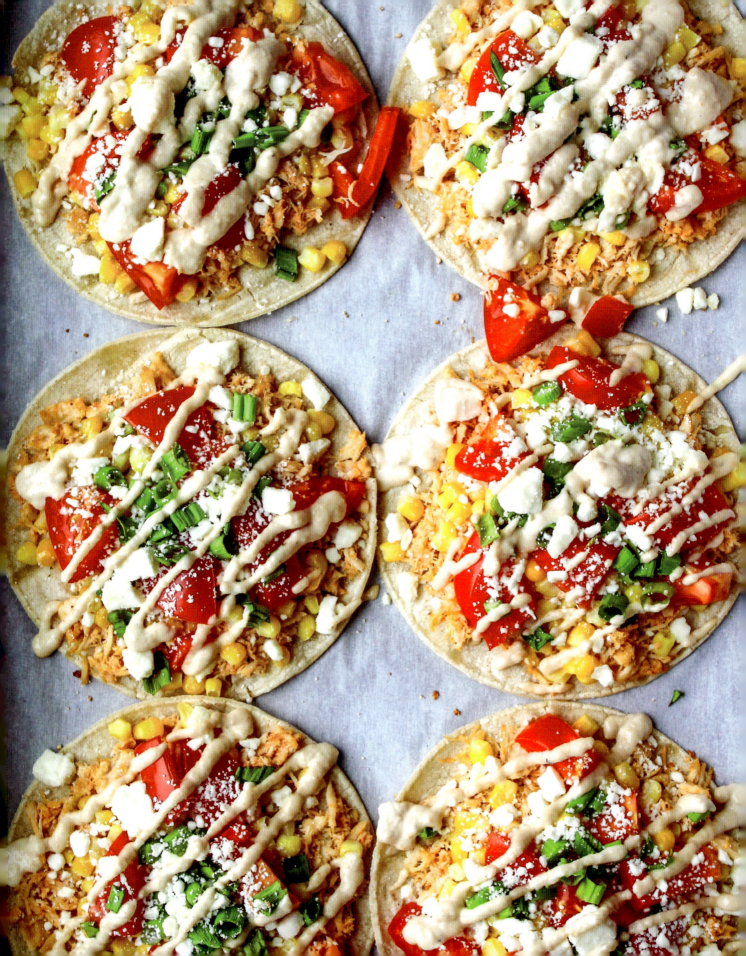

BUFFALO CHICKEN TOSTADAS

Makes 4 servings
350 calories / 12F / 34C / 27P / per serving

Prep: 10 min | **Cook:** 25 min

8 oz. cooked chicken breast (10.6 oz. raw)
4 Tbs. Cashew Sour Cream (recipe on the next page)
8 corn tortillas
2 Tbs. Frank's hot sauce
200g frozen sweet corn
200g diced tomatoes
4 Tbs. bleu cheese or feta cheese crumbles
½ cup sliced green onions

1. Cook or grill the chicken over medium heat until all sides are golden and the chicken is cooked through, about 5-7 minutes per side or until internal temperature reaches 160 degrees. Prepare the Cashew Sour Cream.

2. Preheat the oven to 350 degrees. Place tortillas on a baking sheet lined with parchment paper.

3. In a small bowl, toss the shredded chicken with hot sauce. Top each tortilla with 1 oz. buffalo chicken, 25g corn, 25g tomatoes, ½ tablespoon of cheese and one tablespoon of green onions. Bake for 10 minutes or until all the ingredients are heated through.

4. Top each tostada with ½ tablespoon of Cashew Sour Cream. Enjoy two tostadas per serving.

PRO TIP: Use pre-cooked rotisserie chicken to cut down on your cook time.

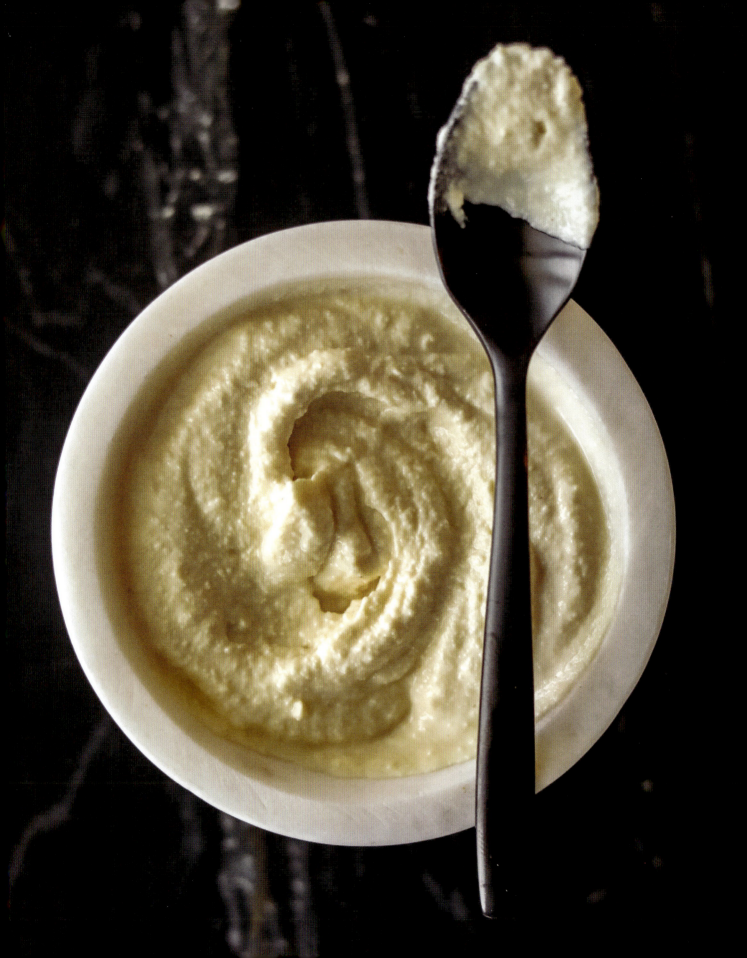

CASHEW SOUR CREAM

Makes 8 servings
50 calories / 4F / 2C / 1P / per serving

Prep: 30 min

½ cup unsalted cashews
1 Tbs. lemon juice
½ Tbs. olive oil
¼ tsp. sea salt
¼-½ cup water

1. Soak the cashews in water for 30+ minutes.

2. Drain the cashews and add to a high-powered blender. Add the lemon juice, olive oil, sea salt and ¼ cup water.

3. Blend on high. Add an additional ¼ cup water if the mixture is too thick. It should be a pourable consistency, but not too runny. Pour into a sealed container and store in the fridge. Use within 5-7 days.

PRO TIP: Freeze single servings of extra Cashew Sour Cream in an ice cube tray and pop out when you are ready to add it to a recipe.

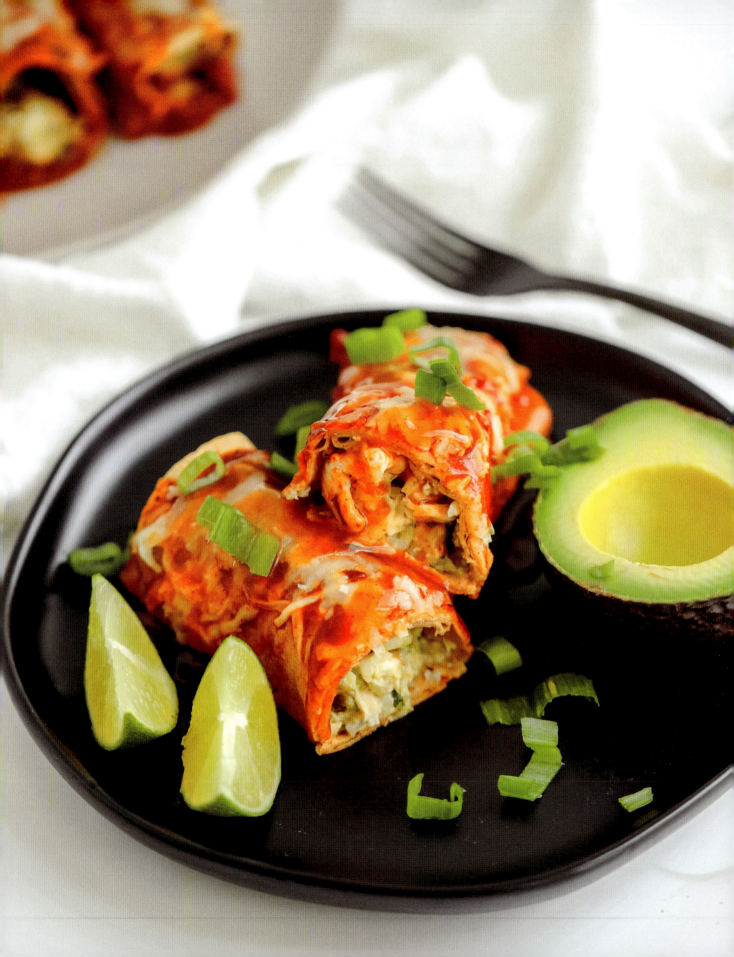

CHICKEN & RICE ENCHILADAS

Makes 4 servings
355 calories / 12F / 32C / 30P / per serving

Prep: 30 min | **Cook:** 45 min

8 oz. raw chicken breast (6 oz. cooked)
¼ cup uncooked white jasmine rice
  (¾ cup cooked)
100g grated zucchini squash
1 tsp. cumin
½ tsp. oregano
½ tsp. onion powder
Dash sea salt
½ lime, juice of

4 Light Laughing Cow cheese wedges
4 oz. canned, diced green chiles
4 Flatout flatbread wraps
1 cup enchilada sauce
½ cup low-fat, shredded mozzarella cheese

Toppings:
120g fresh avocado, chopped
4 Tbs. green onions, sliced

1. Cook or grill the chicken over medium heat until all sides are golden and the chicken is cooked through, about 5-7 minutes per side or until internal temperature reaches 160 degrees. Cook the rice according to the directions on the package.

2. Preheat the oven to 350 degrees.

3. In a medium-sized bowl, combine the shredded chicken, grated zucchini, cumin, oregano, onion powder, sea salt and lime juice. Add Laughing Cow cheese, green chiles and rice. Stir until well combined. Weigh the mixture and divide the weight by four to get the amount needed to fill one serving.

4. Place one serving of the chicken mixture in the middle of each wrap and roll up. Place seam side down in an 8x8 greased baking dish. Pour the enchilada sauce evenly on top of the enchiladas. Top with shredded cheese.

5. Bake for 25-30 minutes or until the cheese starts to bubble. Top each serving with 30g fresh avocado and green onion.

PRO TIPS: Make and freeze uncooked, without toppings. Thaw in the fridge overnight. Bake at 350 degrees for 25-30 minutes. Add the toppings fresh.

Use pre-cooked rotisserie chicken to cut down on your cook time.

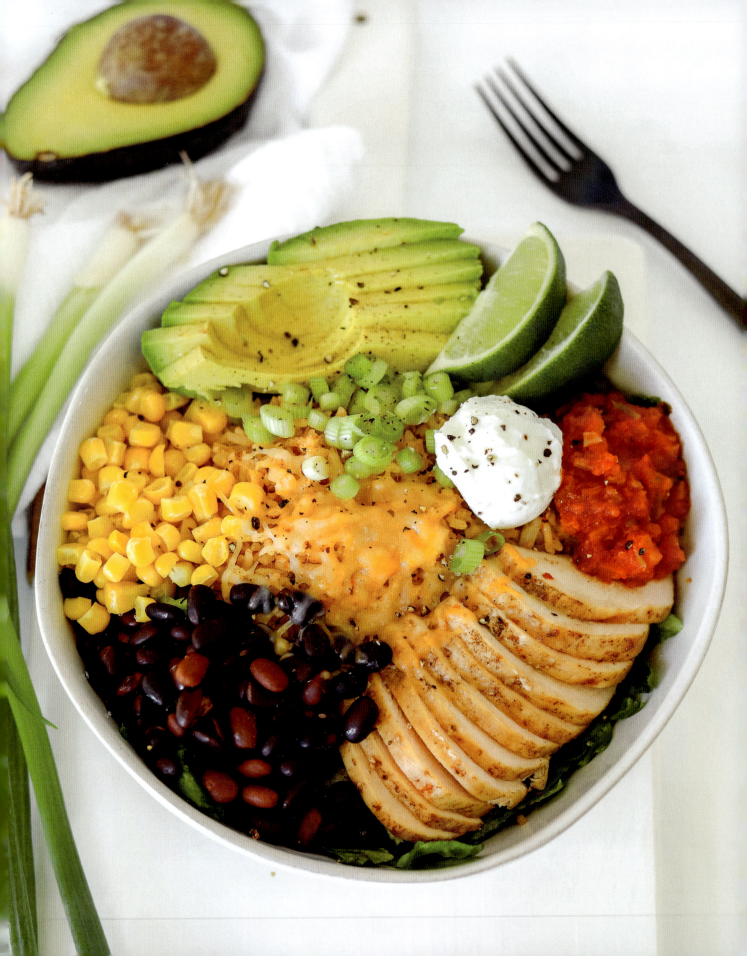

CHICKEN BURRITO BOWL

Makes 4 servings
340 calories / 11F / 33.5C / 27P / per serving

Prep: 20 min | **Cook:** 25 min

8 oz. grilled chicken breast (10.6 oz. raw)
1 cup cooked white jasmine rice (⅓ cups uncooked)
2 cups frozen cauliflower rice
1 tsp. chili-lime seasoning
½ tsp. sea salt
½ tsp. cumin
½ tsp. paprika
Dash garlic powder
2 cups romaine lettuce

1 cup black beans
½ cup frozen corn, thawed
½ cup shredded Mexican blend cheese
160g fresh avocado
4 Tbs. nonfat, plain Greek yogurt
8 Tbs. salsa
Green onions, chopped
1 lime, juice of

1. Cook or grill the chicken over medium heat until all sides are golden and the chicken is cooked through, about 5-7 minutes per side or until internal temperature reaches 160 degrees. Let cool slightly, then slice. Cook the rice according to the directions on the package.

2. Add the cauliflower rice to a greased frying pan. Sauté until tender and warm. Add the jasmine rice, chili-lime seasoning, sea salt, cumin, paprika and garlic powder. Stir until well combined and heated through. Weigh the mixture and divide by four to get the amount needed to fill one serving.

3. Place ½ cup chopped romaine lettuce in the bottom of a bowl and then layer one serving of the rice mixture, 2 oz. grilled chicken, ¼ cup black beans, two tablespoons of corn, two tablespoons of shredded cheese, 40g avocado, one tablespoon of Greek yogurt, two tablespoons of salsa, green onions and lime juice.

PRO TIP: Use pre-cooked rotisserie chicken to cut down on your cook time.

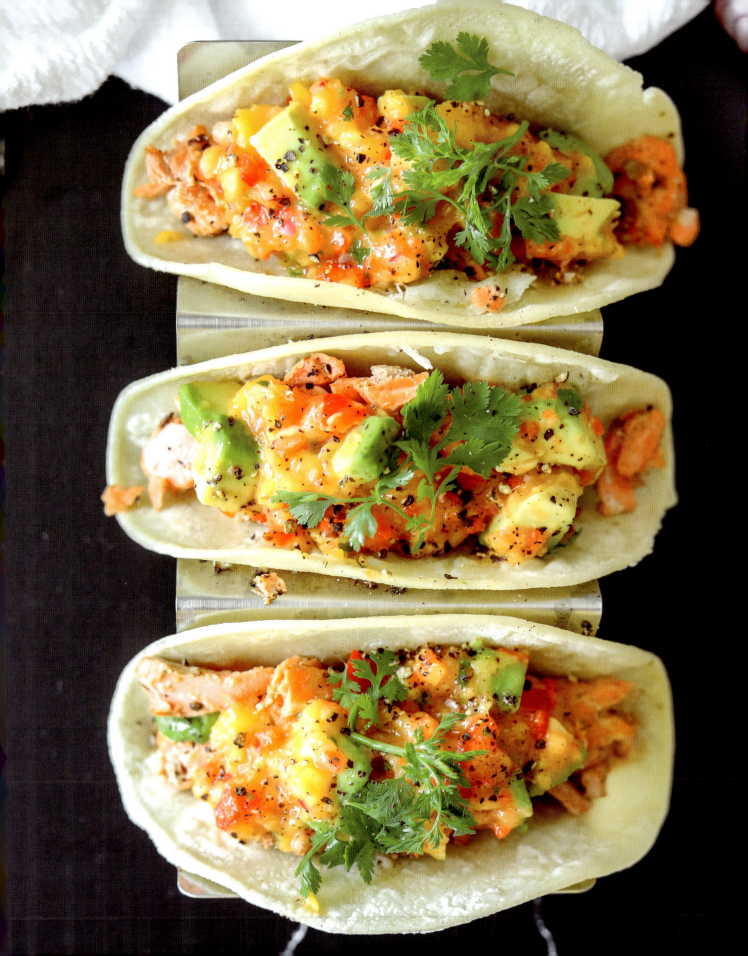

GRILLED LIME SALMON TACOS

Makes 4 servings
350 calories / 12F / 34C / 26P / per serving

Prep: 15 min | **Cook:** 10 min + marination

16 oz. boneless, skinless salmon
Dash sea salt
Dash pepper
8 corn tortillas
Marinade:
1 Tbs. olive oil
1 Tbs. lime juice
1 tsp. minced garlic
1 tsp. lime zest
Dash sea salt
Dash black pepper

Mango Avocado Salsa:
200g mango
100g avocado
½ cup red bell pepper
4 Tbs. red onion
Pinch fresh cilantro
2 Tbs. lime juice
2 tsp. olive oil
Dash sea salt
Dash pepper

1. Add all the marinade ingredients to a large zip top bag. Place the salmon in the bag and let marinate in the fridge for 2+ hours.

2. Heat a grill over medium-high heat. Place a piece of tin foil on the grill and spray with cooking spray. Place the marinated salmon on the foil and cook about 3 minutes per side or until just cooked through.

3. To make the salsa: in a medium bowl, toss together the peeled and chopped mango, avocados, bell peppers, red onions, cilantro, lime juice and olive oil. Season with salt and pepper to taste. Weigh the salsa and divide the weight by four to get the amount needed to fill one serving.

4. Divide the salmon into eight equal portions and add to each tortilla. Enjoy two tacos per serving. Top with one serving of Mango Avocado Salsa.

PRO TIP: Blacken the tortillas by placing them one at a time over the gas stove flame at medium heat. Once the edges begin to blacken, remove the tortilla from the stove with tongs and place on a plate. Repeat with the remaining tortillas.

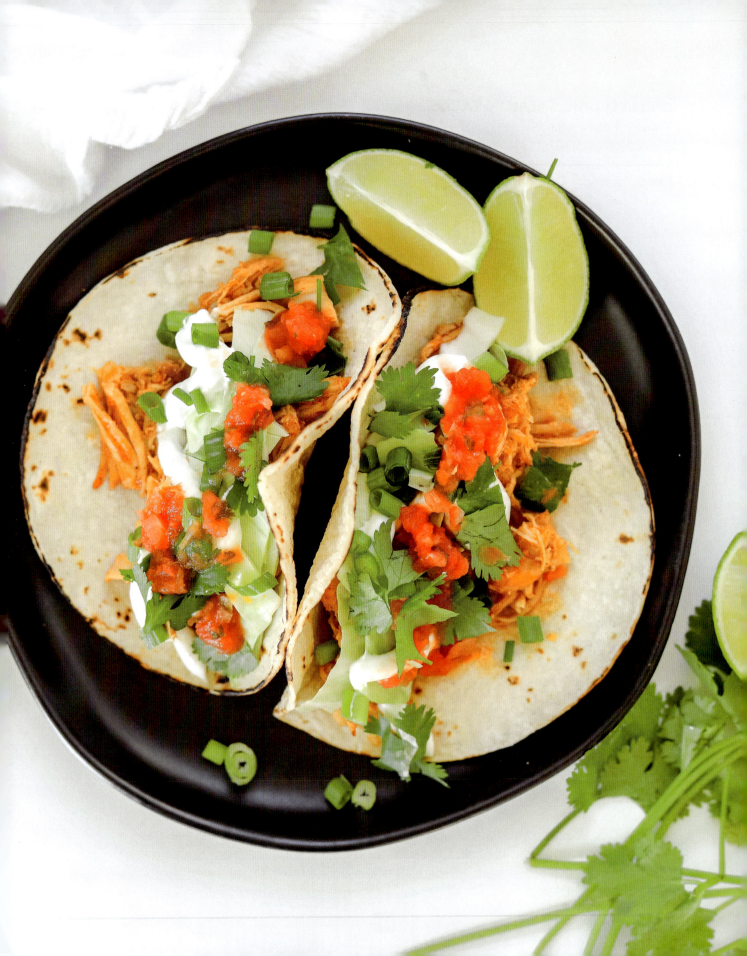

HONEY GARLIC CHICKEN TACOS

Makes 4 servings
340 calories / 10F / 35C / 27P / per serving

Prep: 15 min | **Cook:** 6 hr

2 Tbs. raw honey
1 ½ Tbs. taco seasoning
3 cloves garlic, minced
1 Tbs. melted coconut oil
¼ tsp. sea salt
14 oz. raw chicken breast (10.5 oz. cooked)
8 corn tortillas (6-inch)
1 cup chopped green cabbage
4 Tbs. Cashew Sour Cream (recipe on page 215)
4 Tbs. salsa
1 lime, cut into wedges
Green onions, for garnish
Cilantro, for garnish

1. Spray a crockpot with cooking spray and heat on low.

2. In a large bowl, mix the honey, taco seasoning, garlic, melted coconut oil and sea salt. Add the chicken to the bowl and toss to coat. Add the chicken to the crockpot and pour the remaining mixture over the top. Cook on low heat for 3 hours. Shred the chicken and let cook for another 2-3 hours.

3. Weigh the chicken and divide by four to get the amount needed to fill one serving. Evenly distribute the chicken mixture into the corn tortillas. Top each one with cabbage, ½ tablespoon of cashew sour cream, ¼ tablespoon of salsa, lime juice, green onions and cilantro. Enjoy two tacos per serving.

PRO TIP: Use pre-cooked rotisserie chicken to cut down on your cook time. Shred and mix with the marinade. Skip the crockpot step.

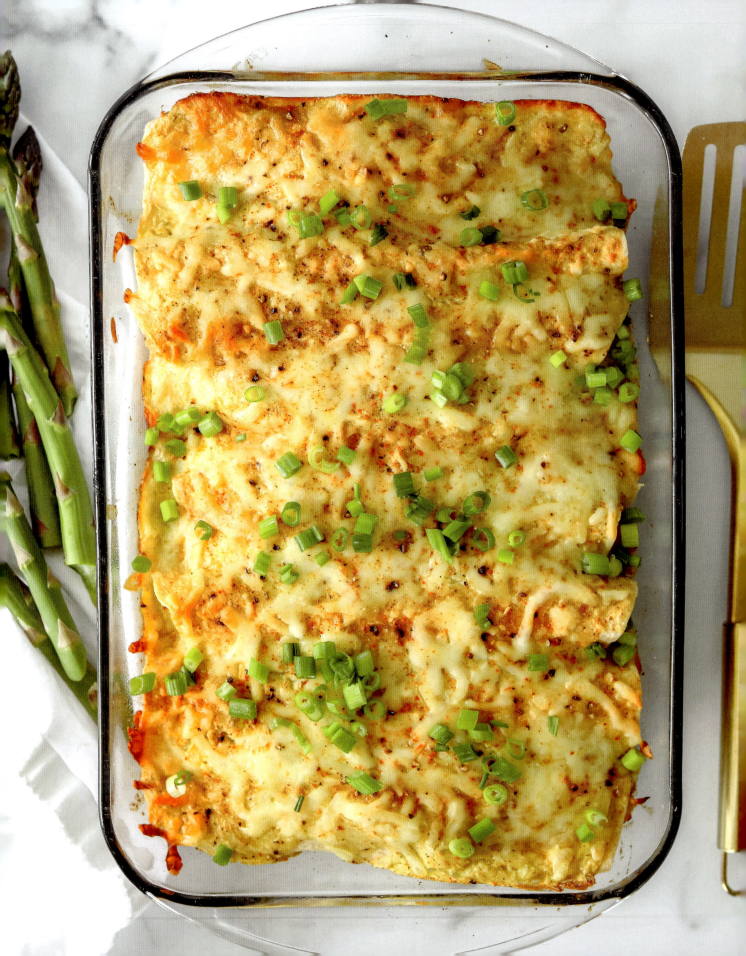

HONEY-LIME CHICKEN ENCHILADAS

Makes 4 servings
340 calories / 8F / 39C / 28P / per serving

Prep: 20 min | **Cook:** 45 min + marination

8 oz. cooked chicken breast
  (10.6 oz. raw)
2 Light Laughing Cow Cheese wedges
¼ cup nonfat, plain Greek yogurt
2 Tbs. raw honey
2 Tbs. lime juice
1 tsp. chili powder
Dash garlic powder
¼ cup fresh minced onion

4 whole grain tortillas
½ cup green enchilada sauce
¼ cup low-fat, shredded mozzarella cheese
4 Tbs. fresh salsa
32 asparagus spears
2 tsp. olive oil
Dash sea salt
Dash black pepper

1. Cook or grill the chicken over medium heat until all sides are golden and the chicken is cooked through, about 5-7 minutes per side or until internal temperature reaches 160 degrees.

2. Beat the Laughing Cow Cheese until smooth. Add the whipped cheese, plain Greek yogurt, honey, lime juice, chili powder and garlic powder to a large zip top bag. Massage ingredients together until well combined. Add cooked, shredded chicken and onion to the bag. Massage all ingredients until well combined. Store in the fridge and let marinate 2+ hours.

3. Preheat the oven to 350 degrees. Weigh the marinated chicken mixture and divide by four to get the amount needed to fill each tortilla. Fill the tortillas with the chicken mixture. Roll up tight and place in a greased 8x8 baking dish.

4. Pour the enchilada sauce over the top of the tortillas and then sprinkle with shredded mozzarella. Bake for 30 minutes. Top with fresh salsa, salt and pepper to taste.

5. Turn the oven heat up to 400. Place asparagus on a baking sheet lined with parchment paper. Drizzle olive oil over the top and sprinkle with salt and pepper. Roast for 8 minutes. Enjoy on the side.

PRO TIPS: Make and freeze without baking, without toppings. Thaw in the fridge overnight. Bake at 350 degrees for 30 minutes. Add the toppings and cook the asparagus fresh.

Use pre-cooked rotisserie chicken to cut down on your cook time.

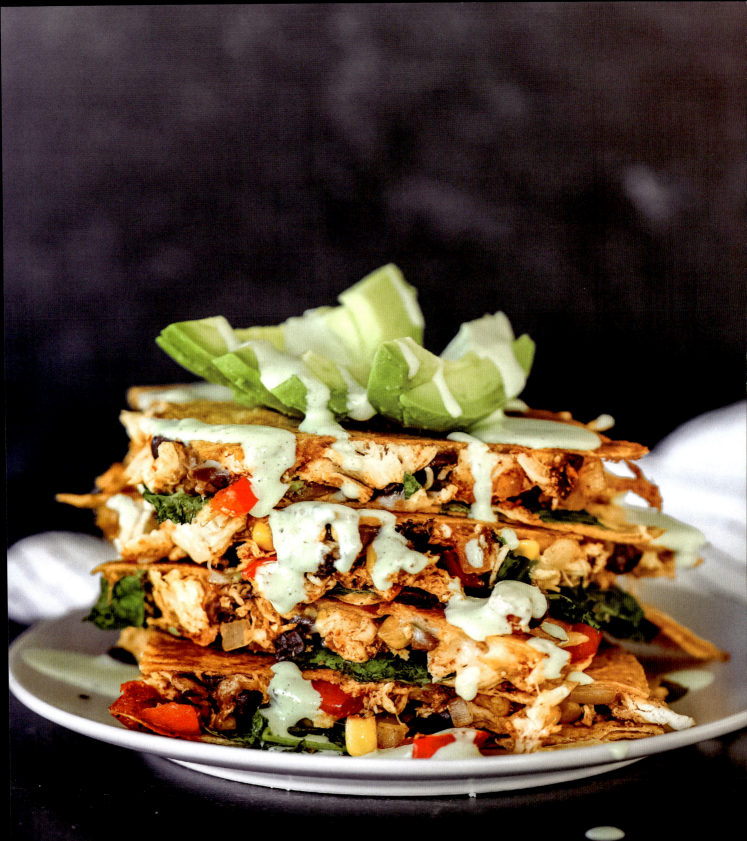

LOADED CHICKEN QUESADILLAS

Makes 4 servings
350 calories / 13F / 33C / 26P / per serving

Prep: 20 min | **Cook:** 35 min

6 oz. cooked chicken breast (8 oz. raw)
½ cup chopped red bell peppers
¼ cup chopped yellow onions
¼ cup chopped jalapeño, optional
¾ cup black beans, rinsed and drained
¼ cup frozen sweet corn
1 cup chopped baby kale
1 Tbs. taco seasoning
2 (70g each) whole grain tortillas
½ cup shredded mozzarella cheese
100g avocado

Cilantro-Lime Crema:
¼ cup nonfat, plain Greek yogurt
2 Tbs. green enchilada sauce
2 Tbs. olive oil mayo
¼ cup chopped cilantro
½ of a lime, juice and zest of

1. Cook or grill the chicken over medium heat until all sides are golden and the chicken is cooked through, about 5-7 minutes per side or until internal temperature reaches 160 degrees. Let cool slightly, then shred.

2. Make the Cilantro-Lime Crema by adding all the ingredients to a blender or food processor. Blend until smooth. Weigh the mixture and divide by four to get the amount needed for one serving. Store in the fridge until ready to use.

3. Add the chopped bell peppers, onions and jalapeño to a greased frying pan over medium heat. Sauté until the veggies are tender. Add the beans, corn, kale, chicken and taco seasoning to the pan. Stir together until well combined. Remove from heat.

4. Spray a large frying pan or skillet with cooking spray and heat over medium heat. Add one of the tortillas to the skillet. Spread the chicken and veggie mixture evenly over the tortilla. Top with cheese and the other tortilla. Once browned on one side, cut the quesadilla into four triangles and then flip each one and cook until brown on the other side. Serve one loaded quesadilla triangle with 25g avocado and one serving of Cilantro-Lime Crema.

PRO TIP: Easily shred the chicken by placing it in a Kitchen Aid Mixer while still warm and beat on medium speed with the paddle attachment.

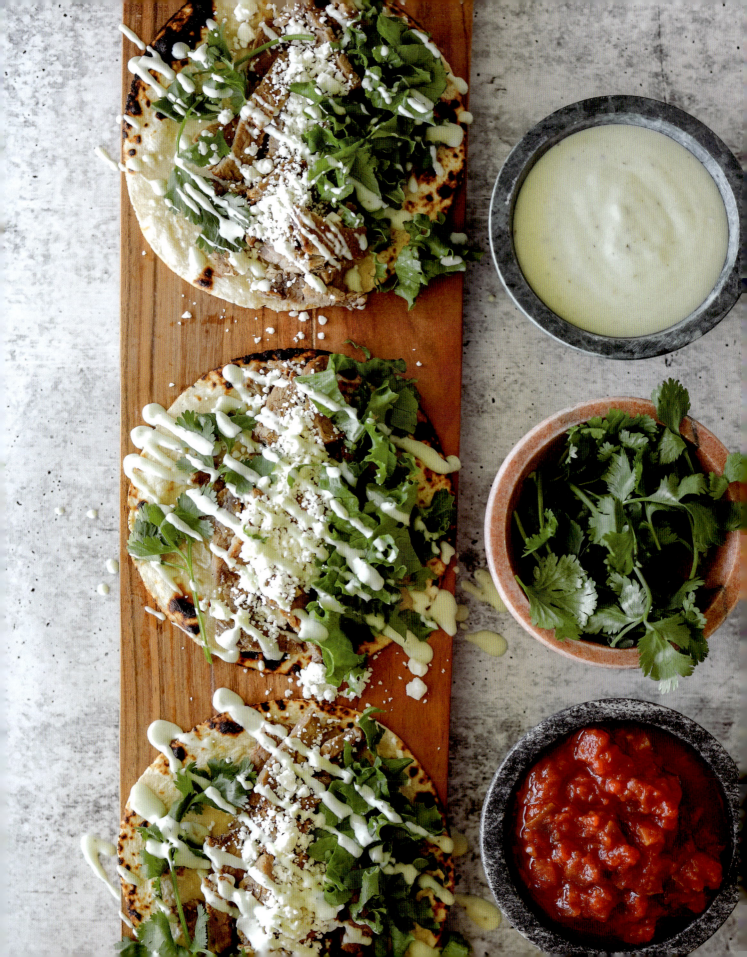

MARINATED STEAK TACOS

Makes 4 servings
350 calories / 14F / 30C / 26P / per serving

Prep: 15 min | **Cook:** 8 min + marination

2 Tbs. lime juice
2 tsp. olive oil
2 tsp. raw honey
1 tsp. minced garlic
Dash cumin
Dash chili powder
Dash sea salt
Dash black pepper
14 oz. raw Sirloin-Tip Steak
8 corn tortillas

Toppings:
Shredded lettuce
½ cup fresh salsa
4 Tbs. Bolthouse Farms Salsa Verde Dressing
4 Tbs. feta cheese crumbles
Cilantro, for garnish
1 lime, juice of

1. Combine the lime juice, olive oil, honey, garlic and seasonings in a large zip top bag. Slice steak into thin strips and add to the bag. Massage until well coated. Let marinate in the fridge 2+ hours.

2. Heat grill to medium heat. Place sliced steak on the grill and cook 3 minutes per side or until you reach your desired doneness.

3. Weigh the steak and divide into eight equal portions. Add one portion to each tortilla. Top each tortilla with shredded lettuce, one tablespoon salsa, ½ tablespoon of Salsa Verde Dressing, ½ tablespoon of feta cheese, cilantro and a squirt of lime juice. Enjoy two tacos per serving.

PRO TIPS: Add marinade and steak to a bag; marinate and freeze. Let thaw in the fridge overnight before grilling. Grill and add toppings fresh.

Use the sous vide, sliced, grass-fed beef sirloin from Costco to shorten your cook time.

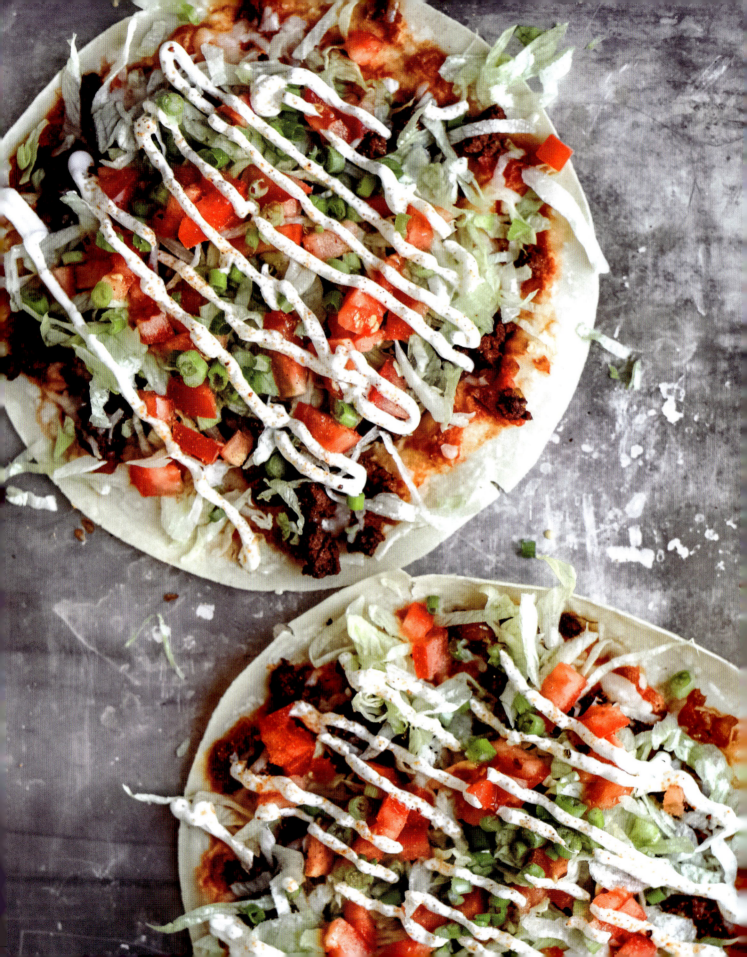

MEXICAN TORTILLA PIZZA

Makes 4 serving
330 calories / 12F / 31C / 24P / per serving

Prep: 10 min | **Cook:** 15 min

- 10 oz. lean ground beef
- 3 Tbs. taco seasoning
- 4 brown rice tortillas
- 8 Tbs. salsa
- 12 Tbs. low-fat, shredded mozzarella cheese
- 4 cups shredded lettuce
- 1 cup fresh vine tomatoes, diced
- 4 Tbs. green onions, chopped
- 4 Tbs. nonfat, plain Greek yogurt

1. Preheat the oven 350 degrees.

2. Brown the ground beef in a pan over medium heat. Once cooked through, add the taco seasoning. Remove from heat.

3. Lay the tortillas out flat on a baking sheet and spread two tablespoons of salsa over the top of each one. Add three tablespoons of cheese and ¼ of the cooked ground beef to each tortilla.

4. Bake for 10 minutes or until the cheese is melted. Top each serving with one cup shredded lettuce, ¼ cup fresh tomatoes, one tablespoon of Greek yogurt and one tablespoon of sliced green onions.

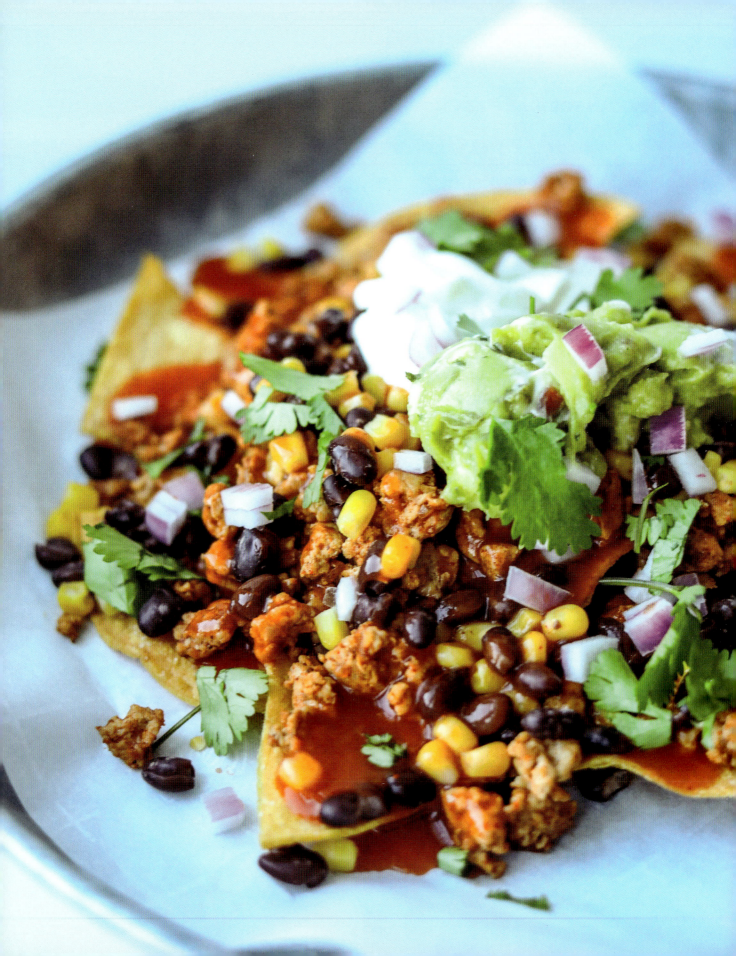

QUEENSTOWN NACHOS

Makes 4 servings
350 calories / 13F / 33C / 26P / per serving

Prep: 15 min | **Cook:** 20 min

8 corn tortillas
15 oz. raw, lean ground turkey
2 Tbs. taco seasoning
½ cup black beans, rinsed and drained
½ cup frozen sweet corn
8 Tbs. red enchilada sauce
4 Tbs. guacamole
4 Tbs. nonfat, plain Greek yogurt
Red onion, chopped for garnish
Lime wedges, for garnish
Cilantro, for garnish

1. Preheat the oven to 350 degrees.

2. Place corn tortillas on a cutting board. Using a pizza cutter, slice each corn tortilla into six triangles and spread out into a single layer on a baking sheet lined with parchment paper. Spray the tops with cooking spray and sprinkle with sea salt. Bake for 20 minutes, flipping halfway.

3. While the chips are baking, place the ground turkey into a pan over medium heat. Cook until browned. Season with taco seasoning. Remove from the pan.

4. Add the black beans and corn to the pan and cook over medium heat until warm. Turn off the heat. Weigh the ground turkey and divide the weight by four to get the amount needed to fill one serving.

5. For one serving, place 12 chips onto a plate. Top with one serving of the ground turkey, ¼ cup of the bean and corn mixture, two tablespoons of enchilada sauce, one tablespoon of guacamole and one tablespoon of Greek yogurt. Garnish with red onion, lime juice and chopped cilantro.

PRO TIP: Great meal for a group! We usually use store bought tortilla chips if we are serving a crowd.

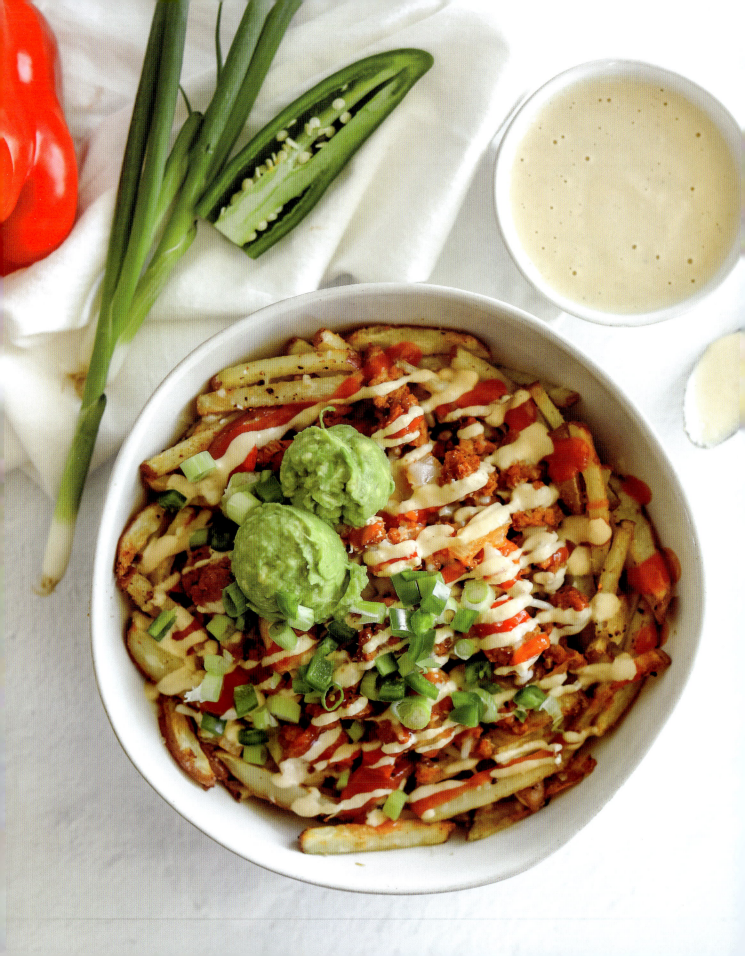

TACO FRIES

Makes 4 servings
350 calories / 12F / 34C / 25.5P / per serving

Prep: 15 min | **Cook:** 40 min

30 oz. baby gold potatoes
Dash sea salt
Dash onion powder
Dash garlic powder
14 oz. raw lean ground turkey
 (10.5 oz. cooked)
2 Tbs. taco seasoning
¼ cup minced onion
¼ cup minced red pepper

Toppings per serving:
1 Tbs. low-fat, shredded mozzarella cheese
1 Tbs. taco sauce
½ Tbs. guacamole
½ Tbs. Cashew Sour Cream (recipe on page 215)
½ of a jalapeño, chopped
Green onions, for garnish

1. Preheat the oven to 425 degrees. Prepare the Cashew Sour Cream.

2. Slice potatoes into fries and lay out in a single layer onto a baking sheet lined with parchment paper. Spray tops with cooking spray and sprinkle with sea salt, onion powder and garlic powder. Bake for 20 minutes, then flip and bake for another 20 minutes.

3. Brown the turkey in a frying pan or skillet over medium heat. Once cooked, add the taco seasoning. Transfer turkey mixture to a bowl. Add the onions and peppers to the pan and cook until tender. Add to the turkey mixture.

4. Weigh the potatoes and turkey/veggie mixture separately and divide by four to get the amount needed to fill one serving. Place one serving of fries onto each plate and top with the turkey mixture, shredded cheese, guacamole, Cashew Sour Cream, taco sauce, jalapeños, and green onions.

PRO TIP: Reheat the potatoes in the air fryer at 400 degrees for 3-4 minutes to make them extra crispy and delicious.

PIZZA & PASTA

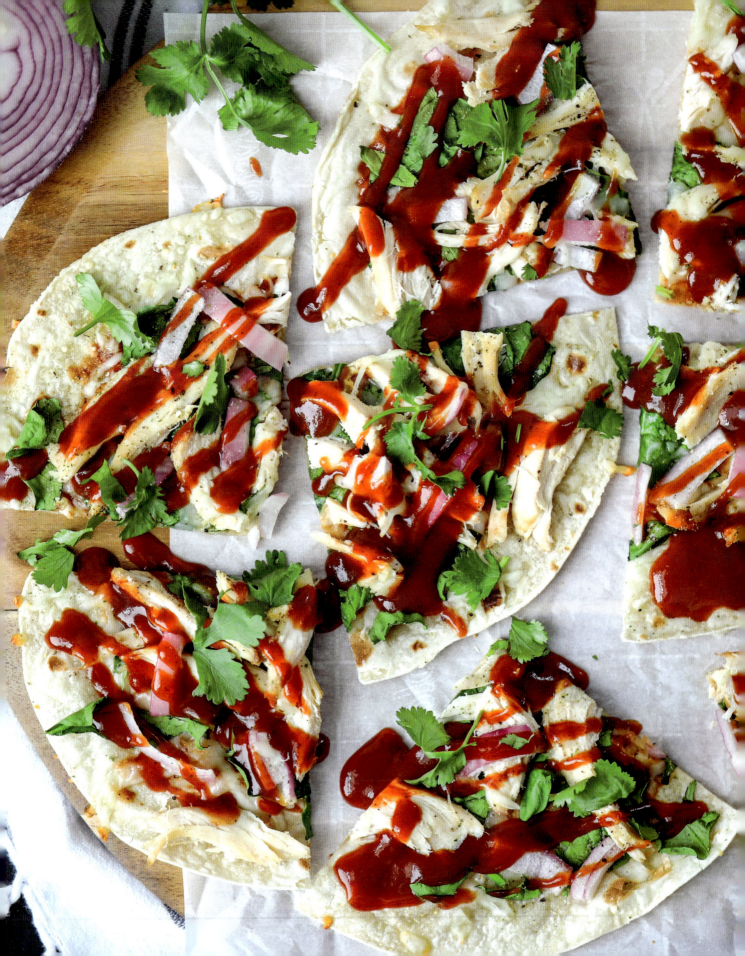

BBQ CHICKEN PIZZA

Makes 2 servings
340 calories / 9F / 37C / 27P / per serving

Prep: 10 min | **Cook:** 25 min

2 whole grain tortillas
4 Tbs. Stubb's Original BBQ Sauce
4 oz. cooked chicken breast (5.2 oz. raw)
½ cup sliced red onions
2 cups chopped spinach
½ cup low-fat, shredded mozzarella cheese
Cilantro, for garnish

1. Heat oven to 375 degrees.

2. Cook or grill the chicken over medium heat until all sides are golden and the chicken is cooked through, about 5-7 minutes per side or until internal temperature reaches 160 degrees. Let cool slightly, then shred.

3. Place tortillas on a baking sheet lined with parchment paper. Spread two tablespoons of BBQ sauce over each tortilla, then layer with ¼ cup shredded cheese, one cup chopped spinach, 2 oz. shredded chicken, ¼ cup onions and cilantro for garnish.

4. Bake for 10 minutes. Enjoy warm!

PRO TIPS: Use pre-cooked rotisserie chicken to cut down on your cook time.

Easily shred the chicken by placing it in a Kitchen Aid Mixer while still warm and beat on medium speed with the paddle attachment.

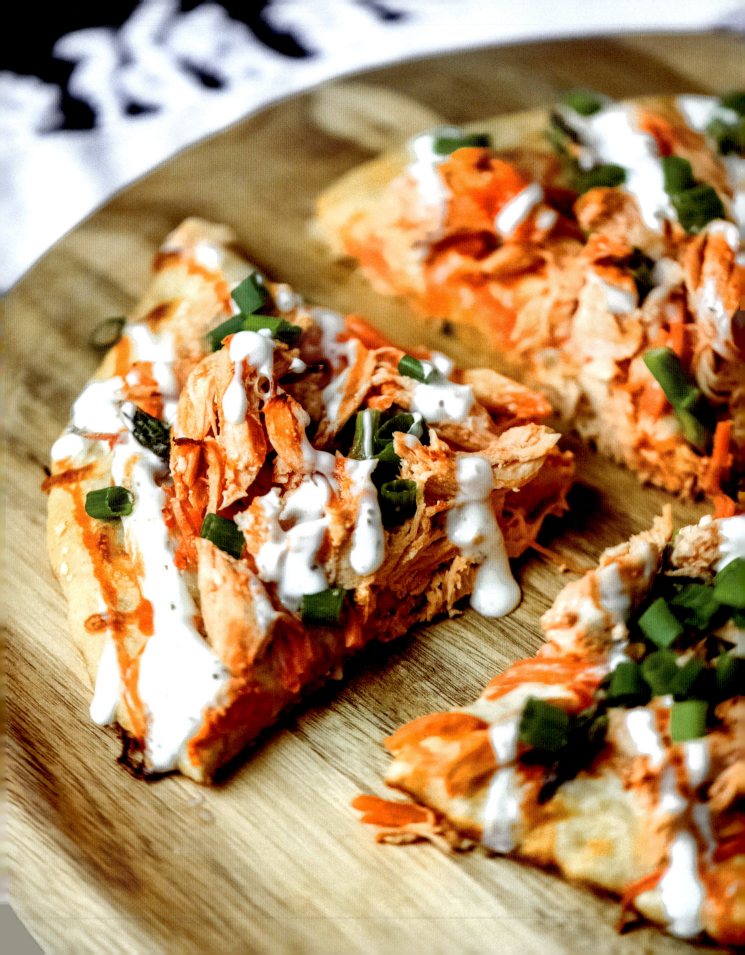

BUFFALO CHICKEN PIZZA

Makes 4 servings
345 calories / 11.5F / 33C / 27P / per serving

Prep: 20 min | **Cook:** 35 min

¼ cup buffalo wing sauce
6 oz. cooked chicken breast (8 oz. raw)
1 cup white whole wheat flour
⅔ cup nonfat, plain Greek yogurt
1 ¼ tsp. baking powder
Dash sea salt
2 Tbs. olive oil
Dash garlic powder
Dash onion powder
½ cup low-fat, shredded mozzarella cheese
2 oz. matchstick carrots
8 chopped asparagus spears
¼ cup Bolthouse Farms Classic Ranch Dressing
Green onions, chopped for garnish

Side per serving:
100g fresh pineapple

1. Heat oven to 450 degrees.

2. Cook or grill the chicken over medium heat until all sides are golden and the chicken is cooked through, about 5-7 minutes per side or until internal temperature reaches 160 degrees. Let cool slightly, then shred. Toss with the hot sauce and set aside.

3. Combine the whole wheat flour, plain Greek yogurt, baking powder and sea salt. Knead until smooth. If the dough is too sticky, add a little more flour until you can handle easily with your hands.

4. Roll out into a circle and place on a baking sheet lined with parchment paper or a pizza stone. Brush the olive oil over the crust and sprinkle with onion powder and garlic powder. Bake for 7 minutes before adding the toppings.

5. Remove from the oven and add the toppings by layering the cheese, carrots, asparagus and buffalo chicken. Return to the oven and bake for another 10 minutes.

6. Drizzle the ranch dressing over the pizza and top with green onions. Add extra hot sauce for an extra kick. Enjoy fresh pineapple on the side.

PRO TIP: Roll the dough out between two sheets of parchment paper for quick clean up.

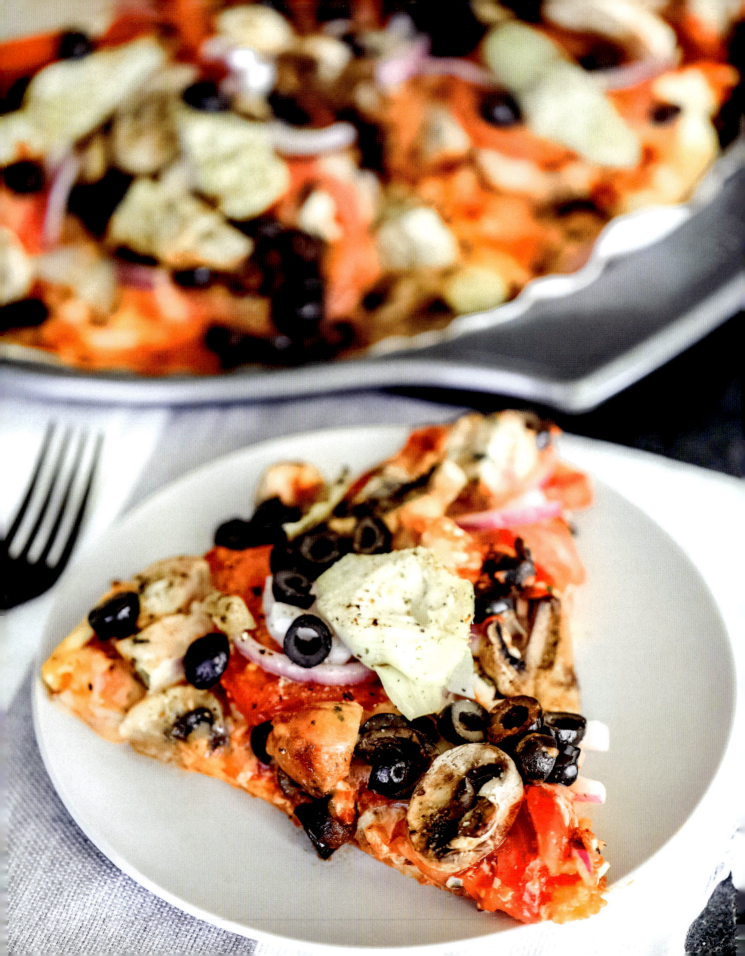

GARDEN VEGGIE PIZZA

Makes 4 servings
335 calories / 12F / 33C / 23P / per serving

Prep: 25 min | **Cook:** 25 min

- ¾ cup white whole wheat flour
- 1 tsp, baking powder
- ¼ tsp. sea salt
- Dash garlic powder
- Dash onion powder
- ½ cup plain, nonfat Greek yogurt
- ¾ cup traditional marinara sauce
- 2 large chicken sausage links (160 cals each), chopped or sliced
- 1 cup low-fat, shredded mozzarella cheese
- 1 tomato, sliced
- ½ cup sliced red onion
- ½ cup sliced mushrooms
- ½ cup canned, chopped, roasted artichoke hearts
- ½ cup sliced olives
- Dash garlic powder
- Dash oregano
- Dash sea salt
- Dash black pepper

1. Preheat the oven to 425 degrees.

2. Whisk the flour, baking powder, sea salt, garlic powder and onion powder together in a bowl. Add the Greek yogurt and use a rubber spatula to fold it in until well combined. If the dough is too dry, add a tiny bit of water; if it's too sticky, flour the surface before rolling out.

3. Roll the dough out into a circle and place on a baking sheet lined with parchment paper. Spray with cooking spray and bake for 6-8 minutes.

4. Evenly spread the marinara sauce over the baked pizza crust. Layer the chicken sausage, cheese and veggies. Sprinkle garlic powder, oregano, salt and pepper on top of the veggies.

5. Bake on the bottom rack of your oven for 10-15 minutes or until the cheese is melted and the veggies are tender. Slice into four equal servings. Enjoy warm.

PRO TIP: Roll the dough out between two sheets of parchment paper for quick clean up.

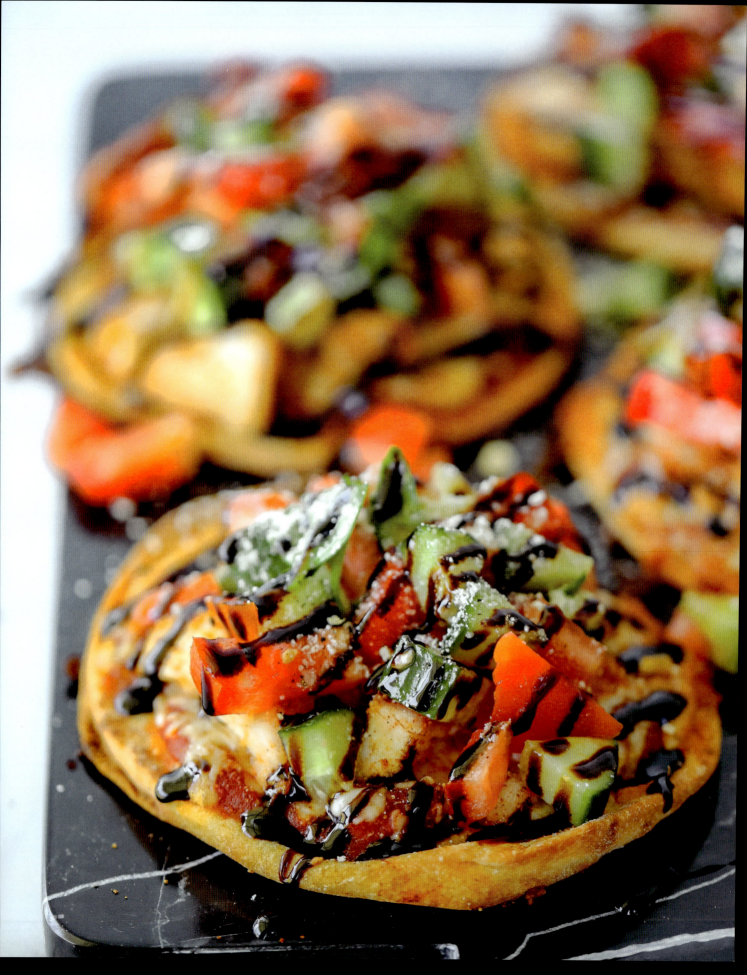

GRILLED BRUSCHETTA PIZZA

Makes 4 servings
350 calories / 12F / 33C / 27P / per serving

Prep: 15 min | **Cook:** 30 min

- 4 pieces Stonefire Mini Naan Bread (about 50g each)
- ½ cup marinara sauce
- ½ cup low-fat, shredded mozzarella cheese
- 8 oz. grilled/cooked chicken breast (10.6 oz. raw)
- Dash paprika
- Dash garlic powder
- Dash onion powder

Bruschetta Salad:
- 6 oz. chopped tomatoes
- 4 oz. chopped cucumbers
- 1 Tbs. olive oil
- ½ tsp. minced garlic
- Dash sea salt
- Dash black pepper
- Pinch fresh basil, chopped

Toppings:
- 2 Tbs. grated Parmesan cheese
- 2 Tbs. balsamic glaze

1. Cook or grill the chicken over medium heat until all sides are golden and the chicken is cooked through, about 5-7 minutes per side or until internal temperature reaches 160 degrees. Let cool slightly, then shred.

2. Heat grill to low heat.

3. Spread two tablespoons of marinara sauce over each piece of naan bread. Add two tablespoons of mozzarella and 2 oz. chopped grilled chicken to each pizza. Sprinkle with paprika, garlic powder and onion powder. Place on the grill and cook until the cheese is melted.

4. Combine the tomatoes, cucumbers, olive oil, minced garlic, sea salt, pepper and fresh basil together in a bowl. Evenly top the pizzas that you are going to eat immediately with ¼ of the bruschetta salad mixture, ½ tablespoon of Parmesan cheese and ½ tablespoon of balsamic glaze.

PRO TIPS: Use pre-cooked rotisserie chicken to cut down on your cook time.

Easily shred the chicken by placing it in a Kitchen Aid Mixer while still warm and beat on medium speed with the paddle attachment.

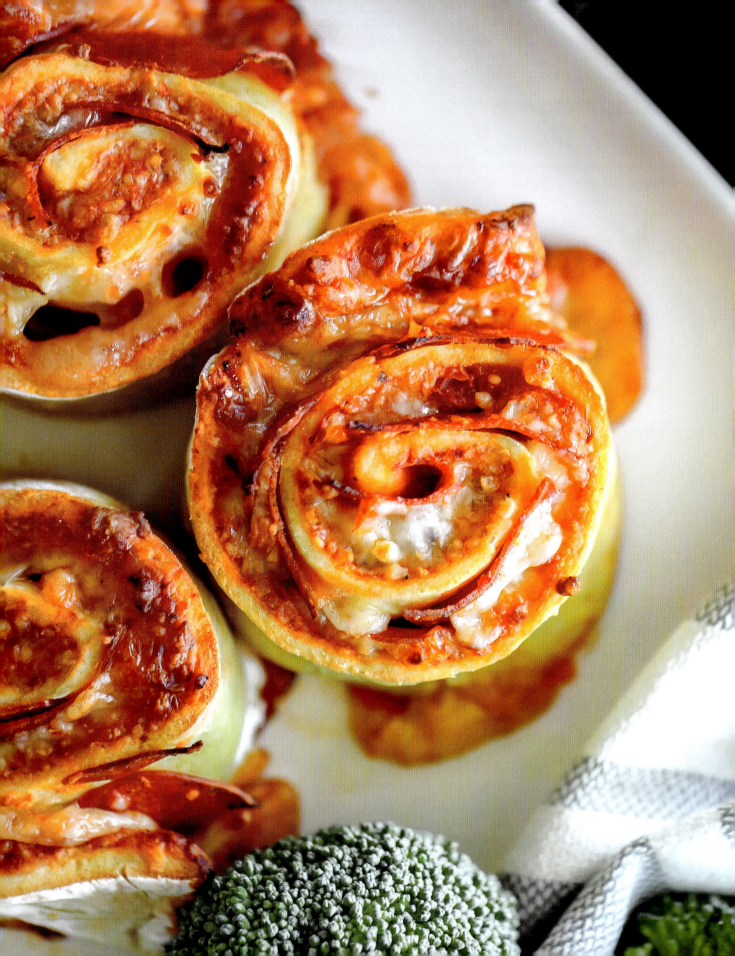

PEPPERONI PIZZA PINWHEELS

Makes 4 servings
335 calories / 12.5F / 32C / 26.5P / per serving

Prep: 30 min | **Cook:** 30 min

¾ cup white whole wheat flour
1 tsp. baking powder
¼ tsp. sea salt
Dash garlic powder
Dash onion powder
4 Tbs. nutritional yeast flakes
½ cup plain, nonfat Greek yogurt

½ cup traditional marinara sauce
2 oz. turkey pepperoni
1 ¼ cups mozzarella cheese, shredded
4 cups broccoli
1 Tbs. olive oil

1. Preheat the oven to 425 degrees.

2. Whisk the flour, baking powder, sea salt, garlic powder, onion powder, and three tablespoons of nutritional yeast flakes together in a bowl. Add the Greek yogurt and use a rubber spatula to fold it in until well combined. If the dough is too dry, add a tiny bit of water; if it's too sticky, flour the surface before rolling out.

3. Roll the dough out into a large rectangular shape. Spread the marinara sauce evenly over the dough, add the pepperoni and cheese. Carefully roll the dough up lengthwise and slice into eight equal pinwheels. Place on a greased baking sheet or muffin tin. Bake for 12-15 minutes. Two pinwheels per serving.

4. Chop the broccoli into florets and place on a baking sheet lined with parchment paper. Drizzle the olive oil over the top, then spray with cooking spray. Sprinkle with sea salt and one tablespoon nutritional yeast (this will give it a cheesy flavor and added nutritional value). Bake for 15-20 minutes. Enjoy on the side of your pinwheels.

PRO TIPS: Roll the dough out between two pieces of parchment paper for quick clean up.

Makes a great freezer meal! Prepare as instructed, without baking, and freeze. Thaw in the fridge overnight before eating. Bake in the oven at 425 for 15-20 minutes.

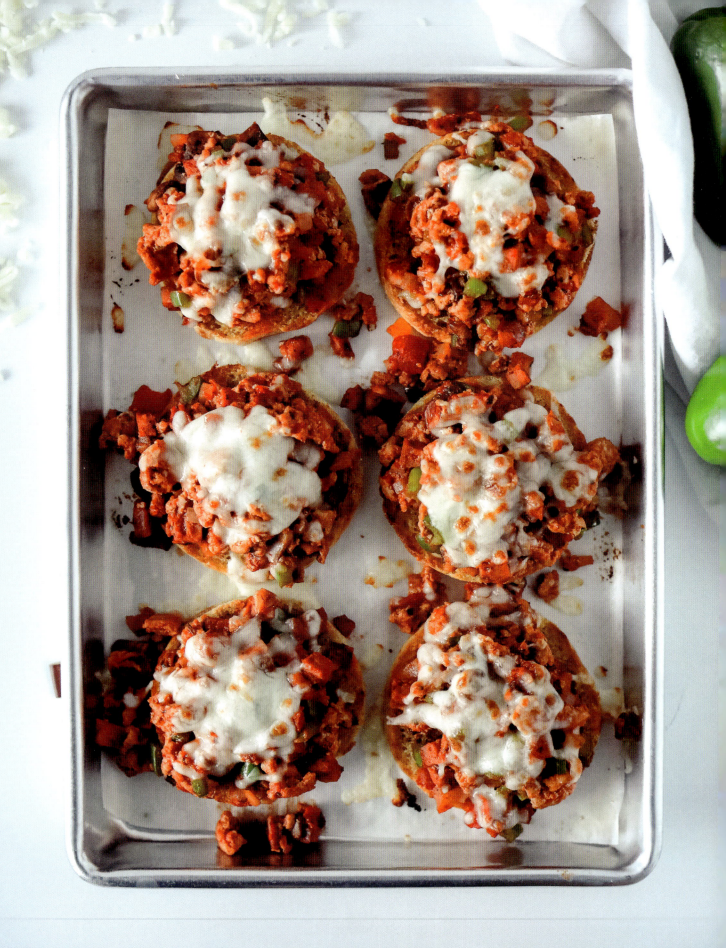

STACKED SUPREME PIZZA BITES

Makes 4 servings
365 calories / 13.5F / 35C / 27P / per serving

Prep: 10 min | **Cook:** 15 min

4 multi-grain English muffins
8 oz. lean ground turkey
Dash sea salt
Dash garlic powder
2 Italian sausage links
½ cup green bell peppers

½ cup white mushrooms
¼ cup yellow onions
¾ cup marinara sauce
½ cup shredded mozzarella cheese

1. Preheat the oven to 350 degrees.

2. Slice the muffins in half and place on a baking sheet lined with parchment paper. Spray the tops with cooking spray and place in the oven for 10 minutes or until crispy and lightly browned.

3. While the muffins are in the oven, add the lean ground turkey to a frying pan over medium heat. Cook until fully browned. Season with sea salt and garlic powder. Remove from the pan and add to a mixing bowl; set aside.

4. Dice the veggies and sausage into small pieces. Spray the frying pan with cooking spray, then add the veggies. Sauté over medium heat until the veggies are tender and the sausage is browned. Add the veggies and sausage and the marinara sauce to the cooked ground turkey. Stir until well combined. Weigh the mixture and divide by eight to get the amount needed to top each muffin half.

5. Remove the muffins from the oven and top each muffin half evenly with the meat and veggies mixture. Sprinkle one tablespoon of shredded cheese over each muffin. Turn the oven up to high broil. Add the muffins back to the oven for 2-3 minutes or until the cheese is melted and starting to brown. Enjoy two muffin halves per serving.

PRO TIP: Swap in different veggies and proteins for a new variation.

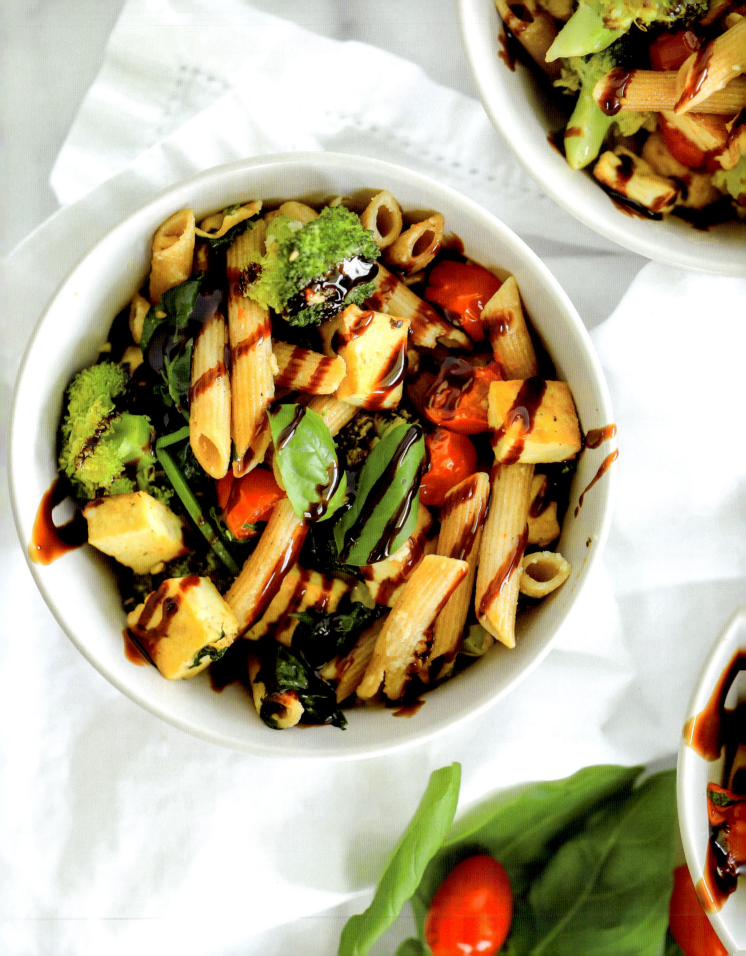

CAPRESE PASTA BOWL

Makes 4 servings
345 calories / 11F / 35C / 26P / per serving

Prep: 15 min | **Cook:** 30 min

- 5 oz. dry brown rice penne pasta (2 ¾ cups cooked)
- 2 cups chopped broccoli
- 7.5 oz. cooked chicken breast (10 oz. raw)
- 1 tsp. minced garlic
- Dash sea salt
- Dash black pepper
- 1 cup cherry tomatoes, halved
- 2 cups chopped spinach
- 1 Tbs. avocado or olive oil
- 4 oz. fresh mozzarella pearls
- Handful of fresh, chopped basil

Toppings:
- Drizzle of balsamic glaze

1. Preheat the oven to 400 degrees. Chop the broccoli into florets and place on a baking sheet lined with parchment paper. Spray the tops with zero calorie cooking spray and sprinkle with sea salt and other seasonings of choice. Roast in the oven for 20 minutes. Cook pasta according to the directions on the package.

2. Chop the raw chicken. Heat a skillet over medium heat. Spray with cooking spray and add the chicken, garlic, salt and pepper. Sauté until the chicken is cooked through; remove from the pan.

3. Halve the tomatoes. Chop the roasted broccoli and spinach. Heat oil in the skillet and then add all the veggies with a little salt and pepper. Sauté for three minutes. Add the cooked chicken, cooked pasta, fresh mozzarella pearls and basil to the pan. Stir until everything is well combined.

4. Weigh the entire recipe and divide the weight by four to get the amount needed to fill one serving. Enjoy warm or cold with a drizzle of balsamic glaze.

PRO TIP: Use pre-cooked rotisserie chicken to cut down on your cook time.

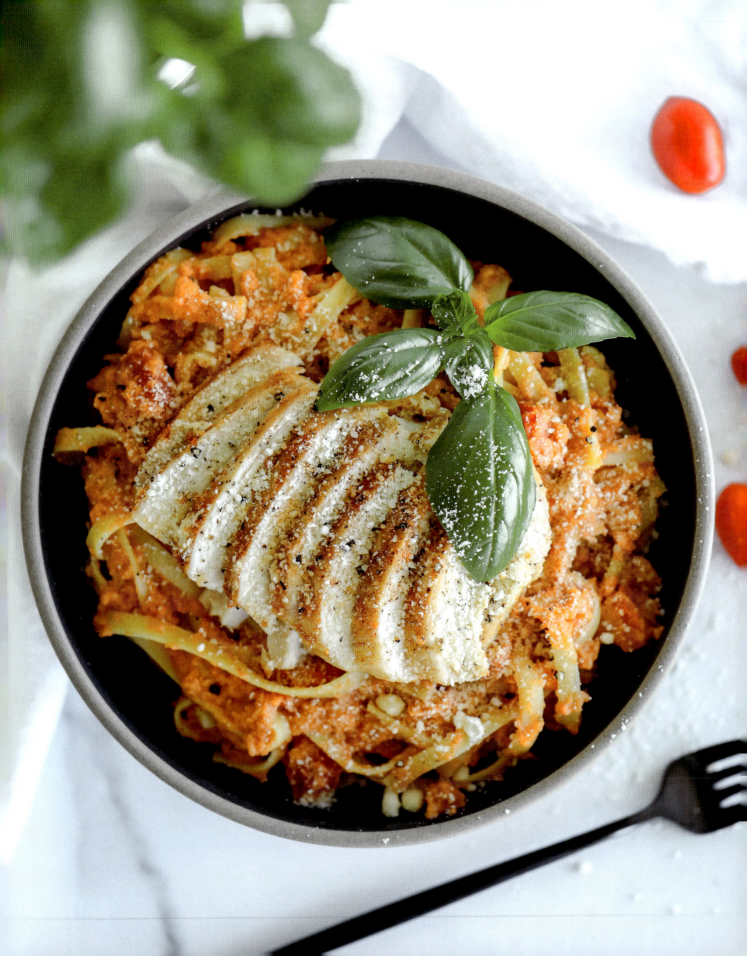

CHICKEN FETTUCCINE ALFREDO

Makes 4 servings
360 calories / 12F / 35C / 28P / per serving

Prep: 10 min | **Cook:** 40 min

6 oz. grilled chicken breast (8 oz. raw)
5 oz. whole wheat fettuccine, dry
2 cups cauliflower florets
Dash sea salt
½ cup unsweetened almond milk
1 Tbs. olive oil
1 Tbs. grass-fed butter
12 cherry tomatoes, halved
2 cloves garlic, chopped
Dash black pepper
¼ cup grated Parmesan cheese
2 Tbs. nutritional yeast flakes
½ cup marinara sauce
⅓ cup low-fat, shredded mozzarella cheese
Fresh basil

1. Cook or grill the chicken over medium heat until all sides are golden and the chicken is cooked through, about 5-7 minutes per side or until internal temperature reaches 160 degrees. Cook the fettuccine according to the directions on the package.

2. Bring a large pot of water to a boil. Add the cauliflower and sea salt. Boil until cauliflower is tender; about 10 minutes. Drain. Place in a blender with the almond milk; blend until smooth.

3. Add the olive oil, butter and tomatoes to a large pot. Cook over medium-low heat until the butter is melted. Add the garlic, black pepper and the creamed cauliflower. Bring mixture to a simmer, stirring constantly. Add the Parmesan cheese, nutritional yeast, and marinara sauce to the pot and simmer for 8-10 minutes. Stir in the mozzarella cheese until smooth. Remove from heat.

4. Add the pasta to the sauce. Weigh the pasta with the sauce and divide the weight by four to get the amount needed to fill one serving. Top each serving with 1.5 oz. grilled chicken breast and fresh basil. Season with sea salt and pepper to taste.

PRO TIPS: Use pre-cooked rotisserie chicken to cut down on your cook time. Leave the marinara sauce out for a classic, white Alfredo sauce.

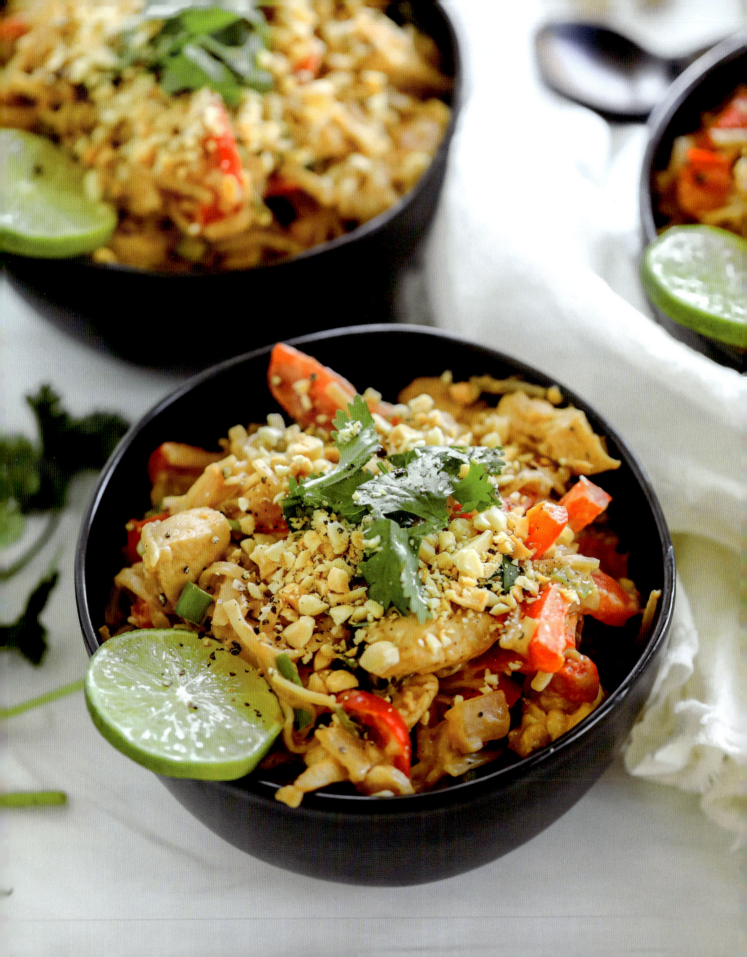

CHICKEN PAD THAI

Makes 4 servings
350 calories / 11F / 36C / 26P / per serving

Prep: 15 min | **Cook:** 20 min

- 4 oz. brown rice Pad Thai noodles, uncooked
- ¼ cup CSE Sweet Classic Peanut Butter or natural peanut butter
- ¼ cup rice vinegar
- 2 Tbs. coconut aminos
- 2 Tbs. raw honey
- 1 Tbs. fresh, minced garlic
- ½ cup fresh, minced yellow onion
- 11 oz. raw chicken breast (8.25 oz. cooked)
- 2 cups chopped red bell peppers
- 1 cup sliced green onions
- 2 cups bean sprouts

Toppings per serving:
- 5g peanuts
- ½ lime, juice of
- Fresh cilantro
- Dash sea salt
- Dash black pepper

1. Cook the noodles according to directions on the package. Drain and set aside.

2. Whisk the peanut butter, rice vinegar, coconut aminos and honey in a bowl. If the sauce is too thick, add a little water until you reach your desired consistency; set aside.

3. Spray a skillet with cooking spray and add the minced garlic and onions. Chop the raw chicken and add to the skillet. Cook until all the sides are golden brown and the chicken is cooked through.

4. Add the veggies and sauce; cook until tender. Add the noodles last. Weigh the entire recipe and divide the weight by four to get the amount needed to fill one serving. Garnish each serving with the toppings listed. Season with salt and pepper to taste.

PRO TIP: Can also be made with any type of pasta noodles.

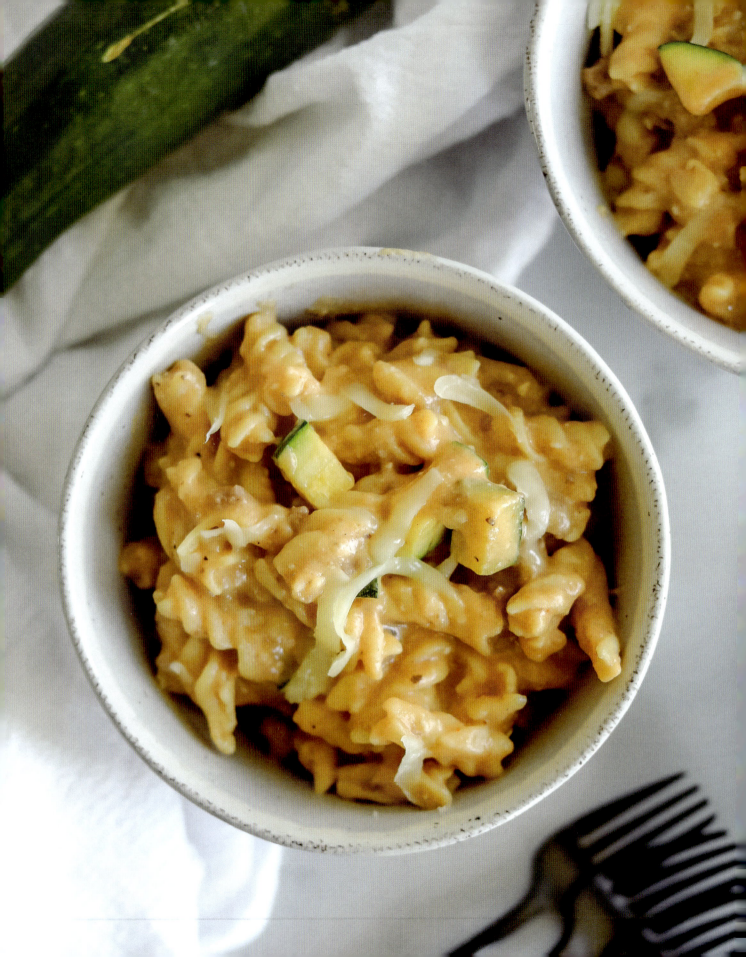

ONE-PAN CHEDDAR BEEF ROTINI

Makes 4 servings
360 calories / 14F / 33C / 26P per serving

Prep: 10 min | **Cook:** 20 min

12 oz. lean ground beef
1 Tbs. ketchup
1 tsp. Dijon mustard
1 tsp. Sriracha sauce or other hot sauce
1 tsp. garlic powder
1 tsp. onion powder
½ tsp. sea salt
Dash black pepper
6 oz. whole wheat rotini pasta
¾ cup beef broth
1 ½ cups water
1 cup zucchini
½ cup nonfat, plain Greek yogurt
⅓ cup shredded cheddar cheese

1. Brown the ground beef in a pan over medium heat. Add in the ketchup, mustard, hot sauce, garlic powder, onion powder, sea salt and black pepper. Stir until well combined.

2. Add the pasta to the pan along with the beef broth and water. Stir. Cover and boil for 8 minutes. Chop the zucchini and add to the pan. Let boil for an additional minute. Remove from the heat.

3. Stir in the Greek yogurt and then the cheese. Weigh the entire recipe and divide the weight by four to get the amount needed to fill one serving. Add extra salt and pepper to taste. Enjoy!

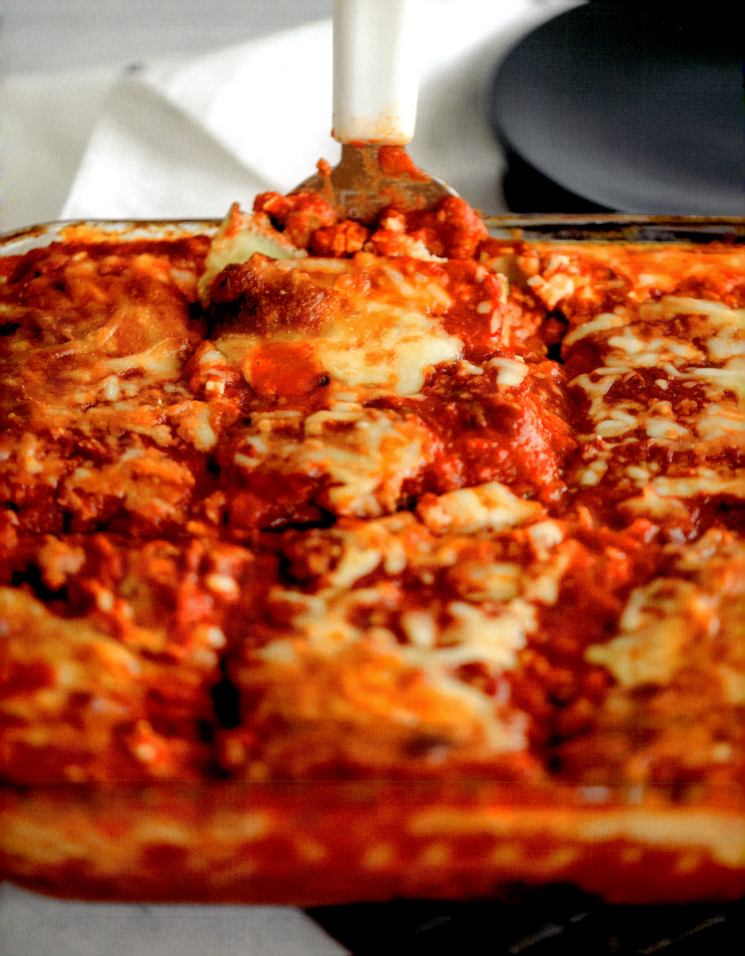

TURKEY SAUSAGE LASAGNA

Makes 4 servings
350 calories / 11F / 35C / 29P / per serving

Prep: 15 min | **Cook:** 70 min

- 1 Italian chicken sausage link
- ¼ cup yellow onion
- 1 cup spinach
- 2 Tbs. fresh basil leaves
- 6 oz. lean ground turkey
- 1 tsp. minced garlic
- 14 oz. crushed tomatoes
- 6 oz. tomato paste
- 8 oz. tomato sauce
- ¼ cup water
- ½ tsp. sea salt
- Dash ground pepper
- ¼ tsp. fennel seeds
- ½ tsp. Italian seasoning
- ½ Tbs. stevia
- 2 ½ oz. whole grain lasagna noodles, dry
- 1 zucchini
- ¾ cup fat-free cottage cheese
- 1 large egg
- ¼ cup shredded mozzarella cheese
- 2 Tbs. grated Parmesan cheese

1. Chop the chicken sausage (link should be 3 oz.), onions, spinach and basil leaves. Add to a large saucepan with the ground turkey and garlic. Cook over medium-high heat until the turkey is fully cooked through.

2. Add the crushed tomatoes, tomato paste, tomato sauce, water, sea salt, pepper, fennel seeds, Italian seasoning and stevia. Stir until combined. Cover and simmer. Grate the zucchini and fold into the turkey mix.

3. Boil the lasagna noodles for 8 minutes. Preheat the oven to 375 degrees.

4. Add the cottage cheese, egg and a dash of sea salt to a bowl. Mix until well combined.

5. Spray the bottom of an 8x8 glass baking dish. Add ⅓ of the meat sauce to the bottom of the pan. Top with the ½ of the cooked lasagna noodles, ½ of the cottage cheese mixture, two tablespoons of shredded mozzarella cheese, one tablespoon of Parmesan cheese, ⅓ of the meat sauce, remaining lasagna noodles, remaining cottage cheese mixture, remaining meat sauce, two tablespoons of mozzarella cheese and one tablespoon of Parmesan cheese.

6. Bake for 45-50 minutes. Slice into four servings and serve warm.

PRO TIPS: Use no-boil, oven-ready lasagna noodles to cut down on cook time.

Makes a great freezer meal! Prepare the recipe without baking. Cover and freezer. Let thaw in the fridge overnight then bake at 375 degrees for 45-50 minutes.

COMFORT FOOD

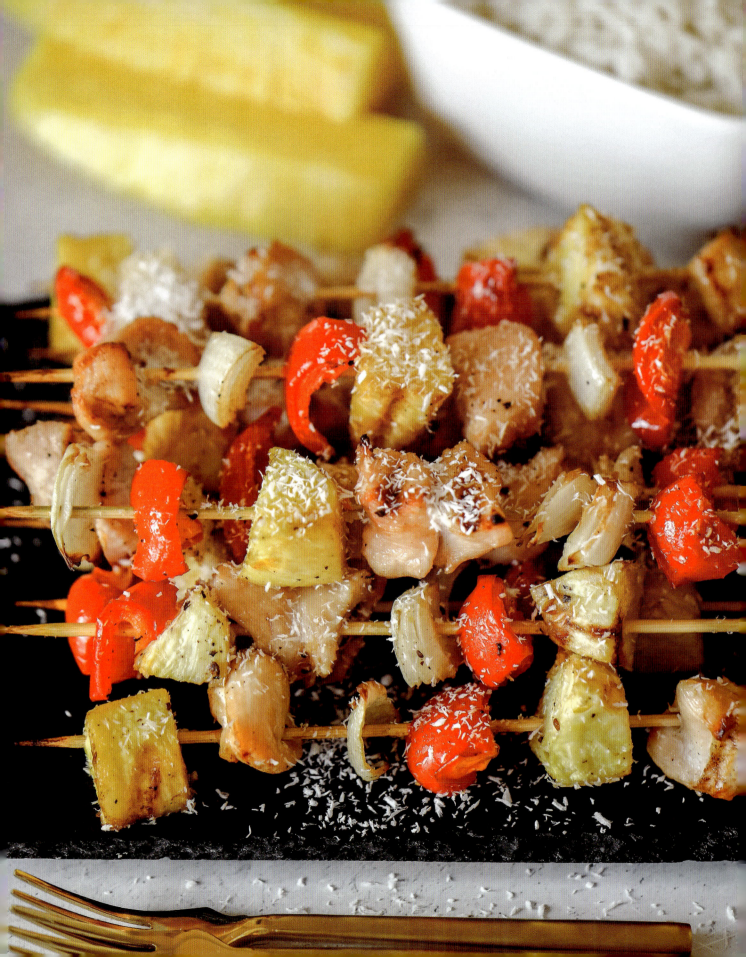

ALOHA CHICKEN KABOBS

Makes 4 servings
350 calories / 11F / 36C / 27P / per serving

Prep: 30 min | **Cook:** 30 min

Wooden skewer sticks
6 Tbs. uncooked white jasmine rice
¾ cup full-fat, canned coconut milk
14 oz. raw chicken breast (10.5 oz. cooked)
1 cup chopped red bell peppers
1 cup chopped yellow sweet onions
4 oz. cubed, fresh pineapple
1 Tbs. coconut aminos
½ Tbs. raw honey
1 tsp. olive oil
1 tsp. rice vinegar
½ tsp. fresh, minced garlic
½ tsp. ground ginger
Dash sea salt
Dash black pepper
2 Tbs. unsweetened shredded coconut

1. Soak the skewer sticks for an hour before cooking.

2. Heat oven to HI broil.

3. Cook the rice according to directions on the package, using coconut milk for the liquid instead of water. Stir in a dash of sea salt. Weigh or measure the rice and divide the weight by four to get the amount needed to fill one serving.

4. Cube the chicken. Measure out 3.5 oz. raw, cubed chicken, ¼ cup peppers, ¼ cup onions and 1 oz. pineapple. Skewer in a pattern, then place onto a greased broiler pan; set aside.

5. Combine the coconut aminos, honey, olive oil, rice vinegar, minced garlic and ground ginger together in a small bowl. Baste the skewers with the mixture and then sprinkle with sea salt and pepper.

6. Broil for 10-15 minutes, flipping halfway. Sprinkle the shredded coconut over the top. Enjoy warm over coconut rice.

PRO TIP: Instead of using skewers, throw the chicken, peppers, onions and pineapple together in a pan. Cook until the chicken is cooked through and the peppers and onions are tender. Add the sauce and cook until heated through. Serve in a bowl over the coconut rice topped with shredded coconut, sea salt and pepper.

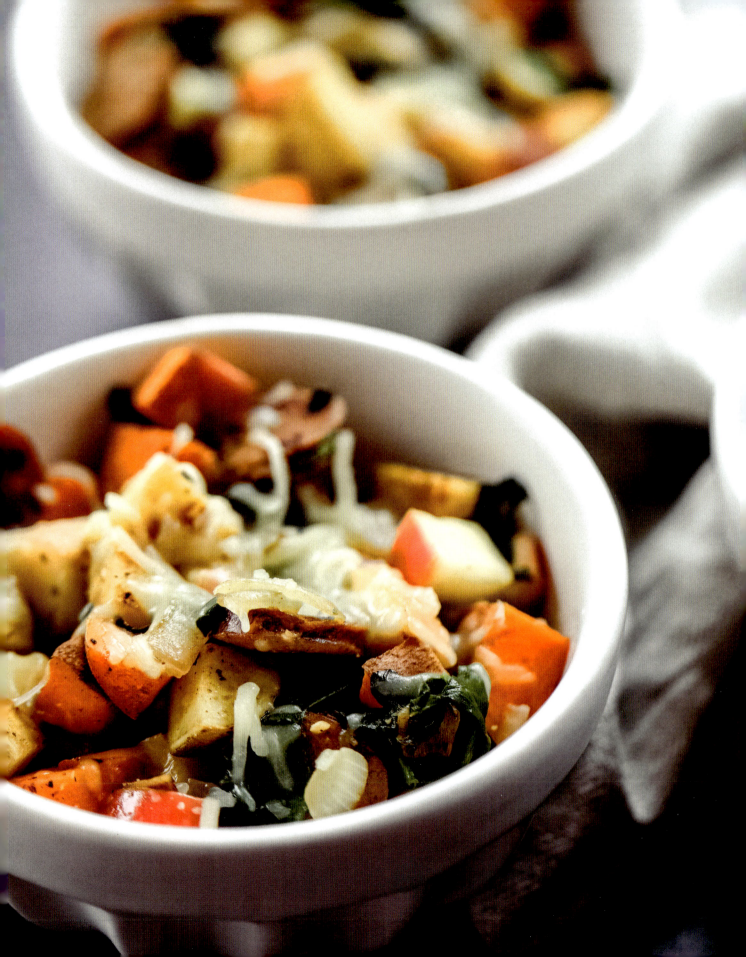

APPLE CHICKEN HASH

Makes 4 servings
345 calories / 12.5F / 31.5C / 27P / per serving

Prep: 15 min | **Cook:** 20 min

4 oz. cooked chicken breast (5.2 oz. raw)
14 oz. raw sweet potatoes
4 large chicken sausages, cut into rounds
1 cup chopped yellow onions
2 cups chopped spinach
Seasonings of choice
140g chopped pink lady apples
¼ cup low-fat, shredded mozzarella cheese

1. Heat a skillet or large frying pan to medium heat. Cube the chicken breast and add it to the greased skillet. Cook until no longer pink and browned on all sides. Remove from the skillet.

2. Cube the sweet potatoes and place on a microwave-safe plate. Spray tops with cooking spray and microwave for two minutes or bake in advance on a baking sheet at 400 degrees for 40 minutes, flipping halfway.

3. Spray the skillet with cooking spray, then add the sausage, sweet potatoes, onion, spinach and seasonings. Cook over medium-high heat for 5-7 minutes or until cooked through. Add the cooked chicken and chopped apples to the pan. Cook for 2 additional minutes or until the apples are tender-crisp.

4. Remove from the skillet. Weigh the entire recipe and divide the total weight by four to get the amount needed to fill one serving. Top each serving with one tablespoon of shredded mozzarella cheese.

PRO TIP: If you don't prefer hot apples, leave them out of the recipe and enjoy them on the side.

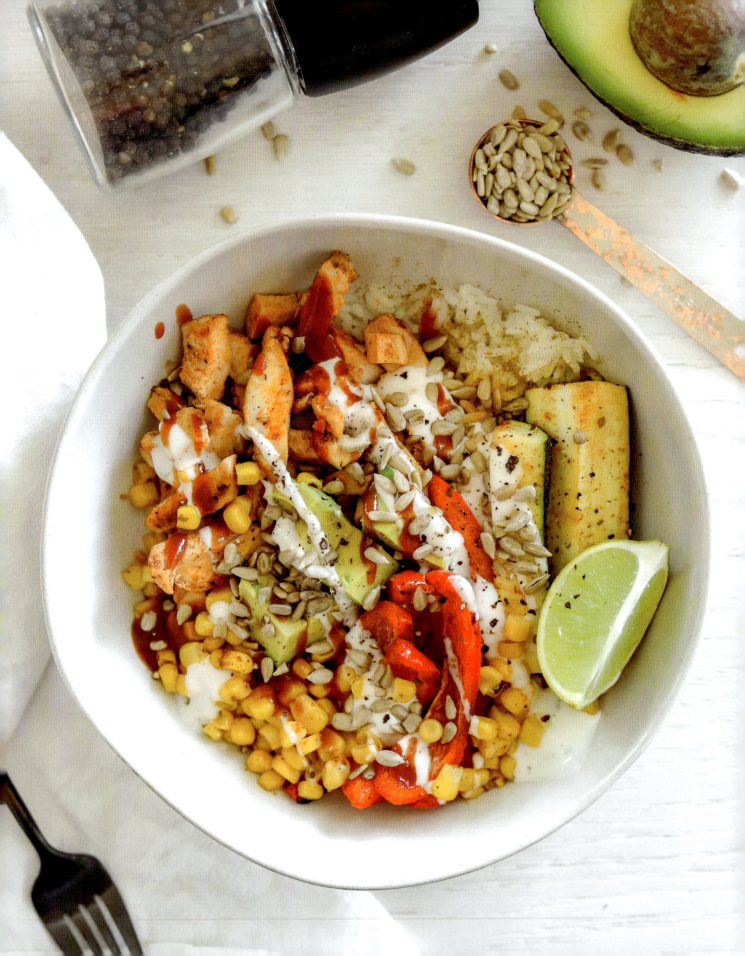

BBQ RANCH GRILLED BOUNTY BOWL

Makes 4 servings
350 calories / 12F / 34C / 27P / per serving

Prep: 10 min | **Cook:** 35 min

- ⅓ cup uncooked white jasmine rice (1 cup cooked)
- Dash cumin
- Dash turmeric
- Dash sea salt
- 13.3 oz raw chicken breast (10 oz. cooked)
- 7 oz. zucchini, sliced into wedges
- 7 oz. bell peppers, seeded and halved
- 2 ears (1 cup) corn
- Dash black pepper
- 120g chopped avocado
- 4 Tbs. Bolthouse Farms Classic Ranch dressing
- 2 Tbs. Stubb's BBQ Sauce, any variety
- 2 Tbs. shelled sunflower seeds
- 1 lime, juice of

1. Cook the rice according to the directions on the package. Season with a dash of cumin, turmeric and sea salt once cooked.

2. Heat grill to medium. Place chicken, zucchini, bell peppers and corn on the grill. Spray corn liberally with cooking spray and make sure to rotate it frequently. Spray tops of other veggies with cooking spray and sprinkle sea salt, pepper and cumin over everything. Cook chicken and veggies for about 5 minutes per side or until chicken is fully cooked through and veggies are tender.

3. Cut the corn off the cobs and set aside.

4. To each bowl add ¼ of the grilled chicken, 50g zucchini, 50g peppers, ¼ cup of corn, ¼ cup cooked rice, 30g chopped avocado, one tablespoon of ranch dressing, ½ tablespoon of BBQ sauce, ½ tablespoon of sunflower seeds and a squirt of lime juice. Enjoy warm.

PRO TIPS: This meal can be cooked in the oven. Place the chicken, zucchini, peppers and corn on a sheet pan, spray the tops liberally with cooking spray and sprinkle with sea salt. Bake at 425 degrees for 18-20 minutes or until the chicken comes to an internal temperature of 160 degrees.

Use microwavable rice pouches to cut down on cook time.

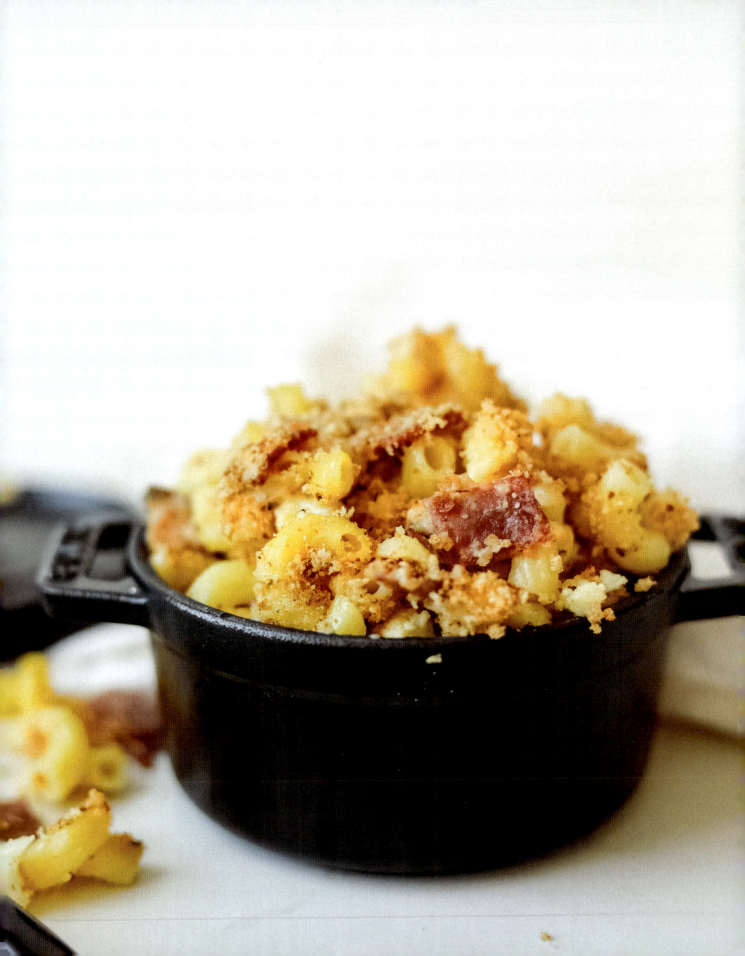

BOSS BAKED MAC & CHEESE
Makes 4 servings
350 calories / 14.5F / 31.5C / 23.5P / per serving

Prep: 15 min | **Cook:** 50 min

- 4 oz. uncooked whole wheat macaroni or elbow pasta
- 1 Italian chicken sausage
- 2 slices turkey bacon
- 1 Tbs. grass-fed butter
- 1 Tbs. CSE Buttermilk or Gluten-Free Buttermilk Pancake & Waffle Mix
- 1 cup fat-free milk
- ¼ tsp. sea salt
- Dash black pepper
- 3 cups frozen cauliflower rice
- ½ cup low-fat, shredded cheddar cheese
- 6 Tbs. grated Parmesan cheese
- 1 slice Ezekiel Bread
- Dash sea salt
- Dash garlic powder
- Dash paprika
- Dash thyme

1. Preheat the oven to 350 degrees.

2. Cook the macaroni according to the directions on the package. Drain and set aside.

3. Slice the chicken sausage into thin rounds and chop bacon into small pieces. Place in a frying pan over medium-high heat. Cook until fragrant and all sides are browned. Remove from heat and set aside.

4. In a large saucepan, melt the butter over low-medium heat. Add the CSE Pancake & Waffle Mix and stir until well combined. Slowly whisk in the milk and stir constantly until slightly thickened. Add in the sea salt, black pepper, cheddar cheese and four tablespoons of the Parmesan cheese. Stir until the cheese is melted into the sauce. Add the frozen cauliflower rice, macaroni, sausage and bacon to the sauce. Stir until well combined. Pour into a greased 8x8 baking dish.

5. Toast the Ezekiel Bread in the toaster until browned on both sides. Break into pieces and place in a blender. Pulse until it turns into bread crumbs. Combine the bread crumbs, two tablespoons of Parmesan cheese, sea salt, garlic powder, paprika and thyme together in a bowl. Sprinkle over the top of the macaroni and cheese. Bake for 25 minutes. Divide into four equal servings and enjoy warm.

PRO TIP: Makes a great freezer meal! Prepare the recipe without baking. Cover and freezer. Let thaw in the fridge overnight, then bake at 350 degrees for 25-30 minutes or until heated through.

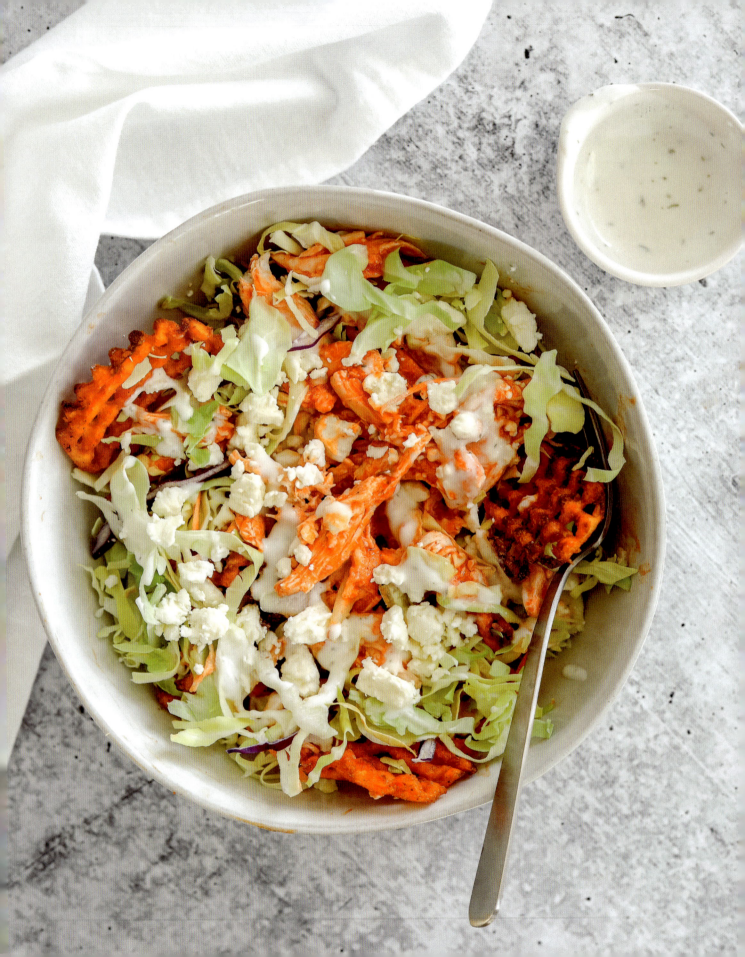

BUFFALO CHICKEN WAFFLE FRIES
Makes 4 servings
350 calories / 11F / 34.5C / 27P / per serving

Prep: 5 min | **Cook:** 20 min

16 oz. Alexia Waffle Cut Sweet Potato Fries
9 oz. pre-cooked rotisserie chicken breast
2 Tbs. Frank's Buffalo Wing Sauce
4 cups tri-color coleslaw
56g feta or bleu cheese crumbles
60g Bolthouse Farms Classic Ranch or Chunky Bleu Cheese Dressing

1. Cook waffle fries according to the directions on the bag. Weigh the fries and divide by four to get the amount needed for one serving.

2. Toss the chicken in the buffalo sauce.

3. Add the waffle fries to a bowl. Top with one cup coleslaw, ¼ of the buffalo chicken, 14g feta or bleu cheese crumbles and 15g dressing.

PRO TIP: Use the air fryer for a quicker method. Place frozen fries in the air fryer and spread out evenly. Heat at 350 degrees for 10-12 minutes, flipping halfway.

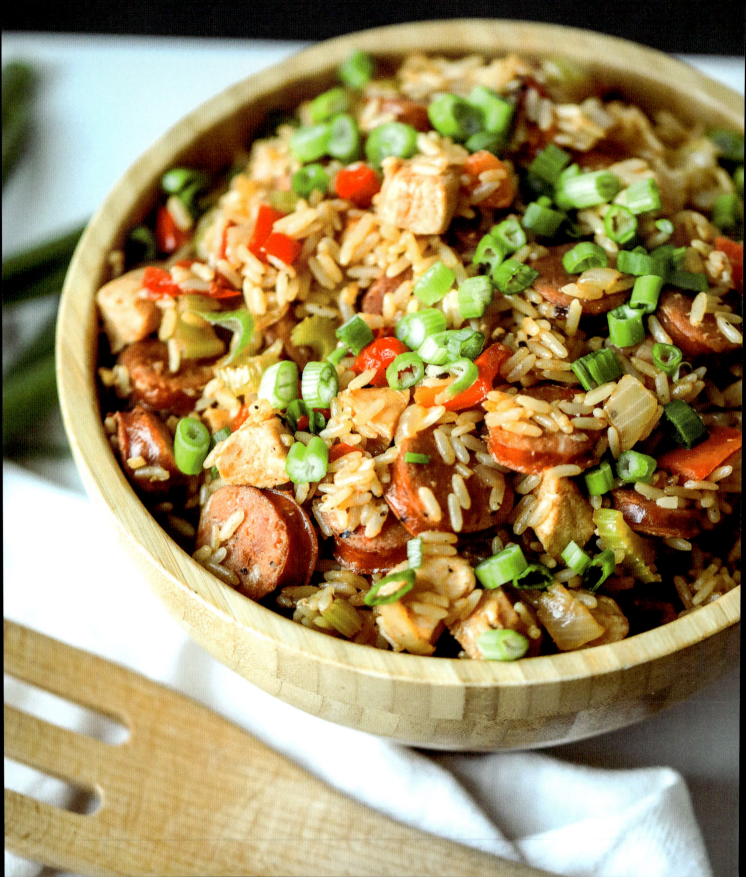

CAJUN CHICKEN SAUSAGE JAMBALAYA

Makes 4 servings
350 calories / 11.5F / 34C / 27P / per serving

Prep: 15 min | **Cook:** 45 min

- 4 Cajun Style Andouille chicken sausage links
- 5 oz. raw chicken breast (3.75 oz. cooked)
- 1 cup chopped yellow onion
- 1 cup chopped red bell peppers
- 2 stalks of celery, sliced
- 1 clove of garlic or 1 tsp. minced garlic
- ½ tsp. cajun seasoning
- 1 bay leaf
- 1 cup uncooked, converted brown or white rice
- 1 cup chicken stock
- ½ cup canned, diced, fire roasted tomatoes
- Green onions, sliced for garnish

1. Slice the sausage into rounds and cube the chicken breast.

2. Spray a skillet with cooking spray. Heat to medium-high heat and add the chicken and sausage. Cook until browned on all sides about 8-10 minutes. Remove from the pan.

3. Add the chopped onion, bell pepper, celery, garlic, bay leaf and Cajun seasoning to the skillet. Cook over medium-high heat until the vegetables are tender, about 5-7 minutes.

4. Stir in the uncooked, converted rice and cook for about 3 minutes. Stir in the chicken broth, tomatoes, chicken, and sausage. Bring to a boil over high heat. Cover and reduce to low-medium heat. Let simmer for about 20 minutes, stirring occasionally, or until rice is tender.

5. Divide into four equal portions and garnish with sliced green onions.

PRO TIPS: Makes a great freezer meal! Make and freeze without garnish. To thaw, place in a crockpot on high for 4-6 hours. Add garnish fresh.

To tone down the spiciness of this meal, swap in another flavor of chicken sausage and omit the Cajun seasoning.

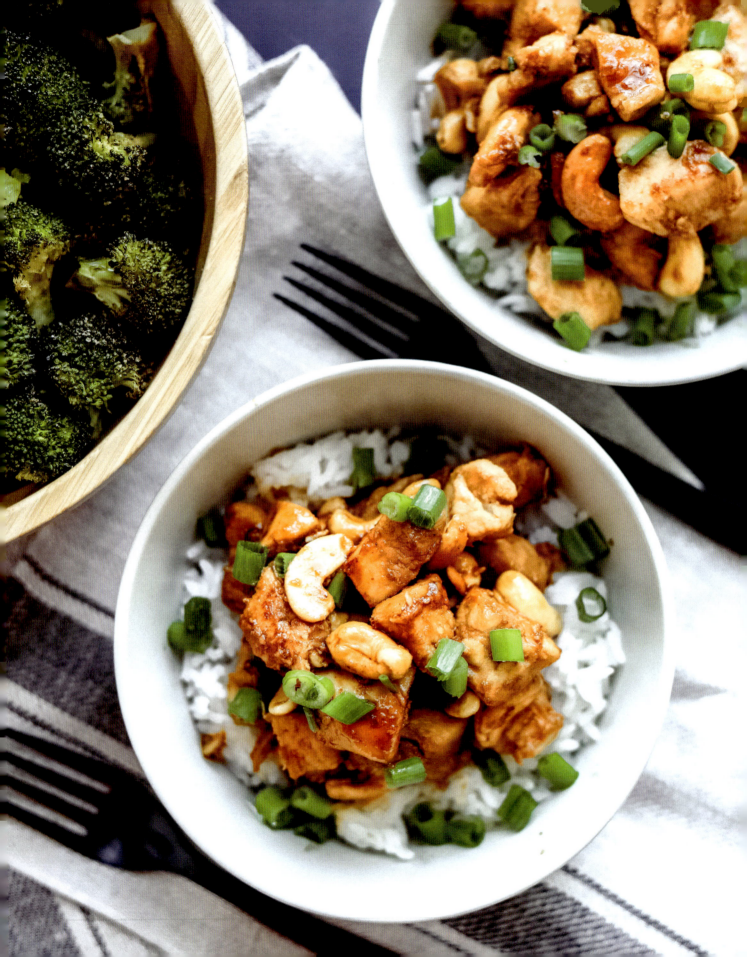

CASHEW KUNG PAO CHICKEN

Makes 4 servings
345 calories / 11F / 35C / 26P / per serving

Prep: 15 min | **Cook:** 30 min

1 cup cooked white or brown jasmine rice (⅓ cup uncooked)
2 cups broccoli florets
12 oz. raw chicken breast (9 oz. cooked)
3 garlic cloves
Dash ground ginger
3 oz. cashews
Green onions, sliced for garnish

Sweet & Spicy Kung Pao Sauce:
4 Tbs. coconut aminos
2 Tbs. raw honey
1 tsp. Sriracha sauce or chili paste
½ tsp. sesame oil

1. Preheat the oven to 400 degrees. Chop broccoli into florets and place on a baking sheet lined with parchment paper. Spray the tops with zero calorie cooking spray and sprinkle with sea salt and other seasonings of choice. Roast in the oven for 20 minutes. Cook rice according to the directions on the package.

2. Cube chicken and place in a greased skillet over medium heat. Add whole garlic cloves and ginger. Cook until all sides of the chicken are golden brown and chicken is cooked through. Add the cashews and cook for another minute. Turn heat off or down to low.

3. Whisk all the sauce ingredients together and add to the skillet. Stir until all the chicken is well coated. Weigh the chicken mixture and divide the weight by four to get the amount needed to fill one serving. Serve one portion of chicken over ¼ cup of cooked rice and garnish with green onions. Enjoy the roasted broccoli on the side or stir in with the chicken and rice.

PRO TIP: Use pre-cooked rotisserie chicken to cut down on your cook time.

Use microwavable rice pouches to cut down on cook time.

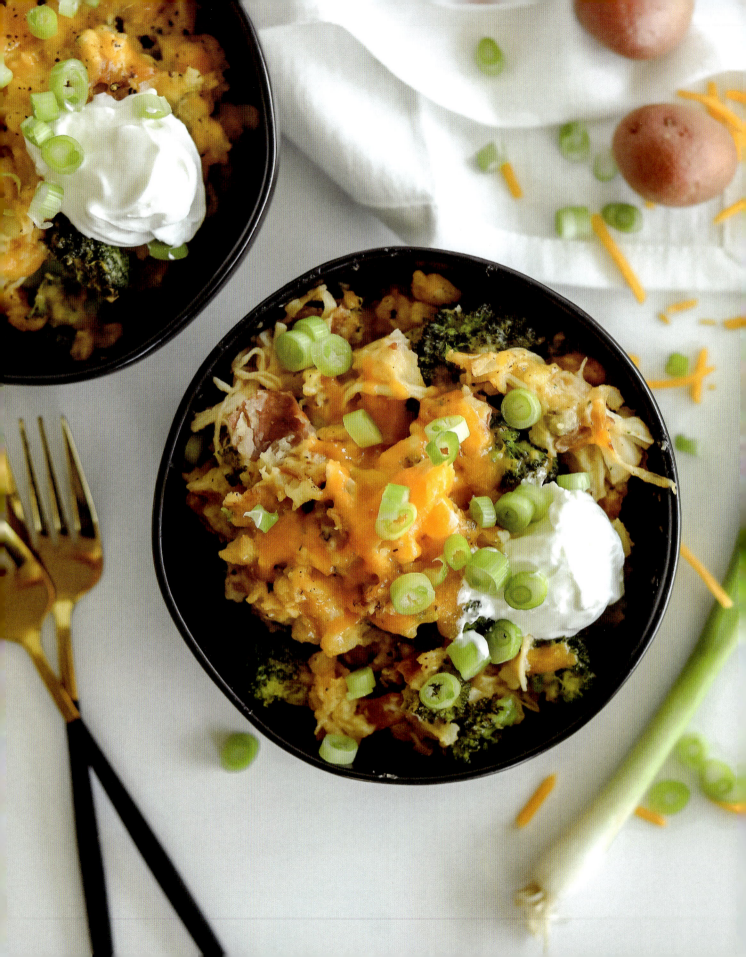

CHEDDAR RANCH CHICKEN & POTATOES
Makes 4 servings
340 calories / 11F / 34C / 26P / per serving

Prep: 10 min | **Cook:** 45 min

4 cups raw broccoli
20 oz. baby gold potatoes
Dash sea salt
Dash black pepper
1 Tbs. grass-fed butter
1 Tbs. CSE Buttermilk or Gluten-Free Buttermilk Pancake & Waffle Mix
1 cup unsweetened almond milk
2 tsp. ranch DIPS powder

6 oz. cooked, shredded chicken breast (8 oz. raw)
1 cup low-fat, shredded cheddar cheese
Toppings per serving:
1 Tbs. plain, nonfat Greek yogurt
Green onions, for garnish

1. Preheat the oven to 400 degrees. Chop the broccoli small and place on a baking sheet lined with parchment paper. Spray the tops with cooking spray and sprinkle with sea salt. Roast in the oven for 20 minutes. Remove from the oven and let cool.

2. Bring a large pot of water to a boil. Add the potatoes and sea salt, then boil for 15-20 minutes or until fork-tender; drain. Smash lightly and set aside.

3. Cook or grill the chicken over medium heat until all sides are golden and the chicken is cooked through, about 5-7 minutes per side or until internal temperature reaches 160 degrees. Shred.

4. Place the pot back on the stove over medium heat and add the butter. Stir until melted, then stir in the CSE Pancake & Waffle Mix. Once combined, add in the milk, ranch powder and a dash of salt and pepper. Bring to a boil then let simmer on medium for 5 minutes. Fold in the shredded chicken, roasted broccoli, smashed potatoes and ½ cup of the cheese.

5. Transfer to a greased 8x8 baking dish and top with the remaining cheese. Bake for 10-15 minutes or until the cheese is melted. Divide the casserole into four equal servings and top each serving with one tablespoon Greek yogurt and sliced green onions. Enjoy!

PRO TIP: Use pre-cooked rotisserie chicken to cut down on your cook time.

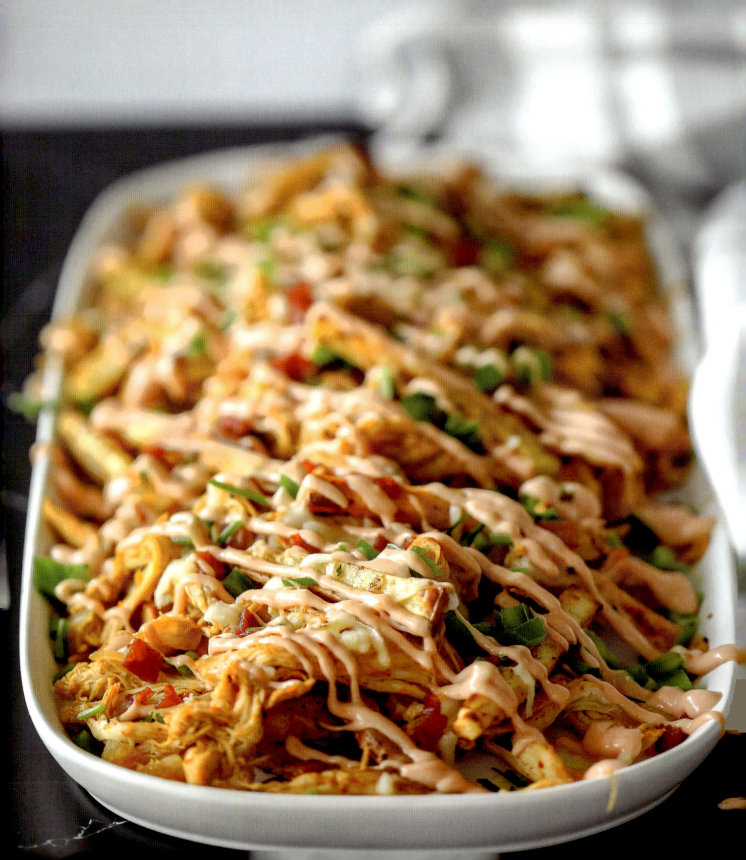

CHILI-LIME JUNKYARD FRIES
Makes 4 servings
350 calories / 12.5F / 34C / 25P / per serving

Prep: 15 min | **Cook:** 45 min + marination

Chili-Lime Chicken:
6.75 oz. cooked chicken breast (9 oz. raw)
½ cup chopped yellow onions
Marinade:
1 Tbs. olive oil
1 lime, juice and zest of
½ tsp. coconut sugar
½ tsp. chili powder
¼ tsp. cumin
¼ tsp. paprika
¼ tsp. garlic powder
¼ tsp. sea salt
Dash black pepper

Junkyard Fries:
19 oz. raw sweet potatoes
¾ cup low-fat, shredded mozzarella cheese
2 slices turkey bacon
1 chopped jalapeño, optional
Chives, for garnish
Fry Sauce per serving:
1 Tbs. olive oil mayo
½ Tbs. ketchup

1. Add chicken and onions to a crockpot. Combine all marinade ingredients together in a bowl and then pour over the chicken and onions. Cook on low for 4-6 hours.

2. Preheat the oven to 425 degrees. Slice the sweet potatoes into fries. Spread fries out in a single layer onto a baking sheet lined with parchment paper. Spray tops with cooking spray and sprinkle with sea salt. Bake for 20 minutes, flip and return to the oven. Bake for another 15 minutes.

3. Chop the bacon and cook in a greased frying pan over medium-high heat. Cook until crispy. Remove from heat and set aside.

4. Top the sweet potato fries with shredded Chili-Lime Chicken and cheese. Return to the oven and cook for 5 minutes until the cheese is melted. Split into four equal portions and top each serving with a ½ slice of crumbled bacon, jalapeños, chives and fry sauce. Enjoy warm with a fork.

PRO TIP: Use pre-cooked rotisserie chicken to cut down on your cook time. Shred the chicken in a bowl and coat with the marinade. Skip step 1.

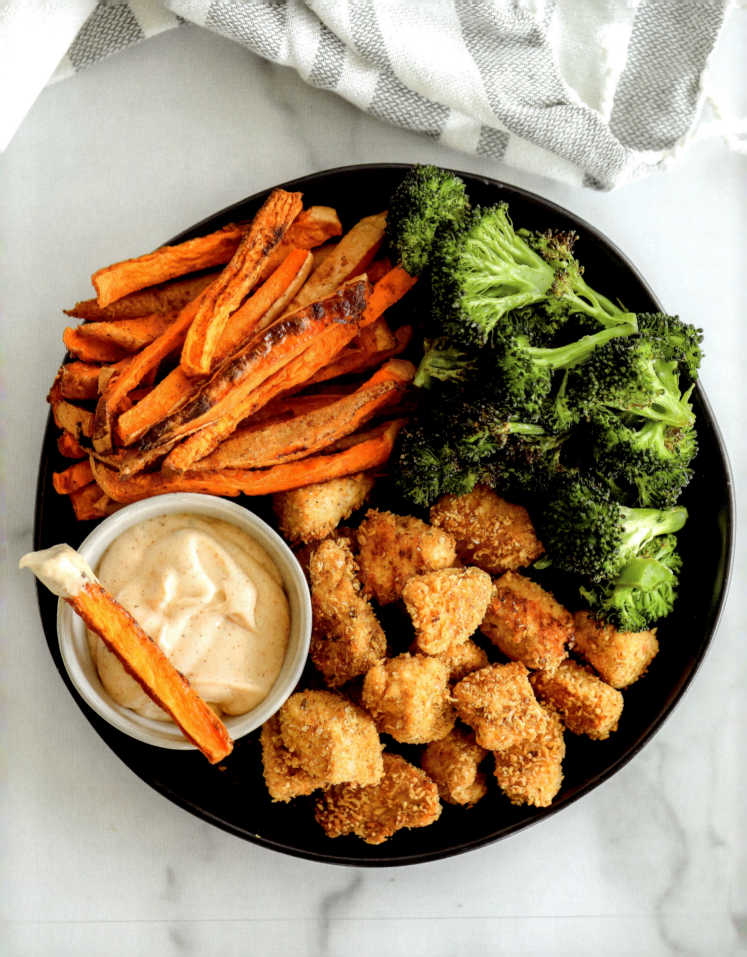

CRISPY CHICKEN NUGGETS

Makes 4 servings
340 calories / 11F / 35C / 25.5P / per serving

Prep: 20 min | **Cook:** 40 min

12 oz. sweet potatoes
6 cups broccoli
4 Tbs. whole wheat breadcrumbs
2 Tbs. flaxseed meal
2 Tbs. grated Parmesan cheese
¼ tsp. sea salt
Dash paprika
Dash garlic powder
Dash onion powder
1 egg white
10 oz. raw chicken breast
  (7.5 oz cooked)

Chili-Lime Mayo:
6 Tbs. olive oil mayo
1 Tbs. ketchup
1 lime, juice of
½ tsp. chili powder
¼ tsp. onion powder
¼ tsp. garlic powder
¼ tsp. paprika
Dash sea salt
Dash black pepper

1. Preheat the oven to 400 degrees. Cut sweet potatoes into fries. Place on a baking sheet lined with parchment paper. Spray tops with cooking spray and sprinkle with sea salt. Bake for 40 minutes, flipping halfway. Turn the oven heat down to 350 degrees.

2. Add the breadcrumbs, flaxseed meal, Parmesan cheese, paprika, garlic powder, onion powder and sea salt to a large zip top bag and set aside.

3. Add the egg whites to a bowl. Chop the chicken breast into bite-sized pieces and add to the bowl with the egg whites. Toss until well coated, then add to a colander and drain. Toss the chicken into the large bag with the bread crumbs and shake until well coated.

4. Spread the nuggets out onto a baking sheet lined with parchment paper. Chop the broccoli and place on the same baking sheet with the chicken. Spray the tops with cooking spray and sprinkle with sea salt. Cook for 20 minutes or until the chicken is cooked through and the broccoli is tender. Weigh the chicken, sweet potatoes and broccoli separately and divide by four to get the amount needed to fill one serving.

5. Combine all the ingredients together for the Chili-Lime Mayo. Weigh and divide by four to get the amount needed to fill one serving. Enjoy the chicken nuggets warm with roasted broccoli and sweet potatoes on the side. Use the Chili-Lime Mayo as a dip for your fries and nuggets.

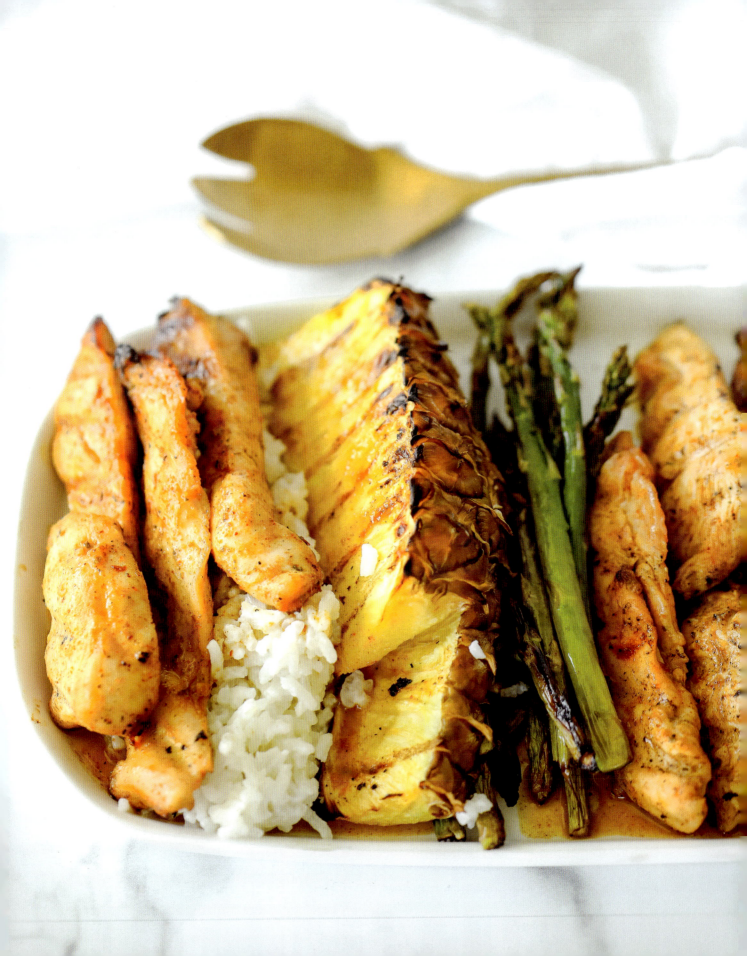

GRILLED COCONUT-LIME CURRY CHICKEN

Makes 4 servings
350 calories / 11F / 36C / 26.5P / per serving

Prep: 20 min | **Cook:** 20 min + marination

1 Tbs. olive oil
1 lime, zest and juice of
½ tsp. ground cumin
1 tsp. ground coriander
1 Tbs. coconut aminos
1 Tbs. raw honey
1 tsp. sea salt
1 tsp. curry powder
4 Tbs. lite canned coconut milk
Dash cayenne pepper
10.5 oz cooked chicken breast
 (14 oz. raw)

Coconut Rice:
½ cup uncooked white jasmine rice
1 ½ cups lite canned coconut milk
¼ cup water
Dash sea salt

Sides and Toppings:
24 asparagus spears, roasted
400g (14 oz.) fresh pineapple
Lime juice
Cilantro

1. Add the olive oil, lime zest and juice, ground cumin, ground coriander, coconut aminos, honey, sea salt, curry powder, coconut milk and cayenne pepper to a small bowl and whisk together. Pour half of the mixture into a large zip top bag. Store the other half in the fridge for later. Slice the chicken into strips and add to the bag. Massage until well coated and let marinate in the fridge 2+ hours.

2. Make the coconut rice by adding the coconut milk, water, rice and a dash of sea salt to a pot. Bring to a boil. Turn the heat down to low, stir the rice, cover and cook for 20 minutes. Stir and remove from the heat.

3. After the chicken has had time to marinate, preheat the grill to medium-high heat. Add the chicken to the grill and cook for about 5 minutes per side. Discard the marinade in the bag.

4. Place a piece of foil on the grill and spray with cooking spray. Add the asparagus and grill for about 8 minutes.

5. Serve ¼ grilled curry chicken over ¼ of the coconut rice. Top with ¼ of the remaining marinade, 100g chopped pineapple, lime juice and cilantro. Enjoy roasted asparagus spears on the side.

PRO TIP: Add the pineapple to the grill with the asparagus!

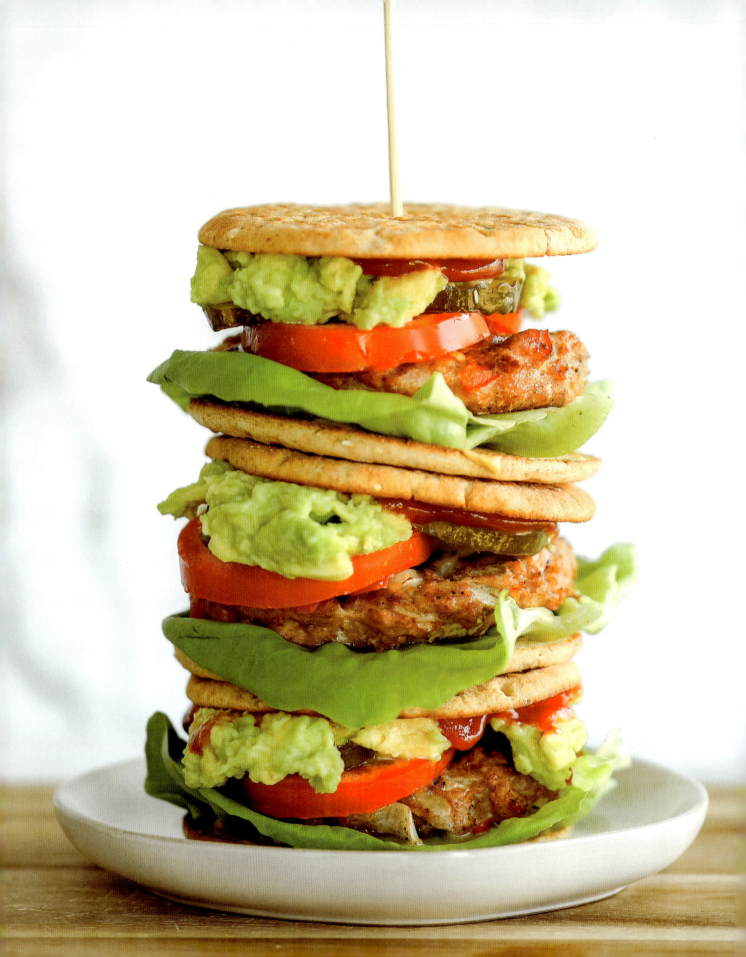

GUACAMOLE TURKEY BURGER

Makes 4 servings
350 calories / 13F / 32C / 26P / per serving

Prep: 10 min | **Cook:** 15 min

16 oz. raw lean ground turkey
½ cup yellow onions
½ cup red bell peppers
1 tsp. minced garlic
1 tsp. ground cumin
½ sp. sea salt
½ tsp. chili powder
4 whole wheat sandwich thins
Toppings:
4 butter lettuce leaves
2 tomato
4 dill pickles
4 Tbs. ketchup
2 Tbs. mustard
4 oz. guacamole

1. In a large bowl, mix the ground turkey, onions, bell peppers, garlic, cumin, sea salt and chili powder together.

2. Form into four equal-sized burger patties. Place on skillet or grill over medium heat for 5-8 minutes per side.

3. Place each burger patty on a sandwich thin and top with butter lettuce, two tomato slices, dill pickles, one tablespoon of ketchup, ½ tablespoon of mustard and 1 oz. of guacamole. Enjoy!

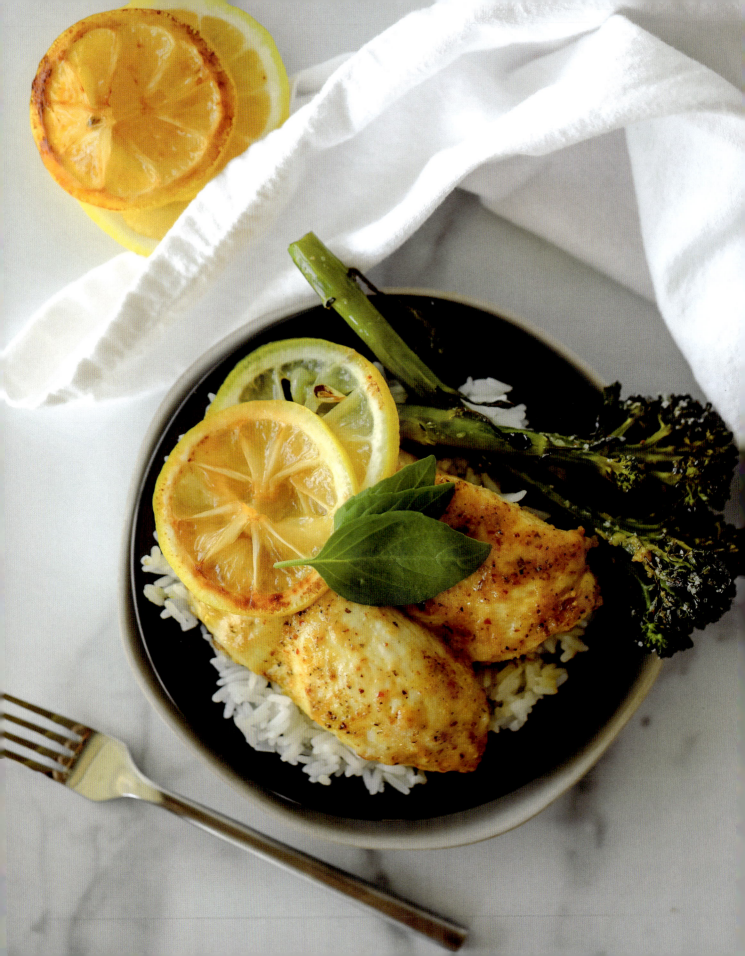

LEMON BUTTER CHICKEN

Makes 4 servings
335 calories / 12F / 32C / 25P / per serving

Prep: 10 min | **Cook:** 35 min

4 cups broccolini
2 cups cooked (⅔ cup uncooked) white jasmine rice
12 oz. raw chicken breast (9 oz. cooked)
2 Tbs. CSE Buttermilk or Gluten-Free Buttermilk Pancake & Waffle Mix
Dash sea salt
1 tsp. lemon pepper
¼ cup grass-fed butter
2 sliced lemons
Fresh, chopped basil leaves

1. Preheat the oven to 400 degrees. Chop the broccolini and place on a baking sheet lined with parchment paper. Spray the tops with cooking spray and sprinkle with sea salt. Roast in the oven for 20 minutes. Cook rice according to the directions on the package.

2. In a small bowl, combine the CSE Pancake & Waffle Mix, salt and lemon pepper.

3. Butterfly-cut chicken and place in a large bowl. Add the mix to the bowl and toss until well coated.

4. Heat a skillet to medium-high heat and add the butter. Once melted, add the chicken to the pan and cover. Cook for about 3-5 minutes per side or until cooked through and juices run clear. Add the lemon slices to the pan and cook for an additional minute.

5. Divide the Lemon Butter Chicken evenly into four servings. Serve each one over ½ cup of cooked rice with lemon slices, fresh basil and ¼ of the roasted broccolini on the side.

PRO TIP: Use microwavable rice pouches to cut down on cook time.

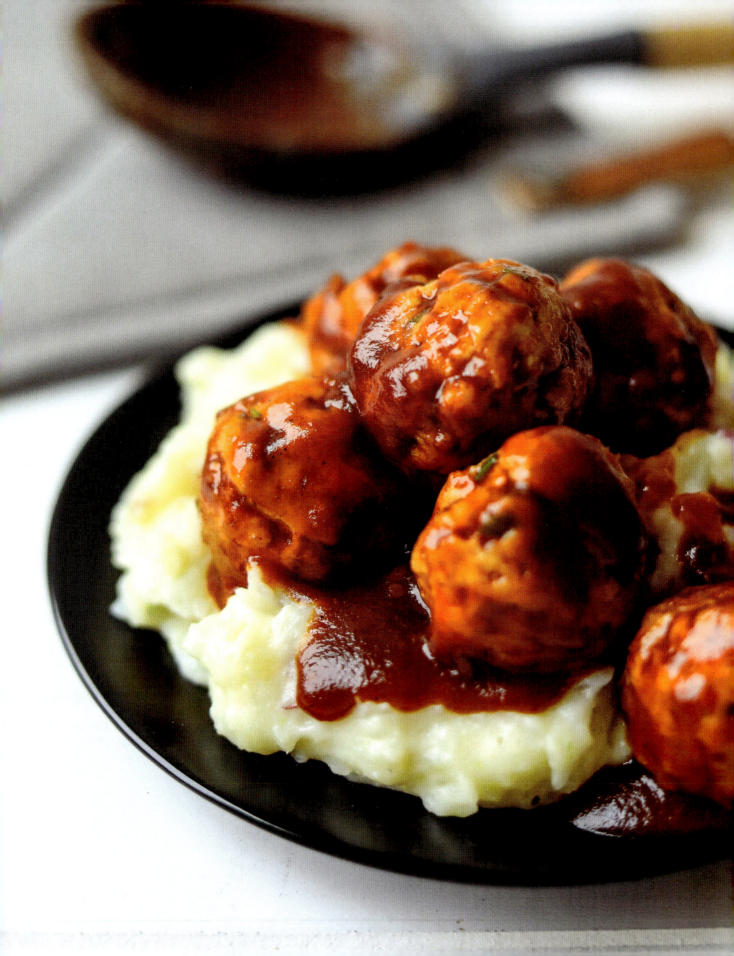

MEATBALLS & MASHED POTATOES

Makes 4 servings
350 calories / 11.5F / 34C / 28P / per serving

Prep: 20 min | **Cook:** 20 min

- 1 slice Ezekiel Bread or Harper's Bran Bread
- 12 oz. raw lean ground turkey
- ¼ cup yellow onions, minced
- 4 Tbs. chives
- 1 tsp. garlic powder
- Dash sea salt
- Dash black pepper
- ½ cup Stubb's BBQ Sauce
- 12 oz. baby gold potatoes
- 4 cups cauliflower florets
- 6 Tbs. nonfat, plain Greek yogurt
- ½ cup low-fat, mozzarella cheese, shredded
- 1 Tbs. grass-fed butter

1. Place the bread in a toaster and toast until lightly browned. Break into pieces and place in a blender. Pulse until bread is broken up into crumbs. Mix thawed ground turkey, breadcrumbs, onions, chives, garlic powder, salt and pepper in a bowl.

2. Heat a skillet to medium heat. Scoop the turkey mixture into balls. Spray skillet with cooking spray and add the meatballs. Flip every few minutes until all the sides are browned and the meatballs are fully cooked through. You can also bake the meatballs in the oven at 375 for 15-20 minutes. Add the BBQ sauce to the meatballs and stir until the meatballs are coated. Turn heat off; cover to keep warm.

3. Bring a pot of water to a boil. Add potatoes. Boil for 10 minutes. Add cauliflower to the pot with the potatoes and boil for another 10 minutes. Drain and remove from heat.

4. Add the Greek yogurt, cheese, butter, salt, pepper and a dash of garlic powder to the potatoes and cauliflower. Beat with a hand mixer until smooth and creamy.

5. Weigh the meatballs and the mashed potatoes separately, then divide the weight by four to get the amount needed to fill one serving. Serve meatballs over mashed potatoes.

PRO TIP: Cook the meatballs and mashed potatoes and freeze separately. Thaw in the fridge overnight. Reheat the potatoes in the microwave or a pot. Reheat the meatballs in a skillet or crockpot for 4 hours on high.

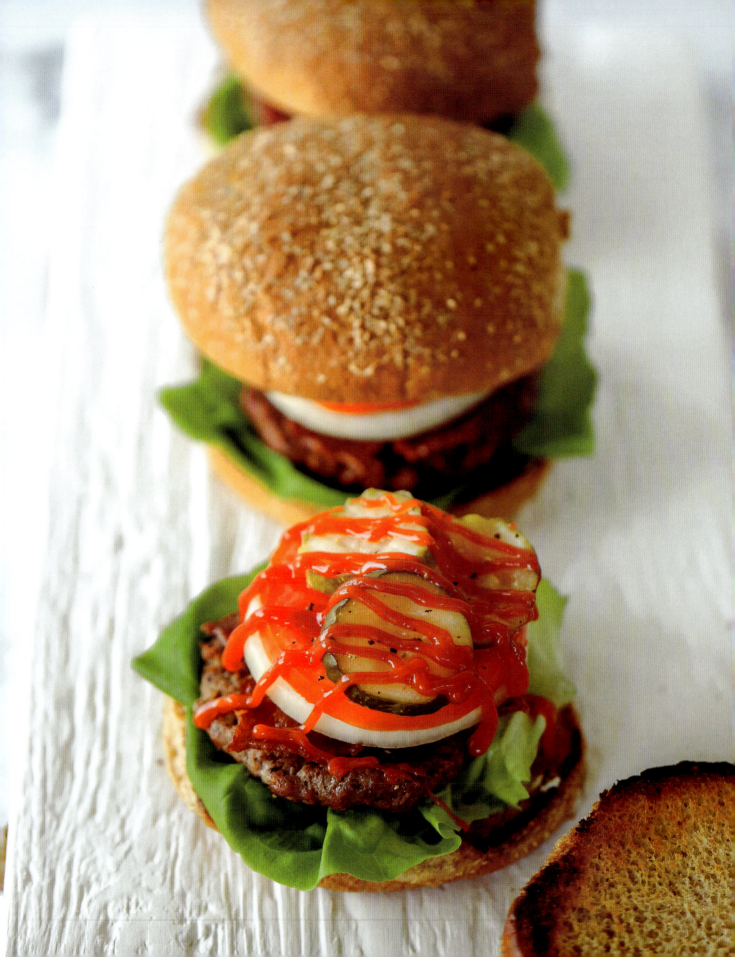

MUSTARD-FRIED BACON BURGER
Makes 4 servings
355 calories / 12F / 35C / 27.5P / per serving

Prep: 10 min | **Cook:** 15 min

10 oz. lean ground beef
2 tsp. Worcestershire sauce
2 tsp. yellow mustard
2 tsp. dried minced onions
½ tsp. garlic powder
½ tsp. sea salt
Dash black pepper
4 slices turkey bacon, chopped
1 sliced sweet onion
4 whole wheat buns
Butter lettuce
8 tomato slices
12 dill pickle slices
Toppings per serving:
½ Tbs. olive oil mayo
½ Tbs. ketchup

1. Heat grill to medium-high heat.

2. Add ground beef, Worcestershire sauce, mustard, dried minced onion, garlic powder, sea salt and black pepper to a bowl. Mix with hands until well combined. Weigh the mixture and divide by four. Form four equal-sized burger patties.

3. Place the burgers and bacon slices on the grill. Cook the burgers for 5-8 minutes per side and cook the bacon until crispy.

4. Heat a frying pan to medium-high heat. Grease and add the onion rings to the pan. Stir and flip until soft and golden on all sides.

5. Assemble burger by layering the bottom bun, lettuce, burger patty, tomatoes, pickles, turkey bacon, and onions. Spread mayo and ketchup on the top bun and place on your burger. Enjoy!

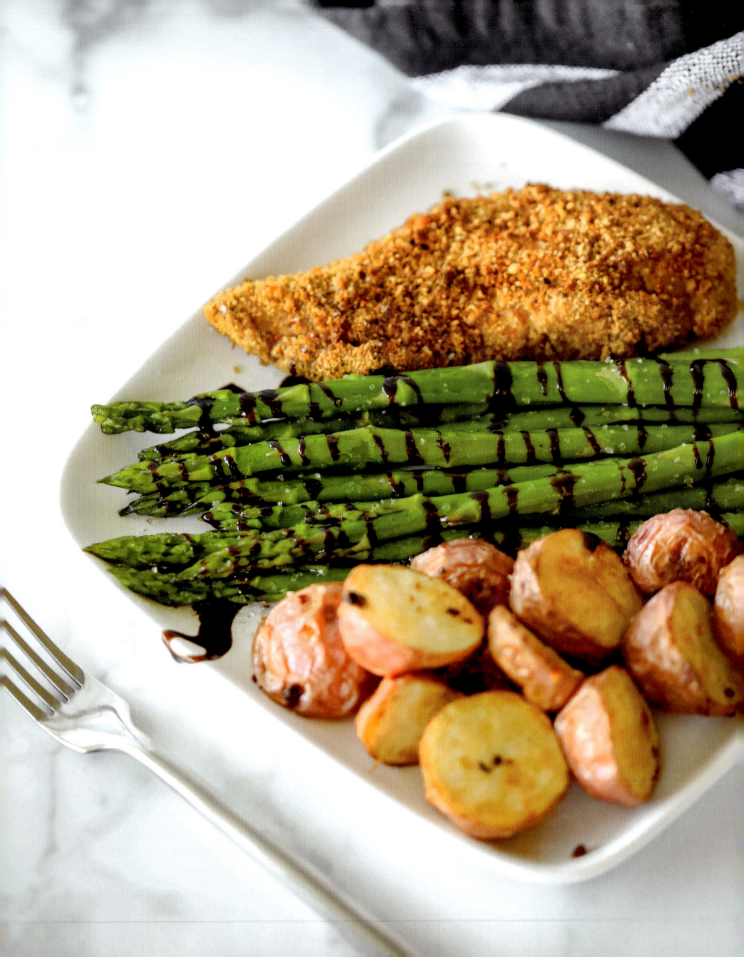

PARMESAN CHICKEN

Makes 4 servings
350 calories / 12F / 36C / 25P / per serving

Prep: 15 min │ **Cook:** 55 min

1 slice Ezekiel Bread or Harper's Bran Bread
1 oz. almonds
2 Tbs. grated Parmesan cheese
¼ tsp. granulated garlic
¼ tsp. dried thyme
½ tsp. sea salt
Dash black pepper
18 oz. baby red potatoes
1 Tbs. olive oil
2 tsp. fresh, minced garlic
9 oz. raw chicken tenderloins (6.75 oz. cooked)
1 egg white
48 asparagus spears
4 tsp. balsamic glaze

1. Toast the bread in the toaster until lightly browned. Place the toast into a blender with the almonds, Parmesan cheese, granulated garlic, thyme, sea salt and pepper. Pulse until broken up into crumbs; set aside.

2. Heat the oven to 400 degrees. Halve the potatoes and place in a large zip top bag. Add the olive oil, minced garlic and a dash of sea salt and black pepper to the bag. Massage until well coated. Pour out onto a baking sheet lined with parchment paper. Bake for 20 minutes; flip and bake an additional 20 minutes. Weigh and divide by four to get the amount needed to fill one serving.

3. Dip the chicken tenderloins in the egg whites and then dip into the bread crumb mixture. Place on a baking sheet lined with parchment paper. Bake at 400 degrees for 8 minutes. Flip the chicken over and add the asparagus to the pan. Spray the tops with cooking spray and sprinkle with sea salt. Bake the chicken and asparagus together for an additional 8 minutes. Weigh the chicken and divide the weight by four to get the amount needed to fill one serving. Serve the chicken with the potatoes and asparagus. Drizzle with balsamic glaze.

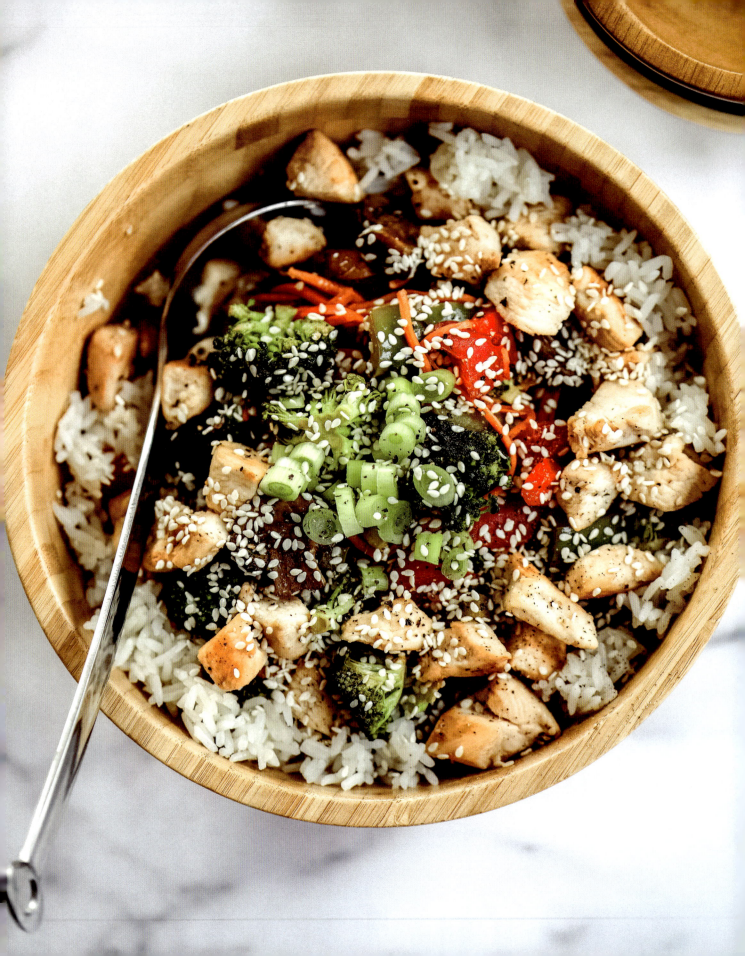

SESAME CHICKEN BOWL

Makes 4 servings
350 calories / 12F / 34C / 26P / per serving

Prep: 15 min | **Cook:** 20 min + marination

2 Tbs. olive oil
2 Tbs. coconut aminos
2 Tbs. raw honey
1 Tbs. fresh lemon juice
2 tsp. Worcestershire sauce
2 tsp. balsamic vinegar
2 tsp. sesame oil
1 tsp. dry mustard
½ tsp. black pepper
Dash sea salt
½ tsp. minced garlic

1 cup chopped bell peppers
1 cup sliced white mushrooms
1 cup chopped broccoli
1 cup matchstick carrots
10.5 oz. cooked chicken breast (14 oz. raw)
1 ⅓ cups cooked white jasmine rice (½ cup uncooked)

Toppings:
Green onions, for garnish
4 tsp. sesame seeds

1. Place olive oil, coconut aminos, honey, lemon juice, Worcestershire sauce, vinegar, sesame oil, dry mustard, black pepper, sea salt and minced garlic in a large zip top bag. Shake and massage mixture until combined. Add all the chopped veggies to the bag and let marinate in the fridge 2+ hours.

2. Cook or grill the chicken over medium heat until all sides are golden and the chicken is cooked through, about 5-7 minutes per side or until internal temperature reaches 160 degrees. After cooking, season as desired and slice. Prepare rice according to the directions on the package.

3. Place veggies and marinade in a large skillet over medium-high heat. Cook and stir veggies constantly for about 5 minutes or until tender-crisp.

4. Serve ⅓ cup cooked rice, with ¼ of the cooked chicken and ¼ of the marinated veggies in a bowl. Top with sliced green onions and one teaspoon of sesame seeds.

PRO TIP: Use microwavable rice pouches to cut down on cook time.

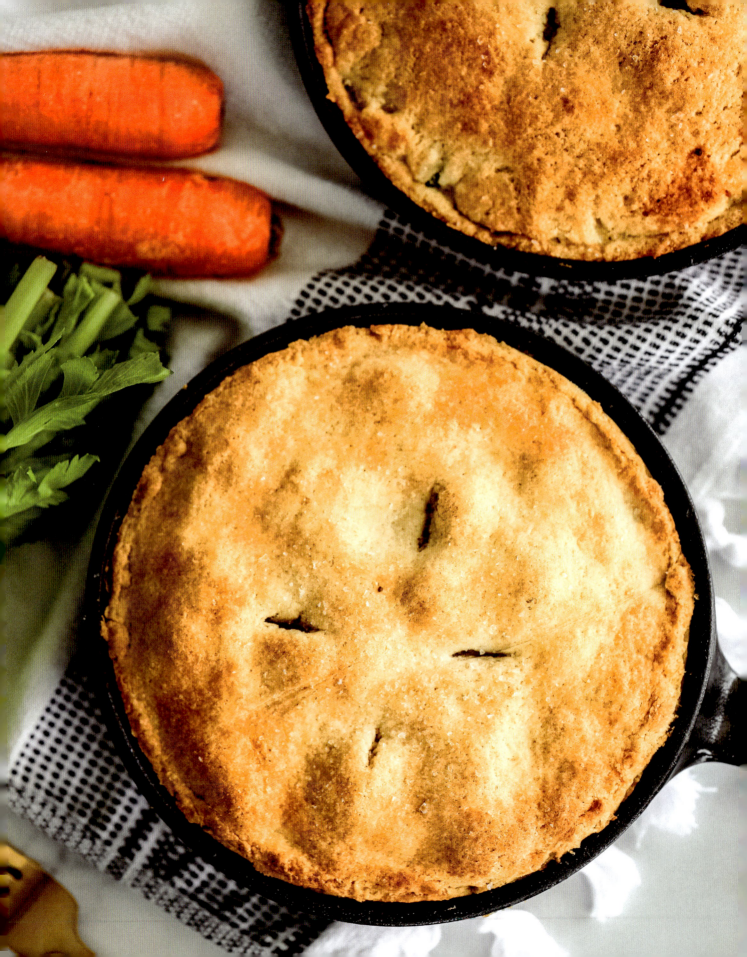

TURKEY POT PIES

Makes 4 servings
330 calories / 13.5F / 32C / 25P / per serving

Prep: 25 min | **Cook:** 30 min

Filling:
½ cup chopped carrots
½ cup thinly sliced celery
¼ cup finely chopped yellow onion
2 Tbs. CSE Buttermilk or Gluten-Free Buttermilk Pancake & Waffle Mix
Dash sea salt
Dash black pepper
¾ cup low-sodium chicken broth
¼ cup unsweetened almond milk
½ cup frozen peas
8 oz. chopped, roasted turkey breast

Crust:
1 ½ cups CSE Buttermilk or Gluten-Free Buttermilk Pancake & Waffle Mix
1 Tbs. grass-fed butter
2 Tbs. olive oil
3-4 Tbs. ice water

1. Preheat the oven to 425 degrees.

2. Spray a small sauce pan with cooking spray and add carrots, celery and onions. Sauté on medium-high heat until onions are translucent. Turn down heat and add two tablespoons of CSE Pancake & Waffle Mix, salt and pepper. Mix well.

3. Slowly stir in the chicken broth and milk. Bring to a boil and then turn down to low and let simmer for about 5 minutes or until sauce begins to thicken. Stir in the peas and turkey. Mix well and set aside.

4. For the crust, pour the CSE Pancake & Waffle Mix into a bowl. Cut butter into the CSE Pancake & Waffle Mix with two knives until butter is in very small pieces. Add the olive oil, then slowly add the ice water until the dough comes together and isn't sticky. You may not need all the water.

5. Roll out the dough into a rectangle between two sheets of parchment paper. Dough should be thin, about ⅛ of an inch, as it will puff when it bakes. Peel the top piece of parchment paper off dough and slice into eight equal portions. Place four pieces of the dough face down into four mini pie dishes. Press the dough to fit the dish and create a crust edge.

6. Evenly pour ¼ of the turkey mixture into each pie dish and cover with the top crust, pinching the edges together. Place the mini pie dishes on a baking sheet. Cut a couple slits in the top of each pie and bake for 20 minutes. Enjoy warm.

PRO TIP: Double the recipe and make one large pie using a 9-inch pie pan instead of four mini pies. Roll the dough out into two equal-sized rounds. Use one for the bottom crust and one for the top crust following the instructions above.

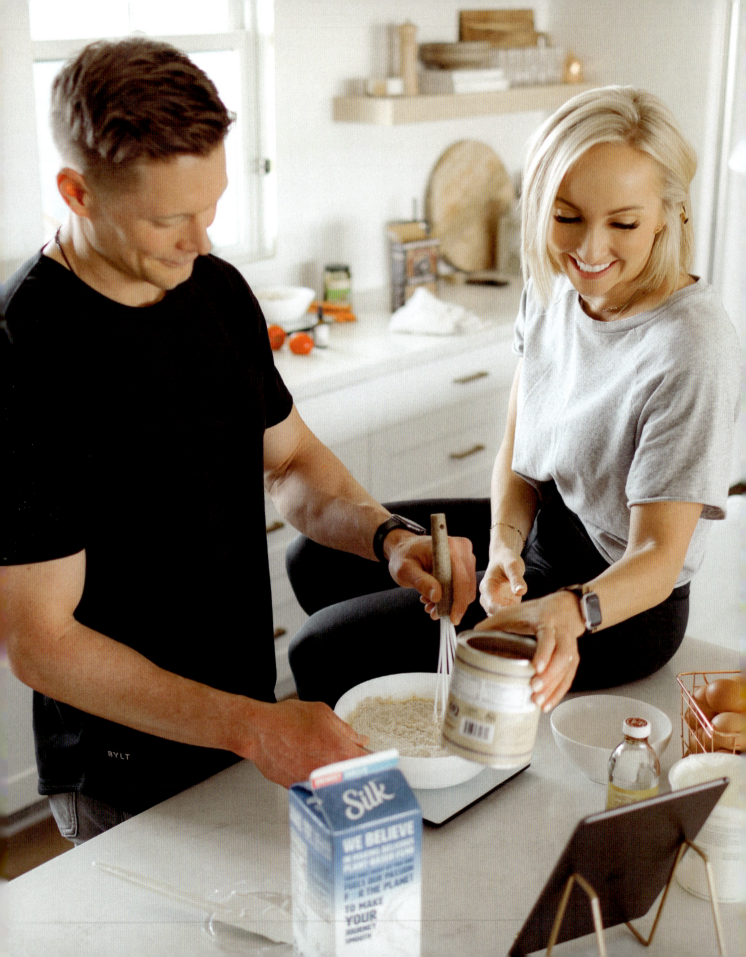

DESSERTS

We know we don't have to tell you how we feel about dessert - that's why we've put a healthier spin on all of our favorites without sacrificing any of that chocolatey, peanut-buttery, sweet-cinna, or fruity goodness. We're bringing you all of the flavor with none of the crash. From **Brownies & Bars** to **Cakes & Crumbles** to **Breads & Rolls**, we've never met a CSE dessert we didn't like. Share the **Cookies** and **Party Treats** with your friends! We're pretty sure they'll be the hit of the party and no one will ever guess they were made with healthier ingredients! Shhh… that's our little secret!

BREADS & ROLLS

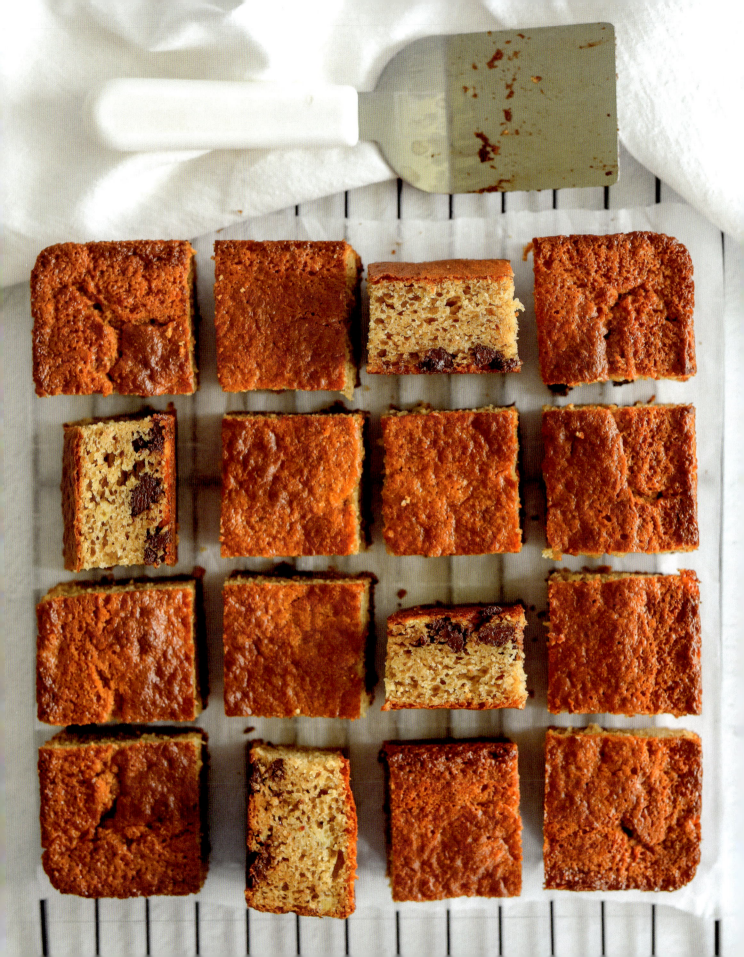

CHOCOLATE CHIP BANANA BREAD SQUARES
Makes 16 servings
145 calories / 5F / 21.5C / 4P / per square

Prep: 10 min | **Cook:** 35 min

2 ripe bananas
½ cup unsweetened applesauce
3 Tbs. melted coconut oil
½ cup raw honey
1 large egg
1 tsp. vanilla extract
1 ½ cups CSE Buttermilk, Gluten-Free Buttermilk,
   or Vanilla Pancake & Waffle Mix
½ tsp. baking soda
½ tsp baking powder
½ tsp. ground cinnamon
¼ tsp. sea salt
½ cup dark chocolate chips

1. Preheat the oven to 350 degrees.

2. Mash the bananas in a large bowl. Beat in the applesauce, melted coconut oil and honey. Add the egg and vanilla; mix well.

3. In a separate bowl, combine the CSE Pancake & Waffle Mix, baking soda, baking powder, cinnamon and sea salt. Add the dry ingredients to the wet ingredients and mix until just combined.

4. Pour the mixture into a greased 8x8 baking pan. Sprinkle the chocolate chips on top. Bake for 30-35 minutes, then let cool. Cut into 16 squares. Store extras in the fridge or freezer.

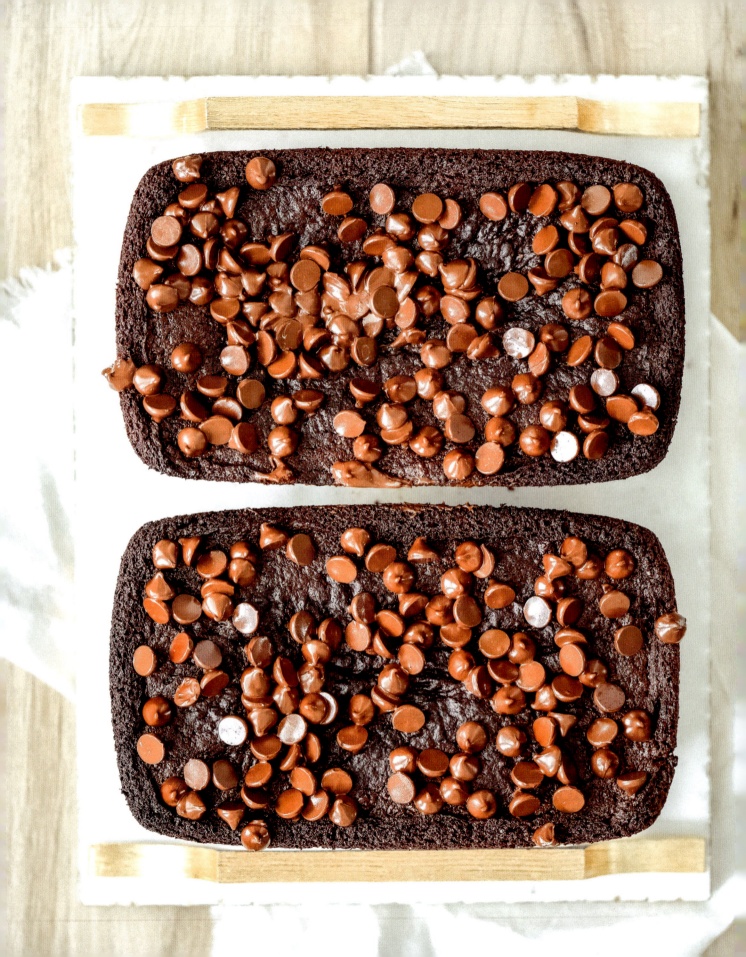

DOUBLE CHOCOLATE BANANA BREAD
Makes 1 loaf / 10 slices
240 calories / 10.5F / 35C / 7.5P / per slice

Prep: 10 min | **Cook:** 55 min

3 ripe bananas
½ cup unsweetened applesauce
½ cup raw honey
¼ cup melted coconut oil
1 large egg
1 tsp. vanilla extract
1 cup CSE Chocolate Chocolate or Gluten-Free Chocolate Chocolate Pancake & Waffle Mix
1 serving CSE Chocolate Brownie Batter Protein Powder
⅓ cup cocoa powder
½ tsp. baking soda
½ tsp baking powder
½ tsp. sea salt
½ cup dark chocolate chips

1. Preheat the oven to 350 degrees.

2. Mash the bananas in a large bowl. Beat in the applesauce, honey and melted coconut oil. Add the egg and vanilla; mix well.

3. In a separate bowl, combine the CSE Pancake & Waffle Mix, protein powder, cocoa powder, baking soda, baking powder and sea salt. Add the dry ingredients to the wet ingredients. Mix until just combined.

4. Pour into a greased 9x5 inch glass loaf pan and sprinkle with the chocolate chips. Bake for 50-55 minutes, then let cool. Remove from the pan and drizzle with extra melted chocolate, if desired. Store extras in the fridge or freezer.

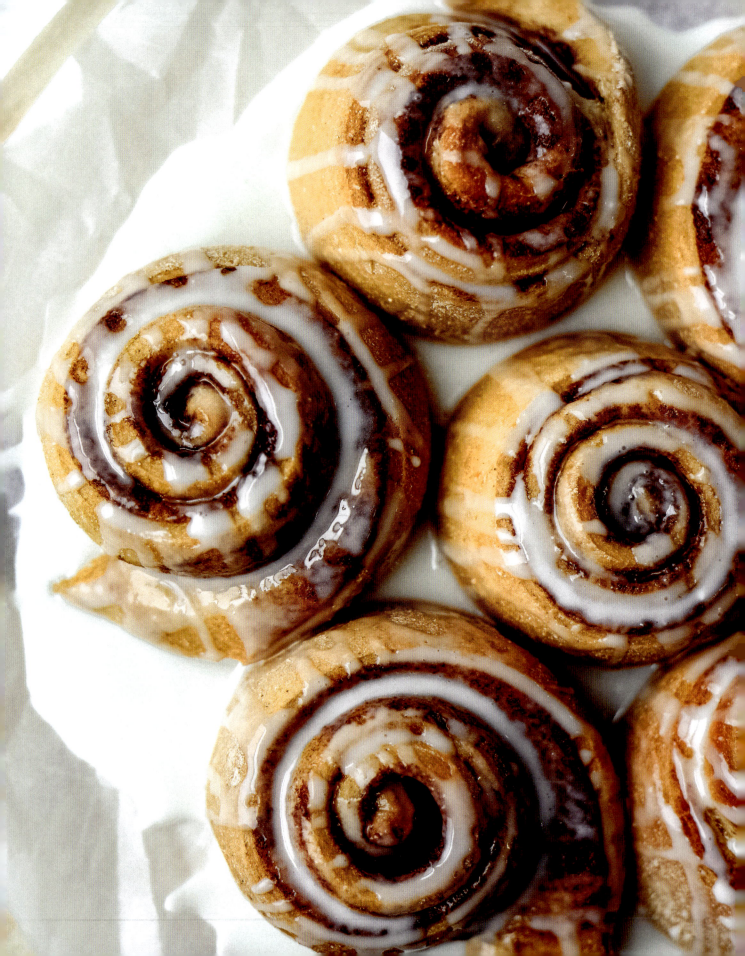

SWEET HONEY CINNAMON ROLLS
Makes 24 rolls
185 calories / 6F / 29C / 4P / per roll with icing

Prep: 30 min | **Cook:** 30 min + rise time

2 large eggs
2 ½ tsp. instant yeast
½ cup warm water (100-115 degrees)
1 cup cooked, peeled & mashed
  sweet potatoes
1 cup unsweetened almond milk
½ cup cold grass-fed butter
½ cup raw honey
1 tsp. sea salt
5 cups white whole wheat flour

Filling:
2 Tbs. grass-fed butter, melted
2 Tbs. coconut sugar
1 Tbs. ground cinnamon
Icing:
1 cup powdered sugar
2 Tbs. pasteurized egg whites
¼ tsp. butter extract

1. Bring a pot of water to a boil. Cube the sweet potatoes and add to the pot. Boil for 20 minutes or until soft. Remove the skins and mash.

2. Beat eggs in a small bowl; set aside. In a separate bowl, dissolve yeast into warm water (100-115 degrees). Once dissolved, pour eggs into water with yeast; set aside. Remove the skins from the cooked sweet potatoes and beat with hand mixers until smooth; set aside.

3. Heat almond milk in a pot over high heat until small bubbles form around the edges. Remove from heat. Add the cold butter, honey, salt and sweet potatoes. Stir until all the butter is melted and the mixture is smooth.

4. Place in a bread or Kitchen Aid Mixer. Add the egg mixture and the flour. Knead for 10 minutes. Cover and let rise in the fridge for 2 hours.

5. Split the dough in half. Place the dough on a floured surface and roll both pieces into large, thin rectangles. Mix the filling ingredients together and then spread evenly over dough. Slice each rectangle into 12 strips and roll up. Place on a greased baking sheet; 12 rolls per sheet. Cover with a dish towel and let rise for 5+ hours or overnight.

6. Bake at 375 degrees for 12 minutes or until lightly browned. Beat icing ingredients together and drizzle over the top. Enjoy!

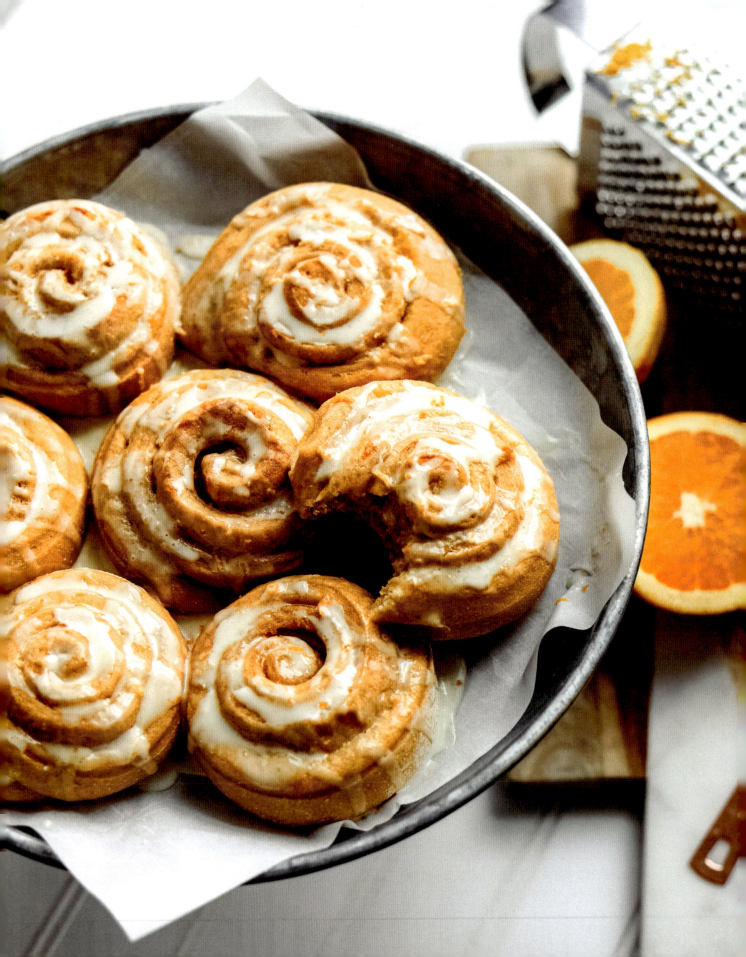

ZESTY ORANGE SWEET ROLLS
Makes 24 rolls
185 calories / 6F / 29C / 4P / per roll with glaze

Prep: 30 min | **Cook:** 30 min + rise time

2 large eggs
2 ½ tsp. instant yeast
½ cup warm water (100-115 degrees)
1 cup cooked, peeled & mashed sweet potatoes
1 cup unsweetened almond milk
½ cup cold grass-fed butter
½ cup raw honey
1 tsp. sea salt
5 cups white whole wheat flour

Filling:
2 Tbs. melted grass-fed butter
2 Tbs. raw honey
1 tsp. orange zest

Glaze:
1 cup powdered sugar
2 Tbs. pasteurized egg whites
1 Tbs. fresh-squeezed orange juice
1 tsp. orange zest

1. Bring a pot of water to a boil. Cube the sweet potatoes and add to the pot. Boil for 20 minutes or until soft. Remove the skins and mash.

2. Beat eggs in a small bowl; set aside. In a separate bowl, dissolve yeast into warm water (110-115 degrees). Once dissolved, pour eggs into water with yeast; set aside. Remove the skins from the sweet potatoes and beat with hand mixers until smooth; set aside.

3. Heat almond milk in a pot over high heat until small bubbles form around the edges. Remove from heat. Add the cold butter, honey, salt and sweet potatoes. Stir until the butter is melted and the mixture is smooth.

4. Place in a bread machine or Kitchen Aid Mixer. Add the egg mixture and flour. Knead for 10 minutes. Cover and let rise in the fridge for 2 hours.

5. Split the dough in half. Place the dough on a floured surface and roll both pieces into large, thin rectangles. Mix the filling ingredients together and then spread evenly over the dough. Slice each rectangle into 12 strips and roll up. Place on a greased baking sheet; 12 rolls per sheet. Cover with a dish towel and let rise for 5+ hours or overnight.

6. Bake at 375 degrees for 12 minutes or until lightly browned. Beat glaze ingredients together and drizzle over the top. Enjoy!

BROWNIES & BARS

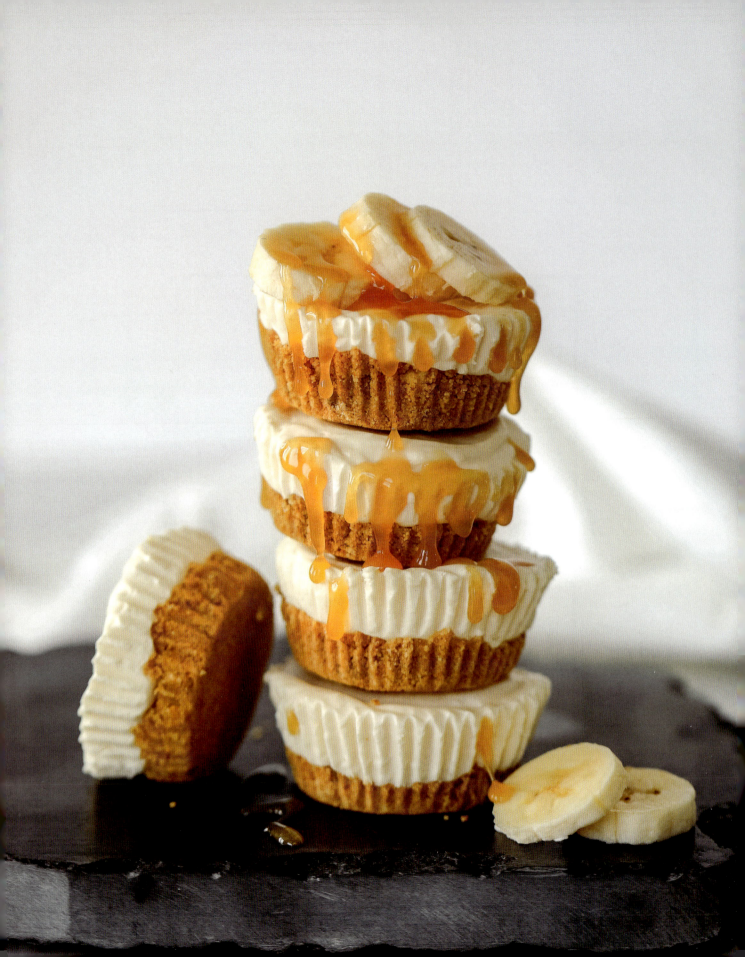

BANANA CHEESECAKE CUPS
Makes 12 servings
165 calories / 10F / 11.5C / 7P / per serving

Prep: 15 min + freezing

Crust:
1 cup (100g) graham cracker crumbs
2 Tbs. (28g) grass-fed butter
1 Tbs. (14g) CSE Monkey Business Butter

Cheesecake:
1 cup (8 oz.) organic cream cheese, room temperature
2 servings (72g) CSE Bananas Foster Protein Powder
1 ½ cups (125g) TruWhip Skinny
⅔ cup (150g) plain, nonfat Greek yogurt

1. Place 12 cupcake liners in a muffin tin. Set aside.

2. Add the Graham cracker crumbs to a bowl. Melt the butter. Add the melted butter and Monkey Business Butter to the bowl. Stir until well combined. Weigh the mixture and divide evenly into the 12 cupcake liners. Press into the bottom and freeze.

3. Add the softened cream cheese to a mixing bowl and beat until smooth. Slowly mix in the protein powder until well combined. Add the TruWhip and Greek yogurt; beat until smooth.

4. Weigh the mixture and divide evenly into the cupcake liners and smooth out the tops.

5. Cover with foil and freeze for 2+ hours. When ready to eat, remove the cupcake liner and let thaw out of the freezer for about 5-10 minutes. Enjoy!

PRO TIP: You can also make this in an 8x8 baking pan. Layer the ingredients, cover with foil and freeze for 2+ hours. When ready to eat, cut into 12 squares.

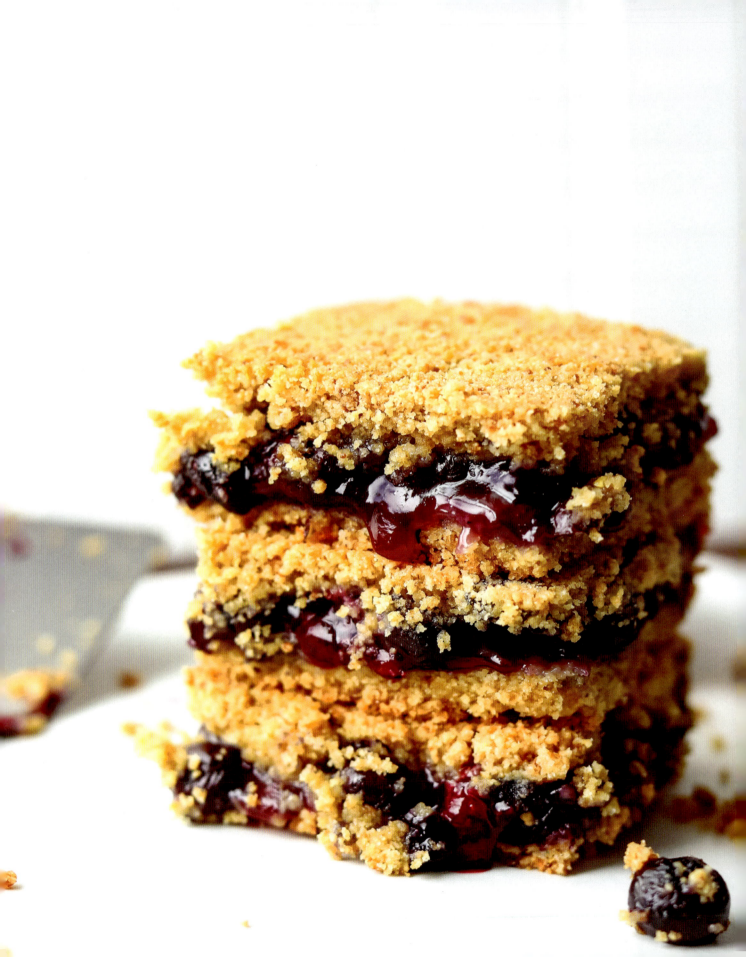

BLUEBERRY CRUMBLE BARS

Makes 18 bars
200 calories / 9.5F / 27.5C / 6P / per bar

Prep: 10 min | **Cook:** 30 min

Crust/Topping:
- ¾ cup xylitol sweetener
- ¼ cup coconut sugar
- 3 cups CSE Buttermilk, Gluten-Free Buttermilk, or Vanilla Pancake & Waffle Mix
- ¼ tsp. sea salt
- 1 lemon, zest of
- ¾ cup grass-fed butter
- ¼ cup flaxseed meal
- 1 large egg

Filling:
- 1 Tbs. cornstarch or arrowroot powder
- 2 Tbs. water
- ¼ cup xylitol sweetener
- ¼ cup raw honey
- 4 cups fresh blueberries

1. Preheat the oven to 375 degrees.

2. Stir together the xylitol, coconut sugar, CSE Pancake & Waffle Mix, sea salt and lemon zest in a bowl. Add the butter, flaxseed meal and egg. Stir together until the mixture begins to ball. Split the mixture in half and press one half of it into the bottom of a greased 9x13 baking pan.

3. Make the filling: In a small bowl, dissolve the cornstarch or arrowroot powder in two tablespoons of water. Add that mixture to a saucepan over low heat with the xylitol and honey; whisk until smooth. Add the blueberries to the pan. Turn the heat up to high and bring to a boil, stirring constantly with a rubber spatula. Remove from heat and continue to stir as the sauce thickens. Pour the blueberry mixture evenly over the top of the crust and then sprinkle the remaining crumble mixture over the top and press down to cover the blueberry filling.

4. Bake for 20-25 minutes or until the top is golden brown. Let cool completely and then cut into bars. Enjoy as is or topped with whipped cream or ice cream. Enjoy! Store extras in the fridge.

PRO TIP: My kids love having these for breakfast too!

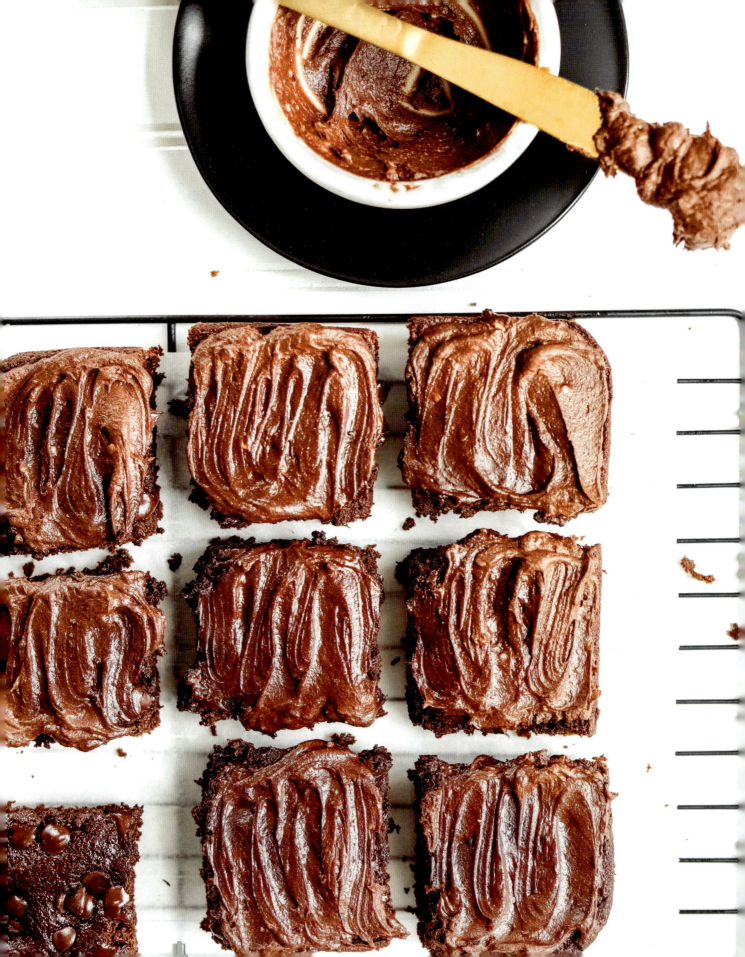

CHOVOCADO BROWNIES

Makes 12 brownies
180 calories / 6.5F / 27C / 4P / per brownie

Prep: 15 min | **Cook:** 25 min + cooling

⅔ cup raw honey
⅓ cup cocoa powder
½ cup unsweetened applesauce
1 tsp. vanilla extract
2 Tbs. light-tasting olive oil
1 large egg
½ cup white whole wheat flour
1 Tbs. flaxseed meal
¼ tsp. baking soda
¼ tsp. baking powder
¼ tsp. sea salt
¼ cup dark chocolate chips

Chovocado Frosting:
¼ (25g) of a ripe avocado
2 Tbs. CSE Sweet Classic or Buckeye Brownie Peanut Butter or natural almond butter
2 Tbs. cocoa powder
1 serving CSE Chocolate Brownie Batter Protein Powder
¼ cup unsweetened almond milk
1 Tbs. raw honey

1. Preheat the oven to 350 degrees.

2. Heat the honey in the microwave for 45 seconds. Stir the cocoa powder into the honey until completely dissolved; set aside.

3. In a separate bowl, beat the applesauce, vanilla, olive oil and egg together. Add the chocolate/honey mixture to the bowl; mix well. Add the flour, flaxseed meal, baking soda, baking powder and sea salt to the bowl and mix until just combined.

4. Pour the batter into a greased 8x8 baking dish. Sprinkle the chocolate chips over the top. Bake for 25 minutes, then let cool.

5. Beat all of the frosting ingredients together in a bowl. Once the brownies are cooled off, spread the frosting over the top and slice into 12 servings. Enjoy!

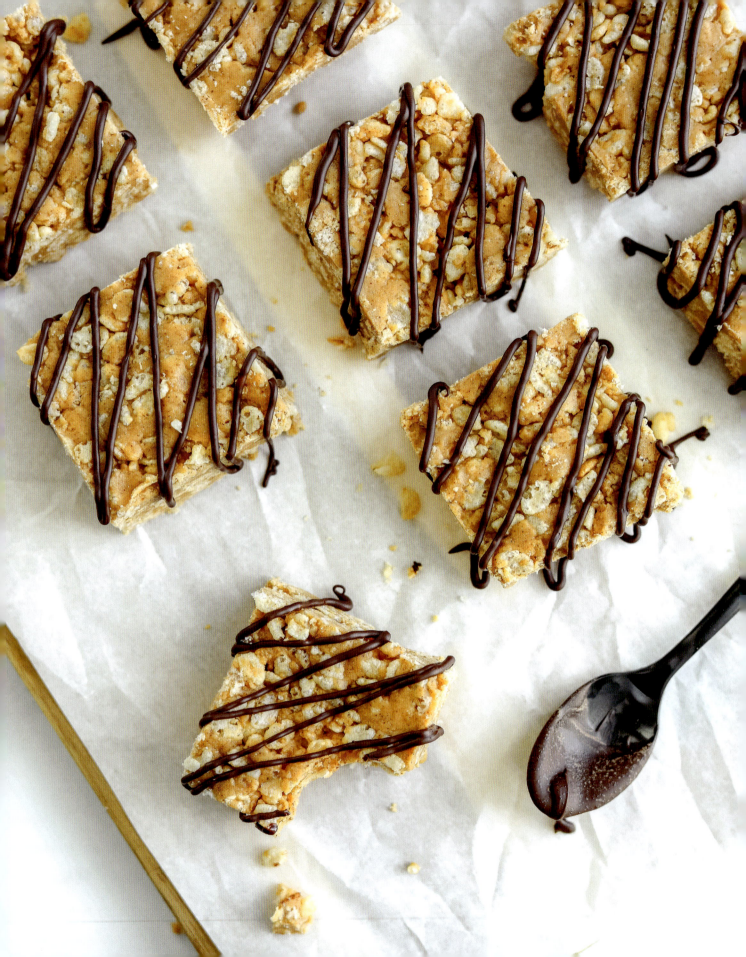

CRISPY CARAMEL BUTTERSCOTCH BARS
Makes 18 bars
225 calories / 12.5F / 23C / 5P / per bar

Prep: 10 min | **Cook:** 5 min

12 oz. CSE Salted Caramel Butter
   or natural almond butter
½ cup raw honey
2 Tbs. unsweetened almond milk
½ cup butterscotch chips
1 serving CSE Caramel Toffee
   or Simply Vanilla Protein Powder
3 ¾ cups Nature's Path Crispy Rice Cereal
Topping:
¼ cup dark chocolate chips

1. Add the nut butter, honey, almond milk and butterscotch chips to a saucepan over low-medium heat. Stir until the butterscotch chips are melted and the mixture is smooth. Remove from heat and stir in the protein powder. Mix until well combined.

2. Pour the cereal into a large bowl and top with the caramel butterscotch mixture. Beat together until the ingredients are well combined. Press into a greased 9x13 pan. Store in the fridge until hardened and cool.

3. Place the chocolate chips in a small bowl. Microwave for 1-2 minutes or until melted and smooth, stirring every 30 seconds.

4. Remove the bars from the 9x13 pan onto a cutting board. Cut into 18 squares. Drizzle the chocolate over the top of the bars. Let the chocolate harden, then enjoy! Store leftovers in the fridge.

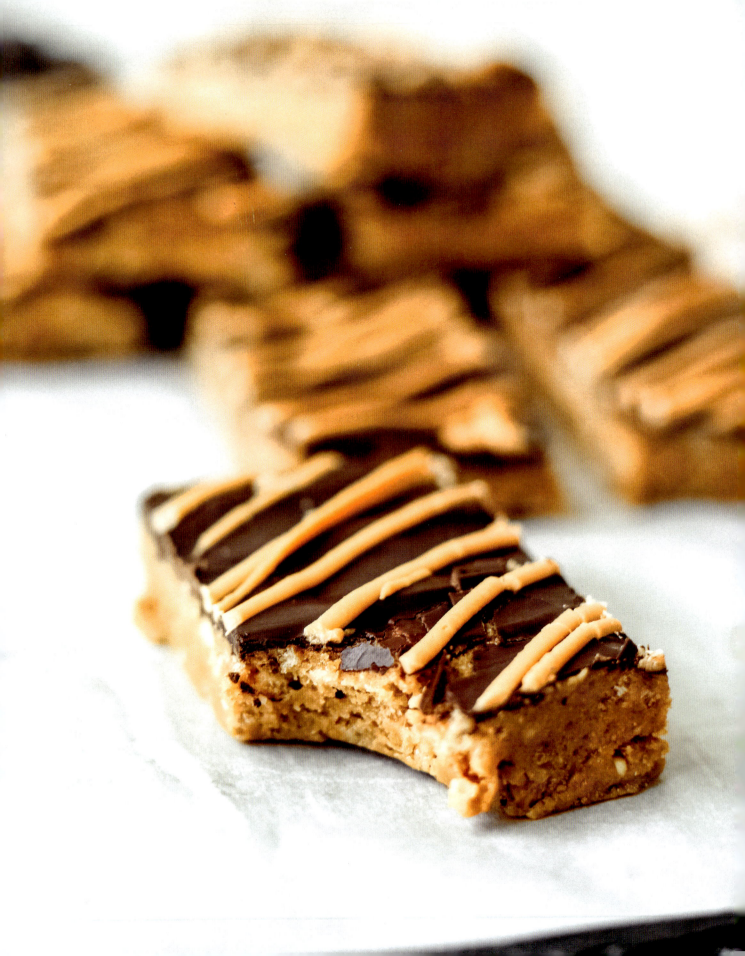

SCOTCHAROO BARS
Makes 18 bars
255 calories / 12.5F / 28.5C / 7.5P / per bar

Prep: 10 min | **Cook:** 2 min + freezing

- 1 cup CSE Sweet Classic Peanut Butter or natural peanut butter
- 1 cup CSE Powdered Peanut Butter
- ¾ cup raw honey
- ¼ cup flaxseed meal
- 2 Tbs. unsweetened almond milk
- 1 tsp. vanilla extract
- ¼ tsp. sea salt
- 1 serving CSE Simply Vanilla Protein Powder
- ¼ cup butterscotch chips
- 2 cups Nature's Path Crispy Rice Cereal

Toppings:
- ¼ cup butterscotch chips
- ½ cup dark chocolate chips

1. Mix the peanut butter, powdered peanut butter, honey, flaxseed meal, almond milk, vanilla extract, sea salt and protein powder together in a bowl. Melt ¼ cup of the butterscotch chips and mix in. Add the Crispy Rice cereal last and gently mix until well combined. Press into a 9x13 pan; set aside.

2. Place the chocolate chips in a bowl and microwave 30 seconds at a time until completely melted and smooth, stirring in between. Drizzle over the top of the bars and spread out smooth. Melt the remaining ¼ cup of butterscotch chips and drizzle over the top of the chocolate.

3. Store in the fridge for 1 hour to allow the chocolate to harden. Cut into 18 bars. Enjoy!

CAKES & CRUMBLES

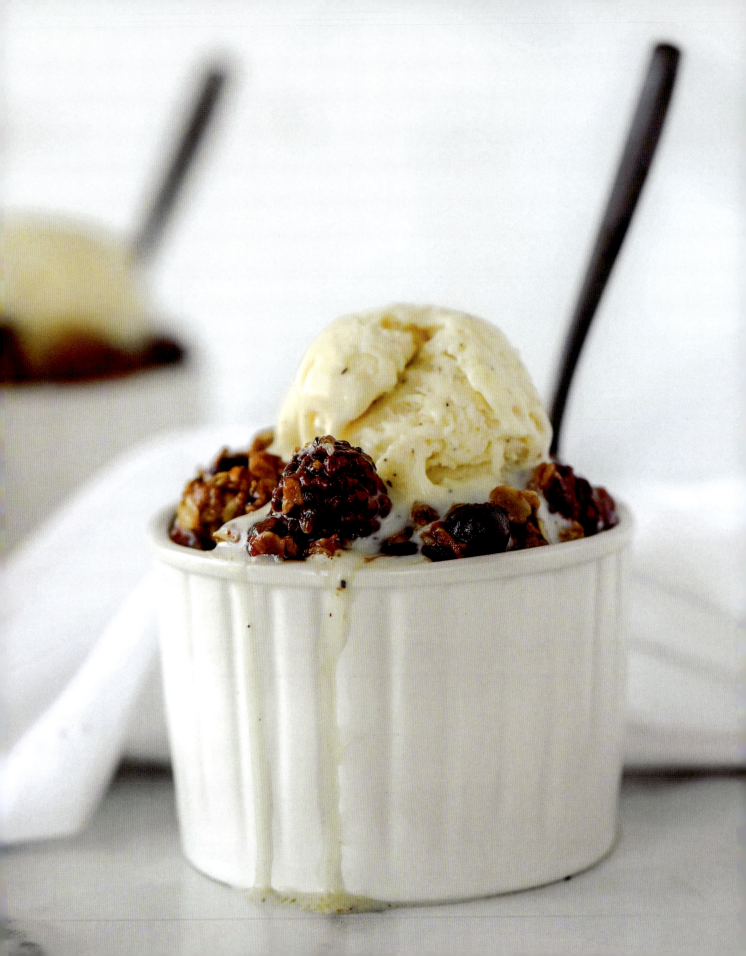

BERRY COBBLER CRUMBLE

Makes 15 servings
290 calories / 13.5F / 37.5C / 4.5P / per serving

Prep: 10 min | **Cook:** 35 min

2 cups blueberries
2 cups blackberries
2 cups raspberries
¼ cup raw honey
2 cups old-fashioned rolled oats
1 cup whole wheat pastry flour
½ cup hemp seed hearts
1 cup coconut sugar
2 tsp. cinnamon
½ tsp. nutmeg
1 cup melted, grass-fed butter or coconut oil

Optional Toppings:
Spray whipped cream
High protein ice cream

1. Preheat the oven to 350 degrees.

2. Add the berries and honey to a large bowl. Stir together until the berries are well coated in the honey; set aside.

3. In a separate bowl, add the oats, flour, hemp hearts, coconut sugar, cinnamon and nutmeg. Whisk together. Add the melted butter or coconut oil and stir until well combined and crumbly.

4. Press ⅔ of the crumble mixture into the bottom of a greased 9x13 baking dish. Pour the berry mixture and all the juices from the bowl over the crust. Top evenly with the remaining crumble mixture.

5. Bake for 30-35 minutes. Serve warm. Enjoy as is or top each individual serving with vanilla high protein ice cream or spray whipped cream (not included in macros). Store leftovers in the fridge.

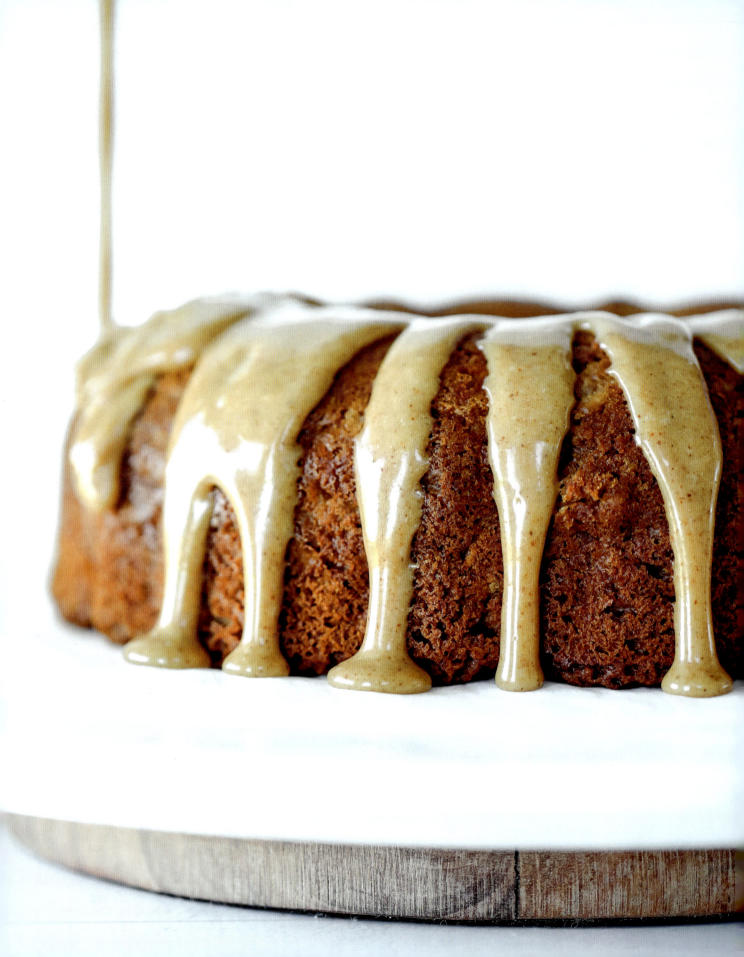

CARAMEL APPLE CAKE

Makes 16 servings
235 calories / 7.5F / 38C / 4P / per serving

Prep: 15 min | **Cook:** 45 min + cooling

1 cup raw honey
2 Tbs. grass-fed butter or coconut oil
2 Tbs. light-tasting olive oil
2 large eggs
1 tsp. vanilla extract
4 cups peeled, shredded apples
2 cups white whole wheat flour
2 tsp. ground cinnamon
2 tsp. baking soda
2 tsp. ground nutmeg
1 tsp. sea salt
½ tsp. ground cloves

Caramel Sauce:
½ cup CSE Salted Caramel, Cinnamon Bun Butter
  or natural almond butter
½ cup raw honey
1 tsp. vanilla extract

1. Preheat the oven to 350 degrees.

2. Beat the honey, butter and olive oil together in a bowl. Beat in the eggs and vanilla. Fold in the shredded apples and mix in all the dry ingredients.

3. Pour the batter into a well-greased Bundt pan. Bake for 45 minutes. Let cool for 30-60 minutes.

4. Make the Caramel Sauce just before serving. In a small saucepan, mix the nut butter, honey and vanilla over medium heat. Stir constantly until all the ingredients melt together. Drizzle the caramel sauce evenly over the top of the cake. Slice into 16 servings. Enjoy!

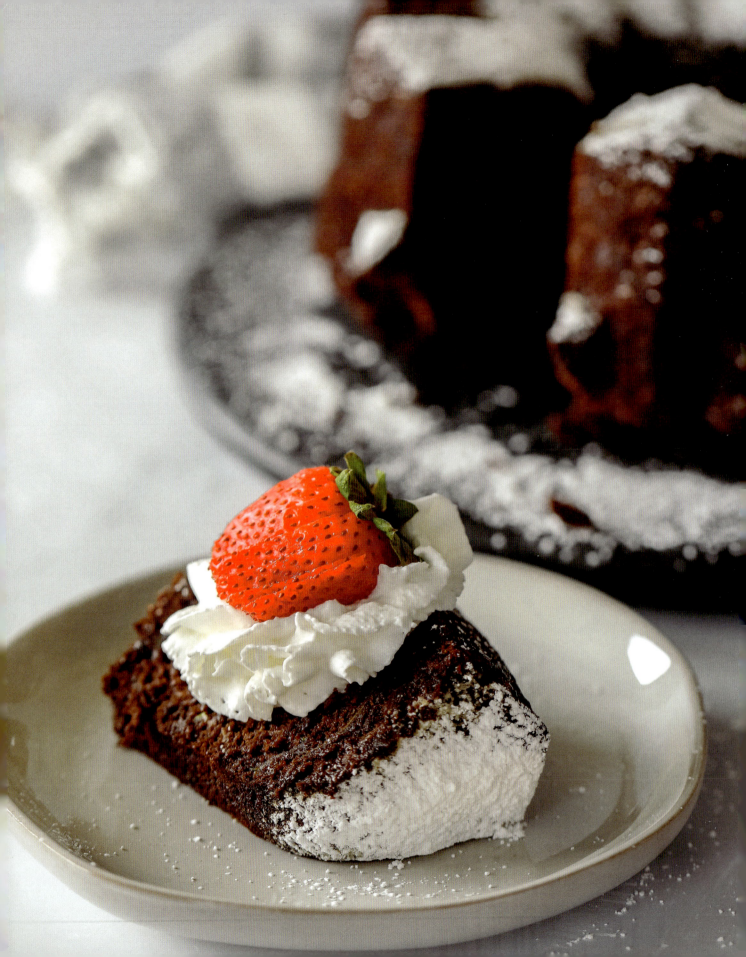

CHOCOLATE ZUCCHINI CAKE
Makes 15 servings
345 calories / 16F / 45C / 5P / per serving

Prep: 15 min | **Cook:** 40 min

2 cups whole wheat pastry flour
¾ cup cocoa powder
2 tsp. baking soda
1 tsp. baking powder
1 tsp. cinnamon
½ tsp. sea salt
1 cup raw honey
¾ cup coconut oil, softened
½ cup coconut sugar
4 large eggs
¾ cup unsweetened applesauce
3 cups grated zucchini
1 cup dark chocolate chips
Optional Toppings:
Spray whipped cream
High protein ice cream
Fresh berries
Chocolate frosting (recipe from the Double Chocolate Donuts on the next page)

1. Preheat the oven to 350 degrees.

2. Combine the flour, cocoa powder, baking soda, baking powder, cinnamon and salt in a large bowl; set aside.

3. In a separate bowl, beat the honey, coconut oil and coconut sugar together. Beat in the eggs and applesauce; add to the dry ingredients and mix until just combined. Fold in the grated zucchini and chocolate chips.

4. Pour the batter into a greased 9x13 baking dish or Bundt cake pan. Bake for 40 minutes. Insert a toothpick into the center of the cake to make sure it is done. Top with optional toppings (not included in the macros). Enjoy!

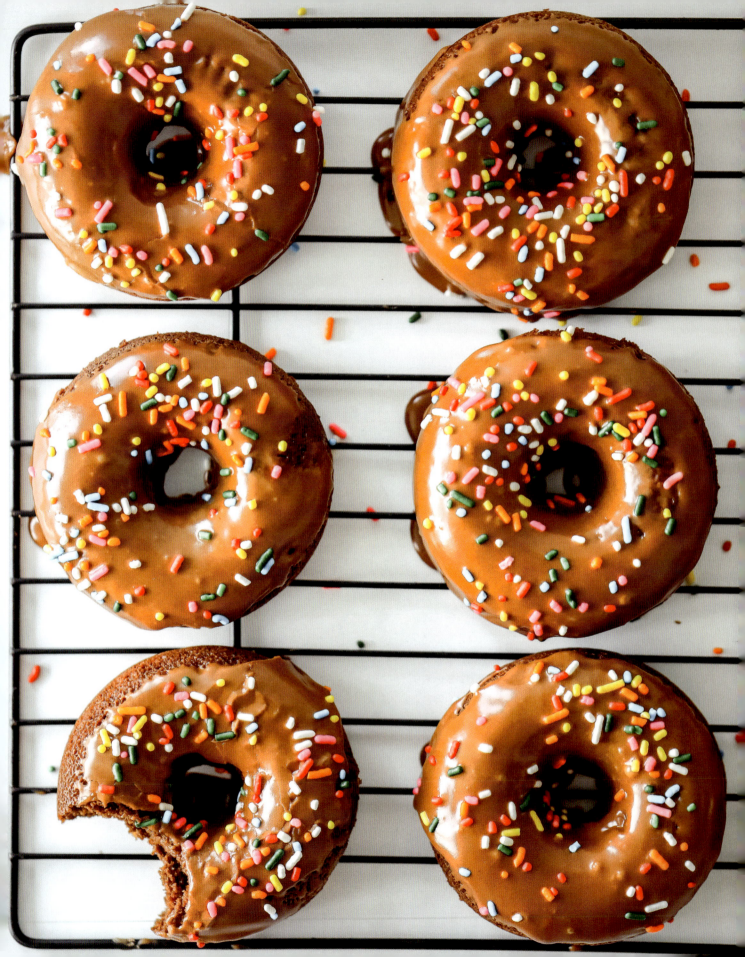

DOUBLE CHOCOLATE CAKE DONUTS
Makes 14 donuts
260 calories / 7.5F / 45.5C / 4.5P / per donut

Prep: 15 min | **Cook:** 40 min

Donuts:
1 cup whole wheat pastry flour
1 serving CSE Chocolate Brownie Batter or Chocolate Peanut Butter Protein Powder
½ cup cocoa powder
1 tsp. baking powder
¼ tsp. baking soda
Dash sea salt
¼ cup melted coconut oil
½ cup raw honey
¼ cup pure maple syrup
¼ cup unsweetened applesauce
½ cup cooked, mashed sweet potatoes
½ tsp. vanilla extract
2 large eggs

Frosting:
2 cups powdered sugar
¼ cup pasteurized liquid egg whites
50g chocolate chips
1 tsp. coconut oil

Optional Topping:
Sprinkles

1. Preheat the oven to 350 degrees.

2. Bring a pot of water to a boil. Cube the sweet potatoes and add to the pot. Boil for 20 minutes or until soft. Remove the skins and mash.

3. Add the flour, protein powder, cocoa powder, baking powder, baking soda and sea salt to a bowl. Stir until combined and set aside.

4. In a separate bowl, add the melted coconut oil, honey, maple syrup, applesauce and mashed sweet potatoes. Beat until well combined. Add the vanilla and eggs; mix. Add the dry mixture to the wet and mix until just combined.

5. Grease a donut pan. Pour the mixture into a large zip top bag. Cut one of the corners off the bag about ½ inch wide. Pipe the batter into the donut molds, filling about ¾ of the way full. Bake for 12-15 minutes. Let cool for a few minutes, then remove from pan and transfer each donut to a cooling rack.

6. Add the chocolate chips and coconut oil to a small mixing bowl. Melt in the microwave for 1-2 minutes, stirring every 30 seconds. Set aside.

7. Add the powdered sugar and egg whites to a mixing bowl and beat until well combined. Add the melted chocolate chip mixture and beat until combined. Dip the top of each donut into the frosting and return to the cooling rack. Top immediately with sprinkles and let the frosting harden. Store leftovers in the fridge or freezer.

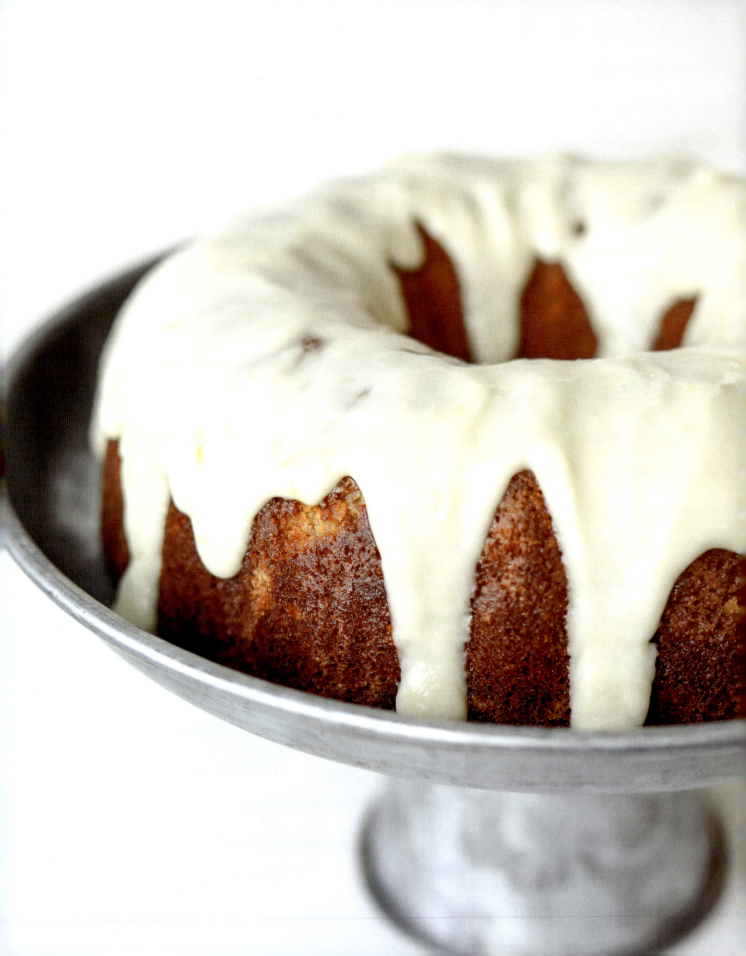

LEMON POUND CAKE

Makes 16 servings
315 calories / 7.5F / 57C / 5P / per serving

Prep: 15 min | **Cook:** 60 min + cooling

1 cup fat-free milk
2 Tbs. lemon juice
2 Tbs. lemon zest
½ cup grass-fed butter
1 ½ cups Swerve confectioners sweetener or xylitol
¾ cup raw honey
3 large eggs
½ cup unsweetened applesauce
3 cups white whole wheat flour
½ tsp. baking soda
½ tsp. sea salt

Syrup:
⅓ cup water
⅓ cup Swerve sweetener
2 Tbs. lemon juice

Glaze:
1 cup powdered sugar
2 Tbs. pasteurized egg whites
1 Tbs. lemon juice
1 tsp. lemon zest
1 tsp. softened CSE Lemon Coconut Bliss Butter or coconut butter

1. Preheat the oven to 325 degrees.

2. Place the milk, lemon juice and lemon zest in a small bowl; set aside.

3. Beat the butter, Swerve and honey together in a large bowl. Add in the eggs and applesauce; set aside.

4. In a separate bowl, combine the flour, baking soda and sea salt together. Add ½ of the dry mixture to the wet mixture, then add the milk and lemon juice mixture and then add the rest of the dry mixture on top. Mix until just combined.

5. Pour the batter into a greased Bundt pan. Bake for 60 minutes. Let cool for 10 minutes in the pan and then transfer to a cooling rack. Place a sheet of parchment paper under the cooling rack. Combine the syrup ingredients and then slowly pour over the cake while warm. Let cool completely.

6. Beat the powdered sugar, egg whites, lemon juice, lemon zest and nut butter together in a large bowl until well combined. Drizzle icing evenly over the cooled cake. Let the icing harden before serving. Slice into 16 servings. Enjoy!

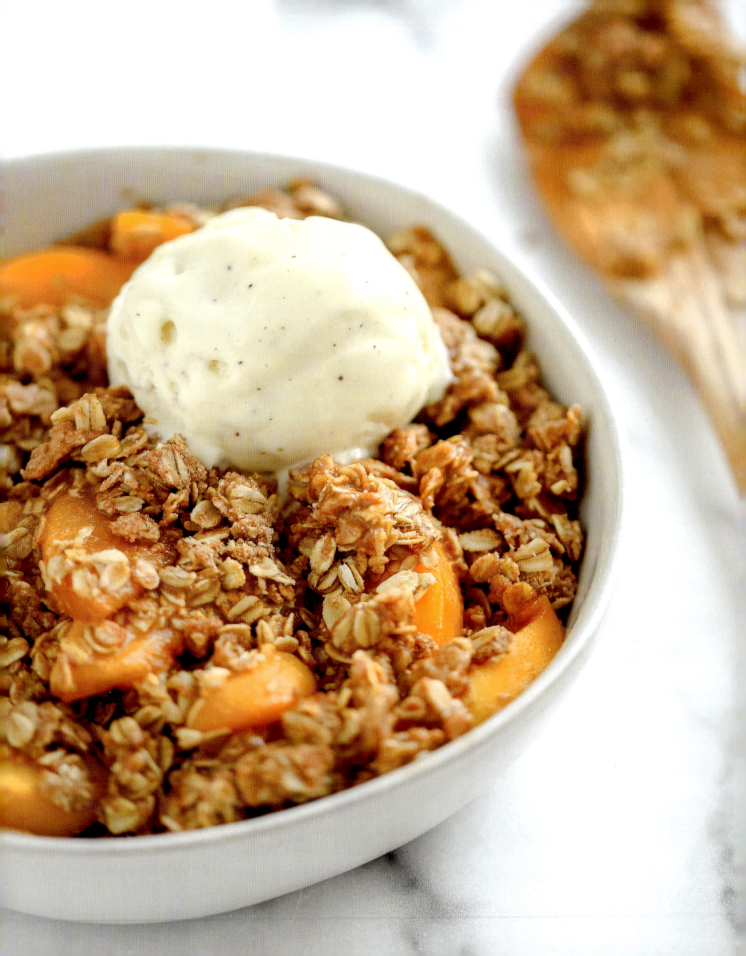

PEACH CRISP

Makes 12 servings
235 calories / 7F / 39C / 6P / per serving

Prep: 15 min | **Cook:** 25 min

2 lbs. ripe peaches, peeled, pitted and sliced
¼ cup coconut sugar
1 Tbs. lemon juice
½ tsp. almond extract

Crumble Topping:
2 cups old-fashioned rolled oats
1 ½ cups CSE Buttermilk, Gluten-Free Buttermilk,
   or Vanilla Pancake & Waffle Mix
½ cup raw honey
1 Tbs. cinnamon
¼ tsp. sea salt
6 Tbs. grass-fed butter or coconut oil, chopped

Optional Toppings:
Spray whipped cream
High protein ice cream

1. Preheat the oven to 375 degrees.

2. In a large bowl, add the peaches, coconut sugar, lemon juice and almond extract. Mix until the peaches are well coated. Pour into a greased 9x13 glass baking dish.

3. Combine all the topping ingredients together in a bowl, using your hands or a pastry cutter, until thick and crumbly. Press on top of the peach mixture.

4. Bake for 20-25 minutes. Serve warm as is or add toppings of choice (not included in the macros). Enjoy!

COOKIES

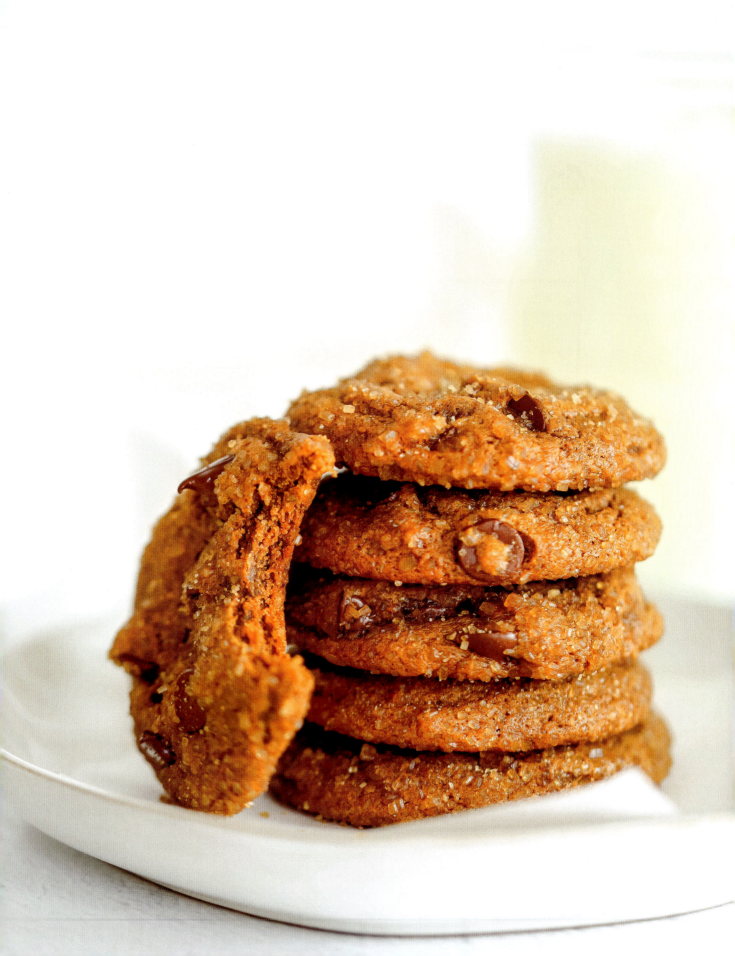

GINGERBREAD CHOCOLATE CHIP COOKIES
Makes 34 cookies
126 calories / 5F / 19C / 2P / per cookie

Prep: 15 min | **Cook:** 10 min + refrigeration

¼ cup CSE Gingerbread Cookie, Cinnamon Bun Butter or natural almond butter
½ cup coconut oil or grass-fed butter
1 large egg
1 tsp. vanilla extract
¾ cup raw honey
⅓ cup molasses
2 ½ cups whole wheat pastry flour
1 tsp. baking soda
½ tsp. sea salt
½ tsp. ground cloves
2 tsp. ground ginger
2 tsp. ground cinnamon
½ cup semi-sweet chocolate chips
½ cup organic sugar in the raw

1. Beat the nut butter and coconut oil/butter together. Add the egg and vanilla. Slowly beat in the honey and molasses; set aside.

2. In a separate bowl, mix the flour, baking soda, salt, cloves, ginger and cinnamon. Add the dry ingredients to the wet ingredients and mix until just combined. Fold in the chocolate chips. Cover and chill in the fridge for one hour.

3. Preheat the oven to 350 degrees.

4. Remove the dough from the fridge. Using a small cookie scoop, drop round balls of dough into the raw sugar one at a time. Roll around until well coated. Place on a baking sheet lined with parchment paper. Bake for 8-10 minutes. Let cool for 2 minutes, then transfer to a cooling rack. Enjoy!

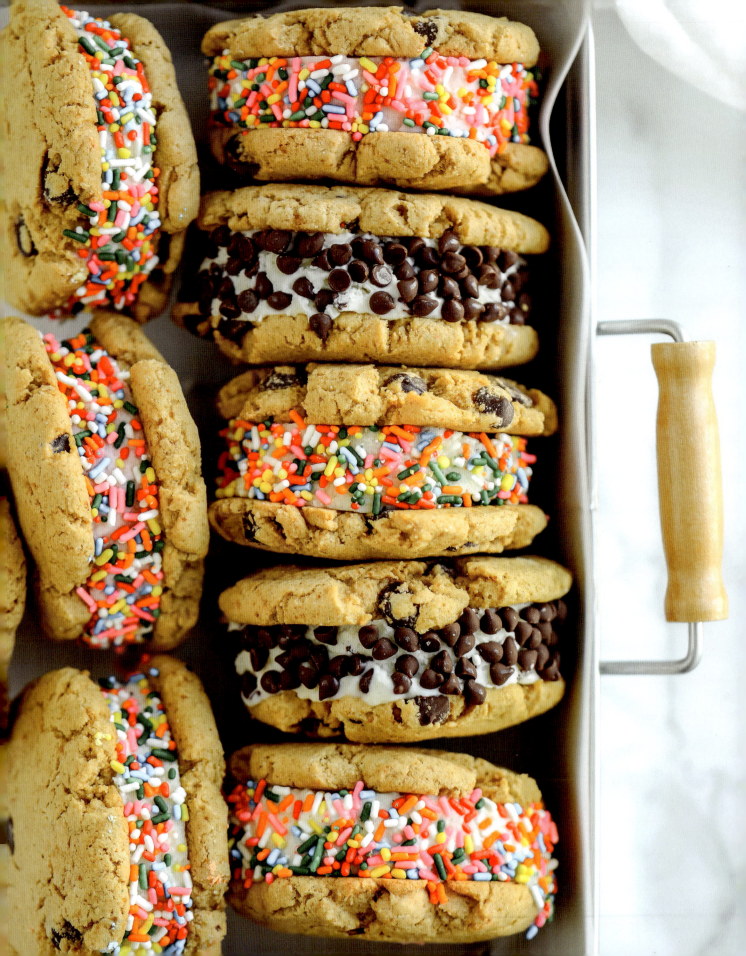

ICE CREAM COOKIE SANDWICHES

Makes 24 cookies / 12 cookie sandwiches
220 calories / 11F / 36C / 5P / per ½ of a cookie sandwich

Prep: 25 min | **Cook:** 10 min + freezing

- 1 cup grass-fed butter
- 1 cup organic brown sugar
- ¾ cup Lakanto Monk Fruit Sweetener
- 2 large eggs
- 1 Tbs. vanilla extract
- 3 cups Cup4Cup Gluten Free flour
- ¾ tsp. baking soda
- ½ tsp. sea salt
- ½ cup dark chocolate chips
- 3 pints of high protein ice cream, any flavor

Optional Toppings:
Sprinkles
Mini chocolate chips
Chopped nuts

1. Preheat the oven to 375 degrees.

2. Add the butter, brown sugar and sweetener in the raw to a mixing bowl. Mix them on medium speed until creamed together and smooth. Add the eggs and vanilla. Mix until combined.

3. Add the flour, baking soda and salt to a separate bowl. Whisk until combined. Add the dry ingredients to the wet ingredients and mix until just combined. Fold in the chocolate chips.

4. Using a large cookie scoop, scoop the cookie dough onto a baking sheet lined with parchment paper. Flatten each cookie with the bottom of a greased cup. Bake for 8-10 minutes. Let cool on the baking sheet for 2 minutes, then transfer to a cooling rack. Once completely cooled, place in a large zip top bag and freeze for 2+ hours.

5. Remove the lid from the ice cream and then cut off the bottom of the carton with a sharp knife. Dump the ice cream out of the carton onto a cutting board, trying to keep the shape intact. Slice each pint of ice cream into three rounds. Sandwich each round, pressing firmly, between two cookies.

6. Pour the toppings of choice into a bowl. Roll the sides of the ice cream sandwich in the toppings and use the backside of a spoon to press the toppings into the ice cream. Return to the freezer until ready to eat.

*Optional toppings not included in the macros listed above.

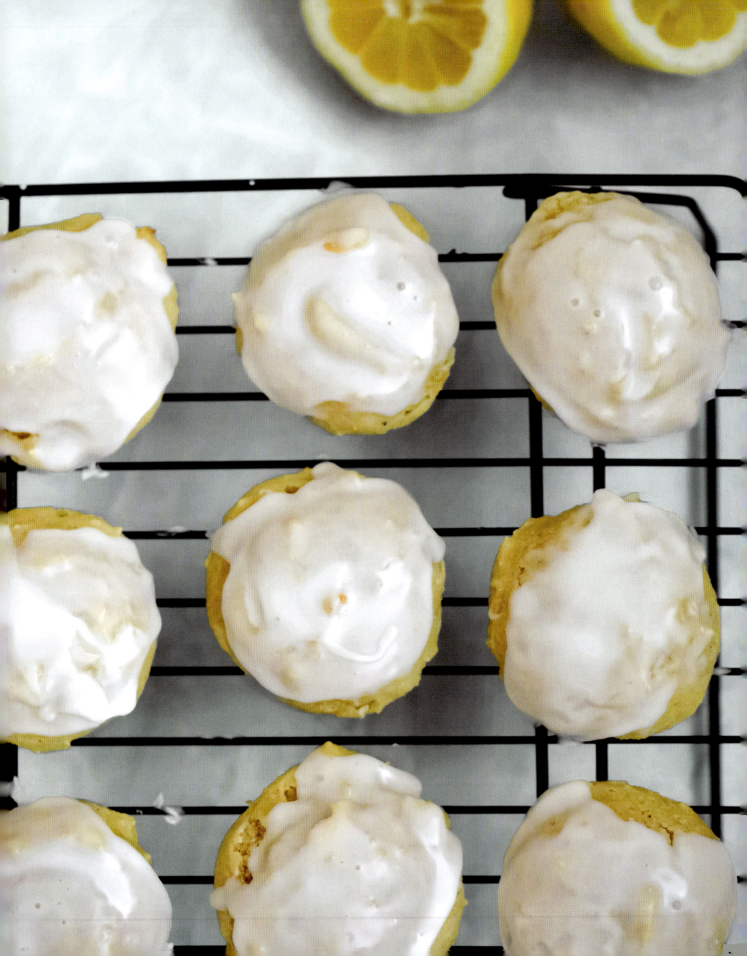

LEMON DROP COOKIES

Makes 16 cookies
140 calories / 6F / 18.5C / 3.5P / per cookie

Prep: 15 min | **Cook:** 6 min

1 large egg
¼ cup unsweetened almond milk
¼ cup raw honey or pure maple syrup
2 Tbs. melted coconut oil
1 Tbs. lemon juice
2 tsp. lemon extract
1 cup whole wheat pastry flour
1 cup almond flour
½ serving CSE Simply Vanilla Protein Powder
1 tsp. baking powder
½ tsp. sea salt
1 Tbs. lemon zest

Icing:
1 cup powdered sugar
2 Tbs. pasteurized egg whites

1. Preheat the oven to 375 degrees.

2. In a large bowl, beat the egg, almond milk, honey/syrup, melted coconut oil, lemon juice and lemon extract together; set aside.

3. In a separate bowl, stir together the flours, protein powder, baking powder and sea salt. Add the wet ingredients to the dry ingredients and mix until well combined. Fold in the lemon zest.

4. Using a small cookie scoop, scoop the dough into balls and place on a cookie sheet lined with parchment paper. Bake for 5-6 minutes or until lightly golden on the bottom. Transfer to a cooling rack.

5. Beat together the powdered sugar and egg whites. Once the cookies are cooled, place a sheet of parchment or wax paper underneath the cooling rack and drizzle each cookie with the icing. Enjoy!

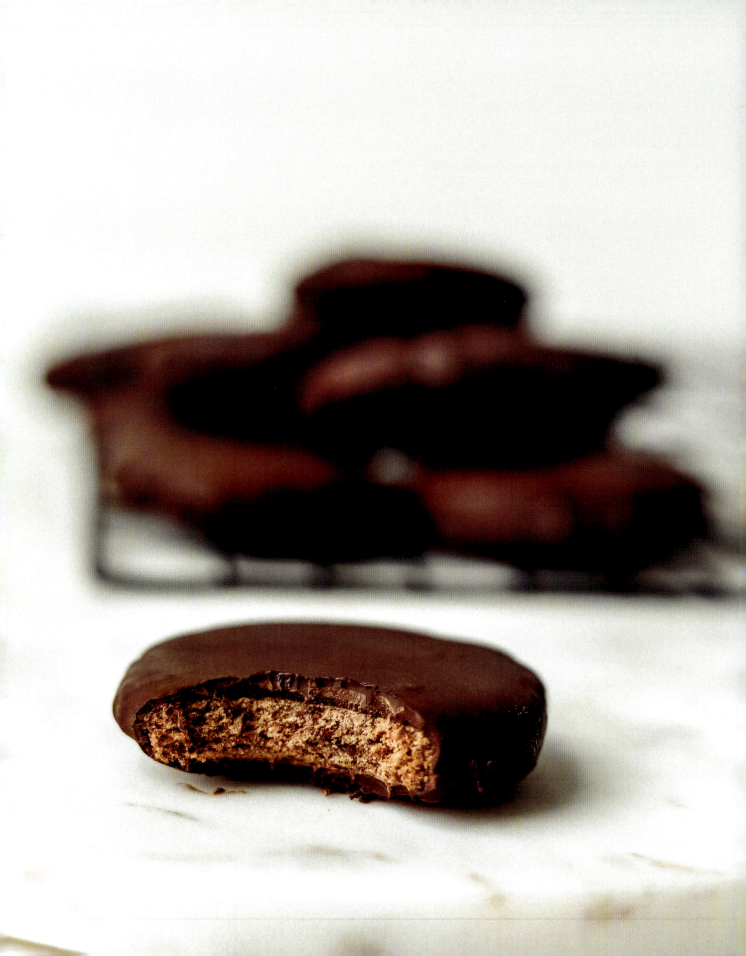

MINT CHOCOLATE COOKIES
Makes 36 cookies
120 calories / 7.5F / 13C / 3.5P / per cookie

Prep: 30 min | **Cook:** 3 min + freezing

12 oz. CSE Mint Chocolate Chip Cookie Butter or chocolate almond butter
½ cup raw honey
2 servings CSE Chocolate Brownie Batter or Mint Chocolate Cookie Protein Powder
1 cup CSE Chocolate Chocolate or Gluten-Free Chocolate Chocolate Pancake & Waffle Mix
½ tsp. vanilla extract
Dash sea salt
2 cups dark chocolate chips
1 Tbs. coconut oil

1. Add the nut butter, honey, protein powder, CSE Pancake & Waffle Mix, vanilla and salt together in a bowl. Mix until well combined. Using a small cookie scoop, scoop the dough onto a baking sheet lined with parchment paper. Using the bottom of a glass cup, smash the balls flat and then round out the edges with your hands to form into a cookie. Place the cookies in the freezer for 30 minutes or until hardened.

2. Place the dark chocolate and coconut oil into a small saucepan over low heat to melt (or melt in a bowl in the microwave). Stir continuously until completely melted, then turn the heat off. Drop each cookie into the chocolate one at a time and scoop out with a fork, letting the excess chocolate drip off into the pan. Place the chocolate dipped cookies back onto the parchment paper and then place them in the freezer to harden.

3. Once frozen, transfer to a storage container or bag. When ready to eat, let cookies sit out 5-10 minutes to thaw before taking a bite. Enjoy!

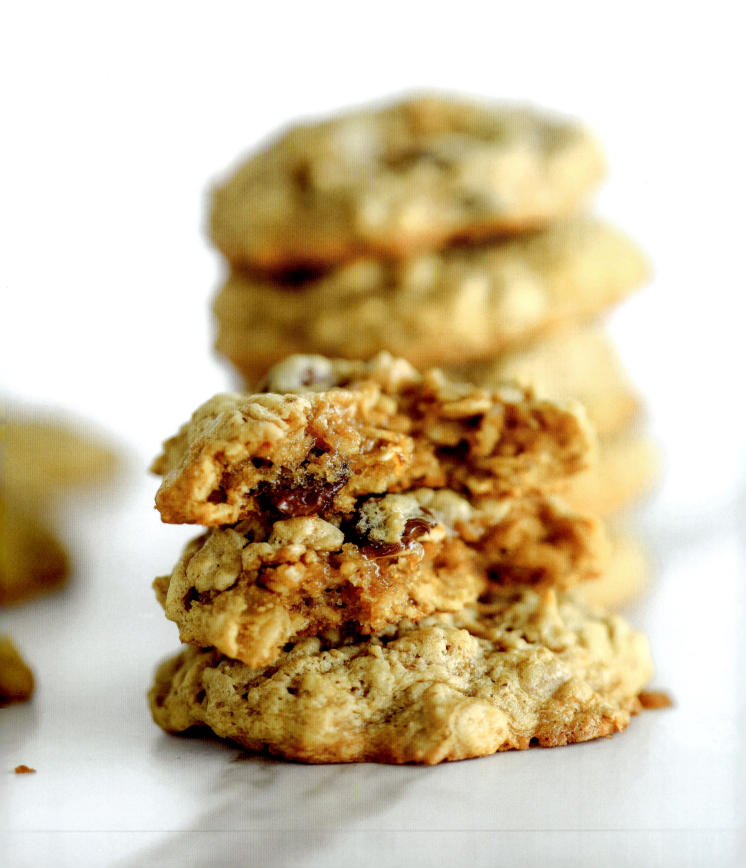

OATMEAL PB CHOCOLATE CHIP COOKIES

Makes 28 cookies
125 calories / 7F / 13.5C / 3P / per cookie

Prep: 10 min | **Cook:** 8 min

½ cup grass-fed butter
½ cup CSE Sweet Classic Peanut Butter
    or natural peanut butter
⅓ cup coconut sugar
¼ cup sugar in the raw
1 serving CSE Simply Vanilla Protein Powder
2 large eggs
1 tsp. vanilla extract
2 ½ cups old-fashioned rolled oats
½ tsp. baking soda
¼ tsp. sea salt
½ cup dark chocolate chips

1. Preheat the oven to 350 degrees.

2. Mix the butter, peanut butter, coconut sugar, sugar in the raw, and protein powder together in a bowl. Add the eggs and vanilla; mix until smooth.

3. In a separate bowl, combine the oats, baking soda and salt. Add the dry ingredients to the wet ingredients and mix until just combined. Stir in the chocolate chips last.

4. Using a small cookie scoop, scoop the cookie dough onto a baking sheet lined with parchment paper. Bake for 6-8 minutes. Let cool 2 for minutes, then transfer to a cooling rack. Enjoy!

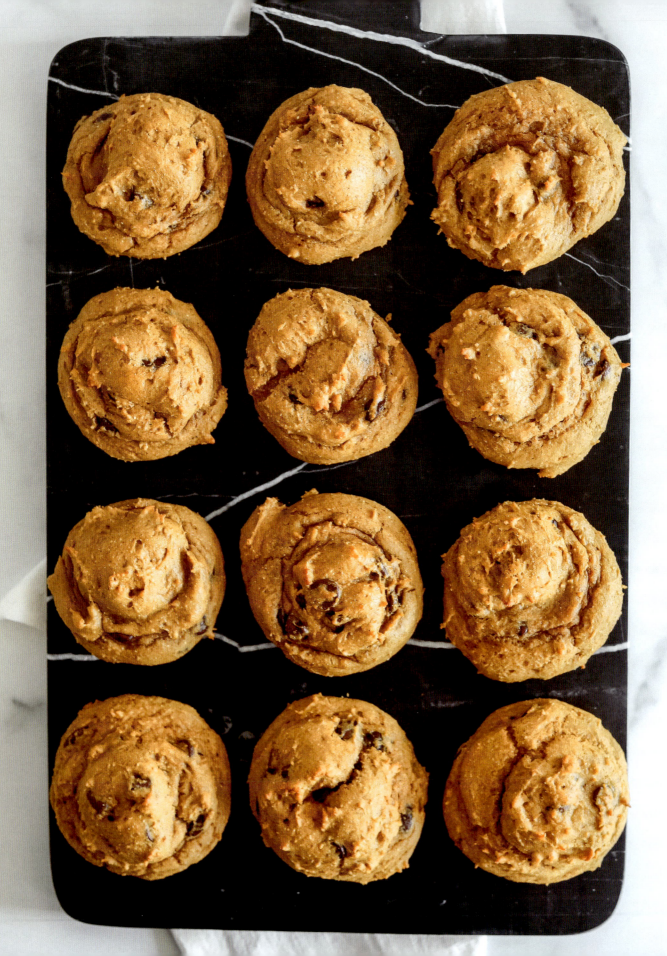

PUMPKIN CHOCOLATE CHIP COOKIES

Makes 24 cookies
170 calories / 7.5F / 22.5C / 5P / per cookie

Prep: 10 min | **Cook:** 8 min

1 cup coconut sugar
½ cup grass-fed butter, softened
1 cup canned pumpkin
1 large egg
1 Tbs. vanilla extract
3 cups CSE Buttermilk, Gluten-Free Buttermilk, or Vanilla Pancake & Waffle Mix
1 tsp. baking powder
1 tsp. baking soda
2 tsp. ground cinnamon
½ tsp. ground cloves
½ tsp. ground nutmeg
¼ tsp. sea salt
1 cup dark chocolate chips

1. Preheat the oven to 350 degrees.

2. Beat together the coconut sugar and butter. Add the pumpkin, egg and vanilla. Mix well and set aside.

3. In a separate bowl, combine the CSE Pancake & Waffle Mix, baking powder, baking soda, spices and sea salt. Add the wet ingredients to the dry ingredients and stir until just combined. Fold in the chocolate chips.

4. Using a large cookie scoop, scoop and drop dough onto a baking sheet lined with parchment paper. Bake for 7-9 minutes. Let cool for 2 minutes and then transfer to a cooling rack. Store extras in the fridge or freezer.

PARTY TREATS

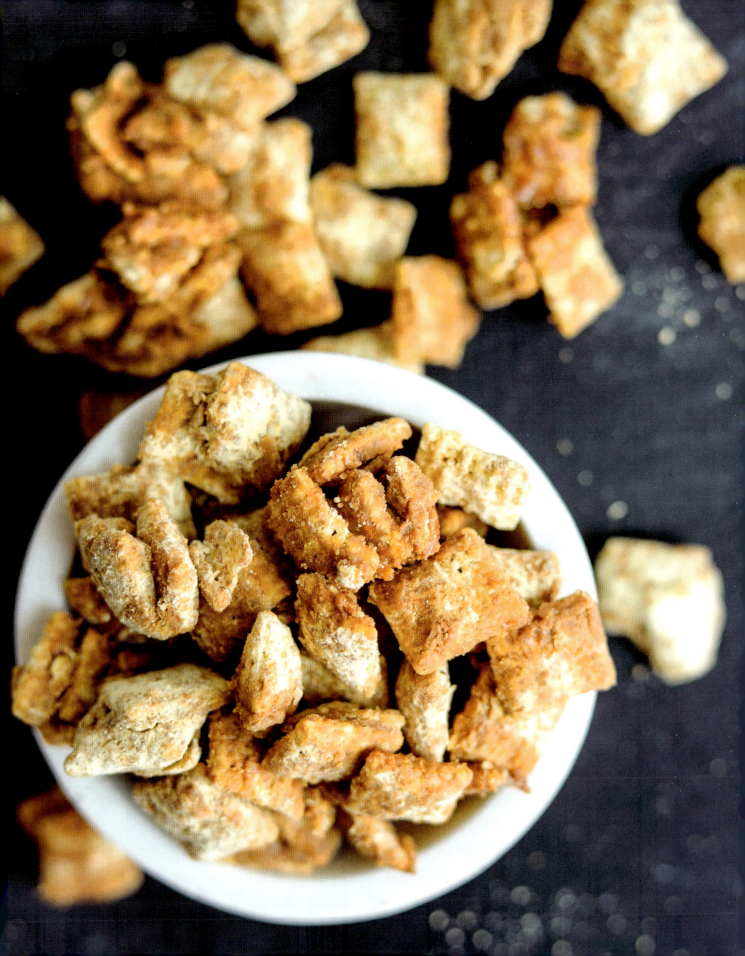

BROWNIE BATTER BUDDIES

Makes 16 servings / ½ cup (45g) per serving
185 calories / 5F / 29C / 7P / per serving

Prep: 10 min | **Cook:** 5 min

¾ cup raw honey
½ cup CSE Sweet Classic Peanut Butter, Buckeye Brownie Peanut Butter
   or natural peanut butter
1 tsp. vanilla extract
1 serving CSE Chocolate Brownie Batter
   or Chocolate Peanut Butter Protein Powder
1 Tbs. cocoa powder
8 cups Rice Chex cereal
1 cup CSE Powdered Peanut Butter

1. In a small saucepan, melt together the honey, peanut butter and vanilla over low heat. Stir until melted together and smooth, then remove from heat. Stir in the protein powder and cocoa powder.

2. Place Chex cereal into a large bowl. Pour the hot mixture over the top and gently stir until the cereal is well coated.

3. Pour the chocolate Chex mixture into a large zip top bag, then dump the powdered peanut butter over the top. Seal the bag and shake until the cereal is well coated. Pour out onto wax or parchment paper to cool. Store leftovers in the fridge. Enjoy!

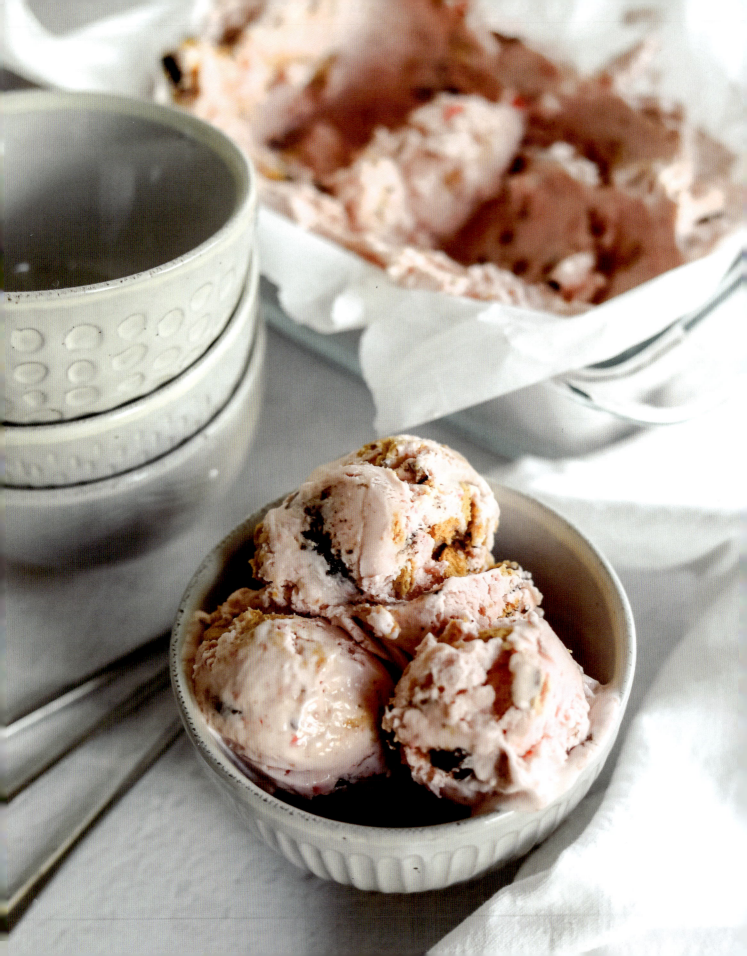

RASPBERRY OREO ICE CREAM

Makes 8 servings
305 calories / 18F / 22C / 15P / per serving

Prep: 40 min + freezing

- 2 cups fresh raspberries
- 1 Tbs. organic cane sugar
- 1 ½ cups fat-free milk
- 1 ½ cups heavy whipping cream
- 4 servings (132g) CSE Simply Vanilla Protein Powder
- 1 tsp. vanilla extract
- Dash sea salt
- 8 Newman-O's Cookies (any variety)

*You will need an ice cream machine for this recipe. Do all the preparation work required of your ice cream machine beforehand.

1. Add the raspberries to a large bowl and sprinkle the sugar over the top. Stir until the raspberries are well coated. Let sit for 15 minutes.

2. Once the juices from the raspberries have released, mash them up to desired texture. Add the milk, heavy cream, protein powder, vanilla extract and sea salt to the bowl. Whisk together until smooth.

3. Start your ice cream machine and turn to low speed. Slowly add the ice cream mixture to the machine. Churn on low speed for 20 minutes or until the ice cream thickens up like soft serve. Remove the bowl from the ice cream machine and remove the mixing paddle from the bowl.

4. Crush the cookies to your desired consistency and add to the ice cream. Stir until well combined. Enjoy as is or follow the next step for a more firm ice cream.

5. Place a piece of parchment paper into a 9x5 loaf pan, covering the bottom and sides of the pan. Scrape the ice cream into the pan and spread out evenly. Place in the freezer for 4 hours to let firm up. Scoop into bowls and serve.

PRO TIP: Store extras in the freezer. If it has been in the freezer longer than 4-6 hours, allow it to soften at room temperature for about 30 minutes before scooping.

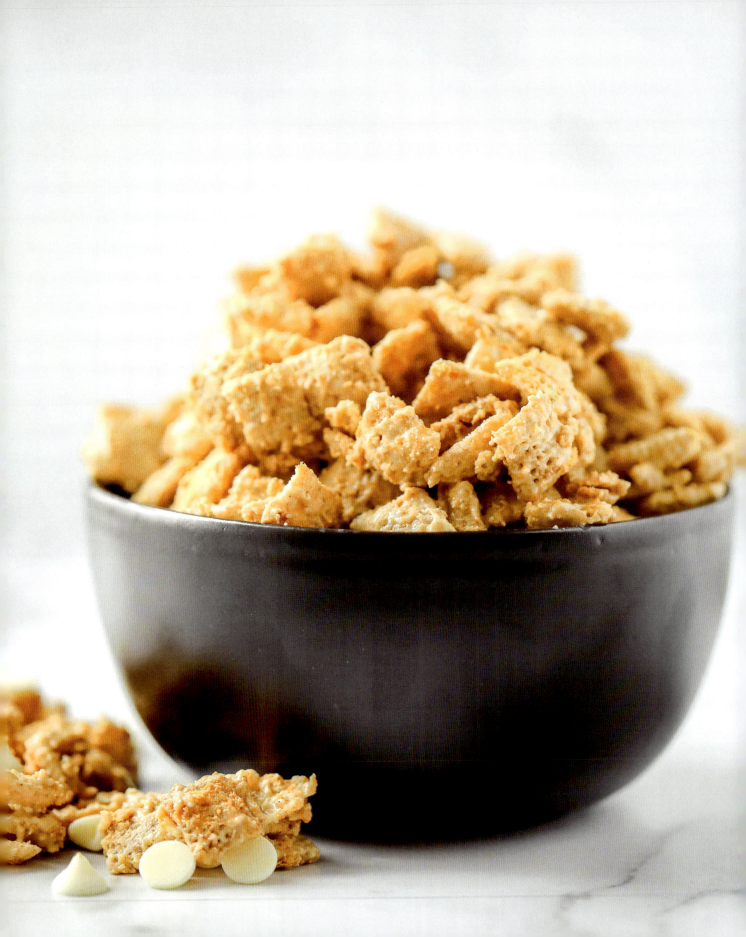

WHITE CHOCOLATE CINNAMON PUPPY CHOW

Makes 16 servings
245 calories / 11F / 29.5C / 6.5P / per serving

Prep: 10 min | **Cook:** 5 min

8 cups Cinnamon Chex cereal
2 Tbs. grass-fed, unsalted butter
1 cup white chocolate chips
½ cup CSE Sweet Classic Peanut Butter or natural peanut butter
1 serving CSE Simple Vanilla or Snickerdoodle Protein Powder
½ cup CSE Powdered Peanut Butter

1. In a small saucepan, melt together the butter, chocolate chips, and peanut butter over low heat. Stir until melted together and smooth, then remove from heat. Stir in the protein powder.

2. Place Chex cereal into a large bowl. Pour the hot mixture over the top and gently stir until the cereal is well coated.

3. Pour the Chex mixture into a large zip top bag, then dump the powdered peanut butter over the top. Seal the bag and shake until the cereal is well coated. Pour out onto wax or parchment paper to cool. Store leftovers in the fridge. Enjoy!

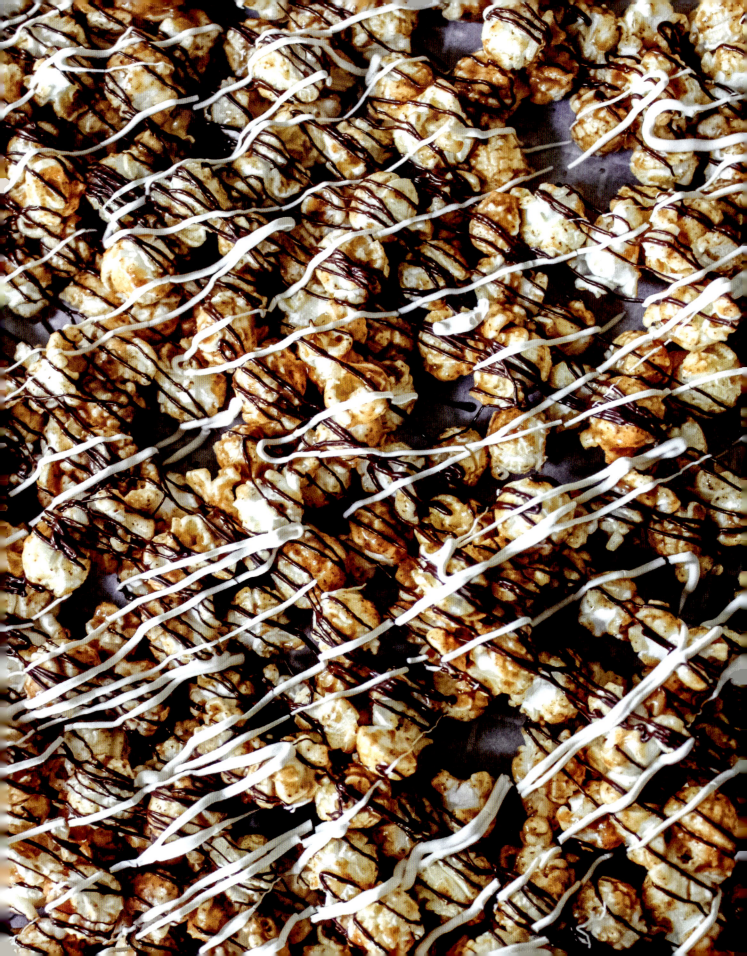

ZEBRA CARAMEL CORN
Makes 8 servings
265 calories / 11F / 38C / 4P / per serving

Prep: 10 min | **Cook:** 5 min

12 cups (½ cup kernels) air-popped popcorn
½ cup CSE Sweet Classic Peanut Butter, Salted Caramel Butter
    or natural peanut butter/almond butter
½ cup raw honey
1 tsp. vanilla extract
¼ cup dark chocolate chips
¼ cup white chocolate chips
Dash sea salt

1. Pour popped popcorn into a large bowl.

2. In a saucepan, melt the nut butter, honey and vanilla over medium heat. Stir until pourable.

3. Pour over the popcorn and stir until well coated. Pour out onto a sheet of parchment paper and let cool.

4. In two separate bowls, microwave the chocolate chip flavors, 30 seconds at a time until completely melted and smooth, stirring in between. Pour the dark chocolate into a zip top sandwich bag. Cut a small hole in one corner and drizzle over the popcorn. Repeat with the white chocolate. Sprinkle sea salt over the top and store in the fridge to cool.

5. Once the chocolate is hardened, separate into eight servings. Enjoy!